Disease Interrupted:

TOBACCO REDUCTION AND CESSATION

CHARL ELS, DIANE KUNYK AND
PETER SELBY
(EDITORS)

Disease Interrupted: Tobacco Reduction and Cessation

COVER IMAGE
"Conceptual Dan" Digitally manipulated painting on vintage suitcase. Ink jet on archival fine art paper. Davida Kidd, 2009.

PROJECT TEAM:
Arvelle Balon-Lyon, William Belyea, Ryan Gullage, Patrick Hlavac-Winsor, and Donna Zazulak.

This book was made possible through a financial contribution from the Drugs and Tobacco Initiatives Program, Health Canada, as well as seed grant funding from CAN-ADAPTT.

Table of Contents

SPECIAL SETTINGS

DISPROPORTIONALLY AFFECTED POPULATIONS

PARTING THOUGHTS

Introduction

WE CAREFULLY SELECTED THE TITLE *DISEASE INTERRUPTED* AS IT REFERS TO TWO fundamental tobacco and disease-related concepts. Following experimentation with tobacco products, their ongoing use may induce the disease of tobacco addiction. Secondly, the use of tobacco is also a risk factor for six of the leading non-communicable diseases globally (including heart diseases, lung diseases and cancers). In fact, tobacco has been identified as the leading preventable cause of death and disease globally. Stopping its use can interrupt the development of disease and is, therefore, a critical health promoting and life saving measure.

Tobacco cessation is possible and there are robust, evidence-based strategies that exist for supporting this process. Furthermore, most individuals that use tobacco want to stop. Yet tobacco use and addiction is considered to be vastly undertreated. The purpose of this book is to provide the background and evidence for healthcare professionals and students in these fields to increase their capacity for closing this healthcare delivery gap. It may also be of interest for individuals who are currently using tobacco, and their families, who are interested in quitting.

This book is primarily focused on tobacco reduction and cessation; it does not explore the other major pillars of tobacco control including prevention and protection. There is a massive and growing body of evidence on strategies to support tobacco reduction and cessation—to the extent that some may become overwhelmed and not always know where to start. In our professional experiences, we have repeatedly been asked for a resource to guide learning and practice. This identified need motivated our successful applications to both CAN-ADAPTT and Health Canada to support the development of this book. To fulfill this purpose, we have been extremely fortunate in that 50 authors from 6 continents have contributed their expertise to this first (that we are aware of) Canadian resource on tobacco reduction and cessation.

In its entirely, the aim of this volume is to portray a multi-faceted approach to tobacco use and cessation. Each chapter is designed to be read either in the context of the book or to stand on its own. The Editors welcomed the divergent styles of writing by each of the respected authors who contributed to a chapter. We also recognize that opinions may vary across different chapters, and believe that strength and value is found by presenting different viewpoints. In places we, as Editors, have added sidebars and highlighted certain parts of the text for the purposes of adding salience to important aspects in the field. The Editors have also added the CAN-ADAPTT Summary Statements to each chapter to allow for an integrated approach in reading the chapter and having the guideline statements readily available. These were reprinted with permission.

In Chapter 1, the Editors elaborate on the differences between tobacco use and addiction—emphasizing that not every person who uses tobacco is addicted to the substance. It provides a broad overview of the treatment of tobacco use and addiction and cites leading Clinical Practice Guidelines for safe and effective interventions. Reduction and cessation are critical steps for improving the health of individuals who use or are addicted to tobacco products.

In Chapter 2, "Legal Duty to Treat Tobacco Use and Addiction, Hlavac-Winsor et al. postulate that tort law is a relevant framework for the issue of tobacco use and addiction treatment. They argue that several aspects of the duty to treat and standard of care look to the medical establishment for guidance on acceptable standards. While the tort framework may not immediately seem to apply to a duty to treat tobacco use and addiction, the reference to accepted treatment by governing medical bodies might serve a patient in making a negligence claim. Based on this argument, it is the authors' belief that the likelihood of a successful tort case for damages sustained as a result of failure to provide treatment is not only possible but also likely under certain circumstances.

In the Foundations Section, Ferrence et al. (Chapter 3, "Health Effects of Tobacco and Secondhand Smoke"), summarize 70 years of research and a wealth of incontrovertible evidence for the major health effects of tobacco and secondhand smoke. The authors conclude that the health effects of tobacco products must not be viewed in isolation as strictly a medical issue, and that current evidence is sufficient to invoke the precautionary principle and develop a plan to eliminate tobacco products from our societies. In Chapter 4, "Evidence for developing and implementing cessation services", Schwartz and colleagues demonstrate that the "data speak for themselves by telling a vivid and chilling story of the dire and urgent need to encourage individuals who smoke to stop and to support them in their quit attempts". They make a compelling case to suggest there is much more work to be done. In Chapter 5 on "Nicotine", Rollema reviews key aspects of nicotine pharmacology, emphasizing current understanding of nicotinic mechanisms underlying tobacco dependence.

The Reduction and Cessation section starts with a stepwise approach to assessment in Chapter 6 "Assessing Tobacco Use in Clinical Practice". Khara et al. recommend a brief and pragmatic approach to comprehensive assessment suggesting that proper assessment guides treatment and lays the foundation for safe and effective therapy. Chapter 7 on "Unassisted Cessation" notes that most individuals stop smoking without assistance and queries whether this is an access issue. In Chapter 8 on "Psychosocial Interventions," Cohen and colleagues provide an overview on evidenced-based treatments through a bio-psychosocial lens and within a harm reduction framework. The chapter provides hands-on skills on how to conduct therapy, enhance coping strategies and problem solving skills, and to optimize outcomes. Chapter 9 addresses "Pharmacotherapy" and the cessation medications are presented in the order they appeared on the market: Nicotine Replacement Therapies is authored by Hughes; Selby et al. discuss the evidence on Sustained-Release Bupropion; and Coe addresses "Varenicline". Els addresses neuropsychiatric considerations, and in "Cardiovascular Complications," Tonstad reminds the reader that all medications used to aid smoking cessation have been questioned in regard to cardiovascular safety. The neuropsychiatric considerations of quitting smoking are also discussed. Pohar designed a range of patient-handouts for use by both practitioners and patients treated in clinical practice.

Special Settings are addressed in the following chapters on detoxification (Els et al.), "Hospital-Initiated Smoking Cessation, the Ottawa Model for Smoking Cessation / OMSC (Reid et al.), "Primary Care Settings" (Kunyk et al.), and finally in the Workplace (Kunyk et al.). The importance of distinguishing between withdrawal management and cessation is emphasized while the section on the OMSC provides one example of effective interventions for treating tobacco use and addiction in hospitalized patients. The authors demonstrate organizational change processes designed to help hospitals create an environment where healthcare professionals can routinely meet hospitalized patients' needs related to the management of acute nicotine withdrawal and/or long-term smoking cessation. Kunyk et al. demonstrate how healthcare professionals in primary care settings are uniquely positioned to intervene and to capitalize on the opportunity to increase the rates and scope of intervention. They argue that integration of tobacco management into routine primary care practice provides opportunities to significantly improve the quality and duration of patients' lives.

In the workplace, tobacco addiction profoundly impacts the environment and the health of employees that smoke. Kunyk et al. suggest that organizations have identified that addressing key employee health issues can boost productivity and positively impact their bottom line.

In the section on "Disproportionally Affected Populations", Wardman and coworkers eloquently describe the "Nontraditional Tobacco Use among Aboriginal Canadians" outlining Canada's Aboriginal peoples' high smoking rate that warrants special attention for many reasons. They argue that the most successful smoking interventions are integrated, flexible, community-based, culturally relevant approaches that increase service access, address negative perceptions and experiences with medications, and are tailored and targeted to local Aboriginal populations. Because of tobacco's traditional sacred role, portraying it as negative or evil, as is often the case in mainstream smoking cessation programs, is neither helpful nor accurate. They make a case for how tobacco can then claim its rightful place as a messenger to and from the spirit world and as a great source of empowerment for Aboriginal individuals and communities. Chapter 15 addresses "Treatment of Tobacco Dependence in Mental Health and Addictive Disorders", and Fillimon et al. review the body of evidence to summarize addressing tobacco dependence in this priority area for clinicians who work with these patients. They cite increasing evidence that standard pharmacological and behavioural treatments, with modest adaptations, can be used safely and effectively in mental health and addictions populations. In Chapter 16: "Imagine: Gender-Specific Tobacco Reduction and Cessation Strategies in Pregnancy and the Postpartum", Bottorff and collaborators argue that during these specific events / times, there are important opportunities to influence both women and men's health by supporting efforts to reduce and stop smoking. They remind the writer that all healthcare providers have a responsibility to intervene with women and men who smoke in ways that reduce stigma and guilt associated with smoking, recognize the influence of relationships and other social factors on smoking cessation efforts, and demonstrate a willingness to tailor approaches to address specific needs. Freeman (Chapter 17: "Youth") suggests that while it is encouraging that smoking rates among young people are at their recorded lowest levels, failing to maintain momentum in implementing effective tobacco control polices will see these rates rise again. She argues it is essential that health groups innovate how they reach and support young smokers and suggests in the future, youth may well view smoking as outmoded as posting a handwritten letter or looking up information in a volume of an encyclopedia.

This volume concludes with "Ethical Contemplations" in which the Editors reiterate that tobacco use and addiction is a critical health issue that deserves urgent and concerted attention. They believe the most reasonable response to the tobacco epidemic is comprehensive tobacco control—a comprehensive, coordinated, and multi-level strategy involving all of the pillars of tobacco control; prevention, protection and cessation. They ask a range of questions in an attempt to promote further discourse on the issues. It is their sincere hope that this chapter and book will encourage further contemplation and discussion in this meaningful field.

The reader is invited to embark on this journey with 50 authors from 6 continents to explore the fascinating and complex field of tobacco reduction and cessation.

The Editors
Fall 2012

1

Disease Interrupted

CHARL ELS, DIANE KUNYK AND PETER SELBY

THE USE OF TOBACCO REMAINS THE LEADING PREVENTABLE CAUSE OF DEATH AND disease worldwide.[1] Tobacco is the only legal consumer product that will kill at least 1 out of 2 of its regular users when used as intended by the manufacturer.[1] The World Health Organization (WHO) has concluded that tobacco killed 100 million people worldwide in the 20th century—a number in excess of the devastating casualties of the First and Second World Wars combined. The WHO also purports that tobacco is responsible for 5.4 million deaths globally each year from lung cancer, heart disease, and other illnesses.[1] It has been estimated that for every person who dies, another 20 individuals will suffer with at least one tobacco-related disease.[2] Without substantial change in the course of this lethal and toxic pandemic, it is predicted that the use of tobacco could kill 1 billion people during the 21st century.[1]

Despite this established and extraordinary scale of suffering and death, and taking into consideration impressive reductions in tobacco consumption over the last few decades, tobacco use remains common in industrialized countries in the 21st century. At the same time, tobacco use has been escalating across the globe in parts of Asia, Africa, and Latin America. The gender gap also appears to be closing with smoking rates for women catching up to those for men in many regions.[3] This increased uptake of tobacco by women and in other parts of the global community is generally considered to be a reflection of the increased efforts by tobacco industries to expand their reach into emerging and profitable markets.[3] Rather than improving economic growth in affected regions, the WHO has noted that although the tobacco industry claims it creates jobs and generates revenues to enhance local and national economies, the industry's net contribution to any country is human suffering, disease, death—and economic losses.[3]

The cigarette has been described as the deadliest artifact in the history of human civilization[4] and remains the predominant nicotine delivery mechanism of tobacco. Its use is a risk factor for other diseases including circulatory system diseases, cancers, and respiratory system diseases.[2] These non-communicable diseases pose a vast challenge to individuals suffering with them, their families, health professionals, policy makers and governments, and the WHO estimates these are the cause of 60% of all deaths worldwide. The rising prevalence of non-communicable diseases, changes in clinical treatment thresholds and recalcitrance, along with an observed plateau in prevalence of smoking, may well translate into even greater demands on the healthcare system in the coming years.[5]

With 1.1 billion people currently smoking worldwide,[6] the global tobacco pandemic is a public health disaster of staggering proportions. This epidemic cannot be reduced solely to a health issue as it involves a complex number of considerations such as business, government, culture, marketing, trade—and politics (among other considerations). As a risk factor for 6 of the 8 leading causes of death in the world,[1] thereby a dominating factor in global preventable illnesses, tobacco has become a priority for concerned public health and political leaders. The first international public health treaty—the Framework Convention on Tobacco Control (FCTC)—was created to mediate the devastation of the tobacco pandemic on global health and is a milestone for public health. While reaffirming the rights of all individuals to the highest standard of health, the FCTC examined demand reduction as well as supply issues and, by doing so, identified critical evidence-based policy instruments for the purposes of dealing well with the tobacco issue. The policy strategies in this treaty include: regulation (i.e. sales, contents, illicit trade, and smoke-free environments); reduction in demand (i.e. cessation, price and tax measures, bans on advertising, promotion, and sponsorship); protection of the environment and the health of tobacco workers; support for viable alternative activities; research, surveillance, and information exchange; as well as legislative action.[7] The WHO, as a part of their MPOWER initiative, describe the 6 key policy strategies that have been demonstrated to denormalize and reduce tobacco use as:

M: Monitor tobacco use and prevention policies,

P: Protect people from tobacco smoke,

O: Offer help to quit tobacco use,

W: Warn about the dangers of tobacco,

E: Enforce bans on tobacco advertising, promotion and sponsorship, and

R: Raise taxes on tobacco.[1]

THE POTENTIAL OF CESSATION POLICIES

The policy strategies identified in the MPOWER initiative are critical measures aimed at halting and potentially reversing the course of the tobacco pandemic. The reduction in smoking rates observed in industrialized nations over the last 4 decades attests to the effectiveness of these tobacco control strategies. However with almost half of lifetime users dying of a tobacco-related disease, and more suffering from non-communicable diseases induced from their tobacco use, it cannot be concluded the current smoking rate of 17% in Canada should be endpoint for success.[1,2] There continues to be an urgent need for reducing these numbers even further for the purposes of saving future lives and suffering. In order to do so, current tobacco control efforts must not only be sustained; they must be enhanced.

Increasing adult cessation is considered a major determinant for reducing smoking-related death and disease over the next few decades.[8] Levy et. al.[9] have used simulation modelling to examine the overall effect of tobacco control policies on estimated population quit rates. Their analysis considered the effects of price increases through taxation, smoke-free indoor air laws, mass media and educational policies, as well as evidence-based and promising cessation treatment policies. The findings from this study have been transposed into a visual display (Figure 1). With a starting point of a 20.1% smoking rate in 2010, it was calculated that continuation with the same combinations of tobacco control policies (status quo) was projected to reduce the smoking rate to 17.5% in 2020. It was estimated that expanded cessation policies that included promising treatments would reduce the rate to 12.8% in the same time period. The authors concluded that evidence-based cessation treatment policies have the strongest effect on population quit rates and could potentially boost these by 78.8% in relative terms.

GRAPH 1: Projected effects of tobacco control policies on US adults' smoking prevalence in 2020.

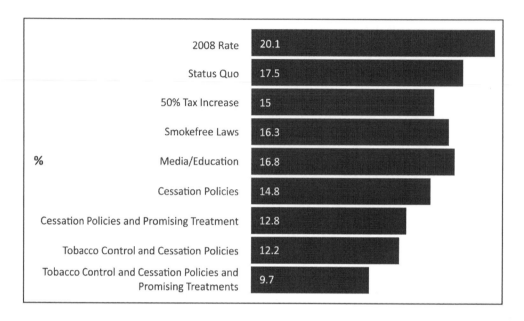

Source: Adapted from: Levy DT, et al. (2010). Reaching Healthy People 2010 by 2013: A SimSmoke Simulation. Am J Prev Med. 2010;38(3S):S373-81.

There is a critical and urgent need for increasing the rates of cessation in order to reduce the burden of tobacco in our society. Yet after a review of approximately 8,700 articles on tobacco treatment for the US Department of Health and Human Services Tobacco Use and Dependence Guidelines, the conclusion was drawn that tobacco presents a unique situation. Although the use of tobacco is a highly significant health threat, there exists a wide array of internationally recognized and robust interventions and most individuals would like to stop their use of tobacco, opportunities for intervention with tobacco use and addiction are vastly neglected.[10]

TOBACCO USE AND ADDICTION

There are differences between tobacco use and tobacco addiction; it is important to note that not every person who uses tobacco is addicted to the substance of nicotine. The disease of tobacco addiction is recognized as a chronic disease by most authorities including Health Canada, the Canadian Medical Association, and the World Health Organization, and it is classified as such in major disease classification systems.[11,12]

Addiction is a preventable and treatable disease as opposed to a *lifestyle choice*, a social problem, or culpable behaviour (in terms of own health and the damage inflicted). Scientific evidence has identified that addiction develops as a result of complex multi-factorial interactions between repeated exposure to substances as well as biological, psychological, spiritual, and environmental factors. Addiction is a primary, chronic, neurobiological disease with genetic, psychosocial, and environmental factors influencing its development and manifestations. It is characterized by behaviours that include 1 or more of the following: impaired control over drug use, compulsive use, continued use despite harm, and craving.[12] Addiction has been described as impaired control over a reward-seeking behaviour from which harm ensues, and as repeated failures to refrain from drug use despite prior resolutions to do so. Addiction refers to a psychiatric syndrome induced by repeated exposure to a particular substance that produces chronic changes in the brain's motivational system as a consequence of which a reward-seeking behaviour has become out of control.[13,14] This complex brain disorder results from the chronic effects of repeated exposure of a specific (addictive) substance on the brain's structure and function. Decision-making and behaviour are subsequently influenced by the underlying pathophysiological changes in the brain. A variety of biological (including genetic), psychological, spiritual, and social contextual factors modulate these changes in the brain.

Cigarettes contain tobacco, and tobacco contains nicotine. Nicotine is a single psychoactive substance that affects the brain and central nervous system, skeletal muscles, cardiovascular system, endocrine system, lungs, and various other organs.[15] Nicotine is addictive and it is the substance that sustains tobacco addiction (nicotine dependence). Although not fully understood, it is recognized that not all persons who use tobacco products will become addicted.

Tobacco (nicotine) addiction is perpetuated by the ability of cigarettes to rapidly introduce nicotine, and a host of other chemicals, to the addiction centres of the brain (i.e. the reward pathways). For the purposes of increasing the addictive nature of nicotine, smoked tobacco through the design of cigarettes delivers nicotine in a free-based format to the brain (i.e. similar to 'crack-nicotine,' see Chapter 4). After nicotine's delivery through the arterial system to the brain, it binds primarily to alpha-4 beta-2 ($\alpha 4\beta 2$) nicotinic receptors. These receptors are central to the initiation and maintenance of addiction. Stimulation of these nicotinic receptors causes the generation of an action potential that stimulates other brain centres resulting in the release of dopamine in the pleasure centre of the brain. When chronically stimulated by nicotine, upregulation and desensitization of these receptors follows. The entire reward pathway can become desensitized with repeated exposure and this represents a second major maladaptive change in brain function in response to tobacco consumption. Chapter 4 describes nicotine in further detail.

The *International Classification of Diseases* (ICD 10)[12] in their definition of nicotine dependence describes a cluster of behavioural, cognitive, and physiological phenomena that develop after repeated tobacco use. These typically include a strong desire to use tobacco, difficulties in controlling its use, persistence in use despite harmful consequences, a higher priority given to tobacco use than to other activities and obligations, increased tolerance, and sometimes a physical withdrawal state. Consistent with this description, the *Diagnostic and Statistical Manual of Mental Disorders* (*DSM-IV-TR*)[11] describes and categorizes nicotine dependence as a mental condition (disorder), specifically belonging to the category of substance-related disorders. A positive diagnosis is made when 3 or more of the following 7 criteria are met within a 1-year time span: tolerance, withdrawal, smoking more than usual, a persistent desire to smoke despite efforts to decrease intake, extensive time spent smoking or purchasing tobacco, postponing work, social, or recreational events in order to smoke, and continuing to smoke despite health hazards.[11]

There are limitations in applying either the *ICD* or *DSM* criteria for diagnosing tobacco addiction as the current criteria do not include validated measures such as the time-to-first cigarette, number of cigarettes smoked per day or measures of craving. Furthermore in these criteria nicotine is deemed harmful due to the physical consequences of its chronic use and not as a result of behavioural or social impairment; this is different than other substances of abuse. The *DSM 5* is anticipated to address some of these current limitations. One of these changes is the possible addition of the criterion of craving as well as the general amalgamation of the categories of abuse and dependence into a single entity (in the *DSM-IV-TR* the diagnostic entity of abuse does not exist for nicotine but does for other substances of abuse). The proposed entity of Tobacco Use Disorder is anticipated to include substantial changes from the current diagnostic entity of Nicotine Dependence. The additional diagnosis of Tobacco Withdrawal is anticipated to replace the current *DSM-IV-TR* nicotine withdrawal diagnostic entity (see also Chapter 5). The current criteria and protocols for the diagnosis and assessment of severity of tobacco dependence are outlined in Chapter 6.

CLINICAL PRACTICE GUIDELINES

The WHO Constitution includes the declaration that "The enjoyment of the highest attainable standard of health is one of the fundamental rights of every human being."[17] This right also belongs to every person who uses or is addicted to tobacco. It is widely acknowledged that the single most important behavioural change for achieving optimal health is to stop using tobacco. Article 14 of the WHO FCTC addresses cessation and recommends the development and dissemination of appropriate, comprehensive, and integrated treatment guidelines based on scientific evidence and best practices.[7]

The US Public Health Service-sponsored Clinical Practice Guideline update identifies the '5-A' model for treating tobacco use and dependence.[10] This includes asking about tobacco use with every patient at every visit, advising tobacco users to quit, assessing willingness to make a quit attempt, assisting those willing to attempt quitting by offering counselling and medication, by motivating future quit attempts in those unwilling, and arranging for follow-up contacts. These Clinical Practice Guidelines offer a framework intended to be utilized in conjunction with the implementation of population-level interventions such as public awareness and mass media campaigns for denormalizing tobacco use and taxation on tobacco products.

Consistent with Article 14, Canada recently released its first federally funded set of Clinical Practice Guidelines through the Canadian Action Network for the Advancement, Dissemination and Adoption of Practice-informed Tobacco Treatment (CAN-ADAPTT). Given the high level of co-occurrence of mood symptoms in persons who use tobacco and/or stop its use, the basic algorithm included in CAN-ADAPTT[18] allows integrated and brief screening of mood in the treatment of tobacco use and addiction (Figure 2). These guidelines conclude that there is strong evidence to support the statement that individuals who utilize treatment in the forms of behavioural counselling and pharmacotherapy have increased odds of quitting their tobacco use compared with those who do not. The overarching goal is that clinicians strongly recommend the use of effective counselling and medication treatments to their patients who use tobacco, and that health systems, insurers, and purchasers assist clinicians in making such effective treatments available.

The CAN-ADAPTT guideline set includes approaches and recommendations for special populations; the Summary Statements are included in the following chapters: psychosocial interventions (Chapter 8), pharmacotherapy (Chapter 9), hospitalized smokers (Chapter 11), Aboriginal populations (Chapter 14), mentally ill persons (Chapter 15), during childbearing years (Chapter 16), and with youth (Chapter 17). The CAN-ADAPTT guidelines advocate for the widespread establishment of supportive infrastructures for promoting tobacco reduction and cessation as well as providing effective treatment specifically in hospital-based settings, primary care settings, and the workplace. These aim to strengthen training programs for health professionals such as physicians, nurses, dentists, pharmacists, practitioners of traditional medicine, and also teachers and community and social workers for the purposes of empowering the provision of safe and effective treatment for tobacco use and addiction.

USDHHS Guideline Key Recommendations for Tobacco Use and Dependence[10]

The overarching goal of these recommendations is that clinicians strongly recommend the use of effective tobacco dependence counselling and medication treatments to their patients who use tobacco, and that health systems, insurers, and purchasers assist clinicians in making such effective treatments available.

1. Tobacco dependence is a chronic disease that often requires repeated intervention and multiple attempts to quit. Effective treatments exist, however, that can significantly increase rates of long-term abstinence.

2. It is essential that clinicians and healthcare delivery systems consistently identify and document tobacco use status and treat every tobacco user seen in a healthcare setting.

3. Tobacco dependence treatments are effective across a broad range of populations. Clinicians should encourage every patient willing to make a quit attempt to use the counselling treatments and medications recommended in the Guideline.

4. Brief tobacco dependence treatment is effective. Clinicians should offer every patient who uses tobacco at least the brief treatments shown to be effective in the Guideline.

5. Individual, group, and telephone counselling are effective, and their effectiveness increases with treatment intensity. Two components of counselling are especially effective, and clinicians should use these when counselling patients making a quit attempt:
- Practical counselling (problem-solving/skills training)
- Social support delivered as a part of treatment

6. Numerous effective medications are available for tobacco dependence, and clinicians should encourage their use by all patients attempting to quit smoking — except when medically contraindicated or with specific populations for which there is insufficient evidence of effectiveness (i.e. pregnant women, smokeless tobacco users, light smokers, and adolescents).

Seven first-line medications (5 nicotine and 2 non-nicotine) reliably increase long-term smoking abstinence rates:
- Bupropion (Sustained Release [SR])
- Nicotine gum
- Nicotine inhaler
- Nicotine lozenge
- Nicotine spray
- Nicotine patch
- Varenicline

Clinicians should consider the use of certain combinations of medications identified as effective in the Guideline.

7. Counselling and medication are effective when used by themselves for treating tobacco dependence. The combination of counselling and medication, however, is more effective than either alone. Thus, clinicians should encourage all individuals making a quit attempt to use both counselling and medication.

8. Telephone quitline counselling is effective with diverse populations and has broad reach. Therefore, both clinicians and healthcare delivery systems should ensure patient access to quitlines and promote quitline use.

9. If a tobacco user currently is unwilling to make a quit attempt, clinicians should use the motivational treatments shown in the Guideline to be effective in increasing future quit attempts.

10. Tobacco dependence treatments are both clinically effective and highly cost-effective relative to interventions for other clinical disorders. Providing coverage for these treatments increases quit rates. Insurers and purchasers should ensure that all insurance plans include the counselling and medication identified as effective in the Guideline as covered benefits.

FIGURE 1: Safety Sensitive Tobacco Use and Addiction Treatment Algorithm

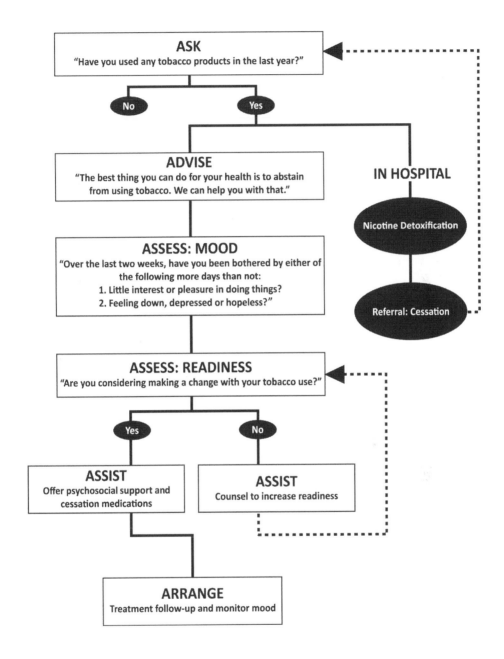

TREATMENT

Among those who currently smoke tobacco, approximately 70% would like to stop and about half of these will try to quit at least once this year.[20] Quitting smoking is possible; there are more individuals that have quit smoking than those currently smoking in Canada today. Many of these achieved abstinence without formal evidence-based interventions (Chapter 7). Others have succeeded with the assistance of evidence-based psychosocial and/or pharmacotherapy interventions.[10] To achieve the goal of the Ottawa Charter for Health Promotion to enable people to increase the control over and improve their health, the question is whether individuals who want to quit are aware of the efficacy of tobacco treatments, are able to access affordable treatment, and whether their treatment options reflect the often chronic and relapsing nature of tobacco addiction.[21]

The use of short-term, acute care models to manage chronic, non-communicable diseases is theoretically inconsistent. Hypertension, hypercholesterolemia, obesity, diabetes, depression, chronic obstructive lung diseases and addiction are some diseases that often require repeated interventions. Following a short-term approach for tobacco-addicted individuals is equally illogical and compromises the chances of long-term cessation success. It is not expected that individuals with diabetes will be able to maintain blood glucose levels within desired parameters without ongoing monitoring and management but individuals with tobacco addiction are often expected to quit without formal assistance or with interventions limited to a few months.

Many individuals with tobacco addiction are often precluded from treatment. This is dissimilar to the situation for the treatment of many other chronic disease conditions. In the case of hypertension, about 80% of Canadians receive evidence-based treatment and 66% are considered to be successfully treated for this chronic condition.[22] For tobacco addiction, the treatment numbers are substantially lower and not as well covered for their related costs, nor are these as readily available, accessible, or affordable. Evidence-based treatments for tobacco use and addiction are considered safe, effective, and cost-effective, and smoking cessation has been described as the gold standard of preventive clinical interventions.[23] Only 9 individuals need to be successfully assisted with cessation in order to prevent 1 premature tobacco-related death.[24] No other interventions are known to be as robust as preventive strategies: for example, the control of hypertension or treatment of dyslipidemia requires vastly more patients to show a similar effect. Yet the rate of individuals managed for the disease of tobacco addiction falls far behind that for many other chronic disease conditions.

Aveyard and Raw (2012) have noted this disparity for tobacco-related interventions when compared with the treatment by healthcare professionals for other chronic and relapsing diseases. They observed that healthcare professionals are often tasked with a range of preventive and treatment interventions in their everyday practices. With other medical conditions, such as diabetes or hypertension, it may also be possible for the individual to improve their health status with advice alone regarding lifestyle change. In these situations, there is also substantive evidence indicating that medical interventions may improve health outcomes. Their conclusion is that it seems reasonable to identify and intervene as often for tobacco addiction as would be the case for those with other chronic medical diseases.[25]

Contemporary best practices are shifting to reflect a far more realistic understanding of the nature of tobacco use and addiction and the processes required for its successful management. The most rational approach is reflected in a dovetailing of various interventions within a broader tobacco control strategy that includes treatment across the continuum of healthcare delivery. Such strategies can be developed and implemented in a highly time-efficient manner and have demonstrated clinical effectiveness.[26] A systematic review determined that full coverage of smoking cessation medications significantly improved 1-year abstinence rates among all smokers (RR 2.45; 95% CI 1.17-5.12), with the potential for almost 2 million life-years gained in Canada.[27] Smoking cessation appears to be one of the most robust and clinically meaningful interventions healthcare professional can offer.

SOCIAL JUSTICE

While the population-level impacts of tobacco control policies have demonstrated success in reducing the rates of smoking in Canada, there is concern that social inequalities are increasingly differentiating those individuals who use tobacco from those who do not. The demographic profile of individuals who use tobacco use has been changing over time. The greatest reductions in smoking have been demonstrated to be among those with the most resources: the wealthy and educated. Those with the least resources, the poor, uneducated, mentally ill and addicted, and other marginalized populations, carry a disproportional amount of the burden of tobacco (Chapter 4). What has been concluded is that there is little doubt that the poorest soccio-economic groups suffer the consequences of tobacco use more than the richest.[28]

Anderson et al. (2009) have claimed that social justice is a matter of life and death; that it affects the way people live, their chance of illness, and their risk of premature death.[29] It does not appear as though the existing levels of tobacco control interventions are narrowing the gap between those who are advantaged and those who are more vulnerable. Is it possible that tobacco control itself may, unintentionally, have increased the social inequities for those who are addicted to tobacco? Treatment use is particularly limited among those with the highest smoking prevalence such as those with comorbid psychiatric and substance abuse problems and lower levels of income and education, thereby contributing even more strongly to poor outcomes to disparities in disease burden and mortality.[30]

Inequalities and smoking are closely related. It is concerning that smoking has been reduced substantially among the more affluent but not at the same rates among the more disadvantaged groups. Smoking has become increasingly concentrated among the poor. Tobacco-related disease, disability, and death results in lost economic opportunities as these occur during prime, productive years. As a result, the net economic effect of tobacco is to exacerbate poverty. For the poor, the costs of tobacco are taken from shelter, food, education, and health care. The poor are more likely than the rich to become ill and die prematurely from tobacco-related illnesses. This creates greater economic hardship and perpetuates the cycle of poverty and illness. Docherty and McNeil (2012) conclude, "If we are serious about reducing health inequalities, we need to improve our efforts to reduce smoking among the disadvantaged in society."[31] (p.267) If this is the case, it is time for tobacco control and health professionals to ensure that our interventions are assisting all tobacco users and not just those who are easiest to reach.

CONCLUSIONS

The use of tobacco remains the leading preventable cause of death and disease worldwide and, having taken into consideration impressive reductions in tobacco consumption over the past few decades, current smoking rates (as an endpoint) cannot be regarded as a success. Yet the problem of tobacco is not an intractable one; the tobacco control policies identified in the FCTC have been proven to be effective. It has been estimated that some of the greatest declines in smoking-related death over the next few decades will come from increasing adult cessation.

There are differences between tobacco use and addiction; not every person who uses tobacco is addicted to the substance. Tobacco (nicotine) addiction is recognized as a chronic disease that is responsive to evidence-based treatments. Clinical Practice Guidelines exist and these endorse a range of safe and effective interventions. These typically include a combination of pharmacotherapy and counselling in a longitudinal context reflective of the chronic disease nature of tobacco addiction. Despite the highly significant health threat of tobacco, the existence of robust interventions, and the desire of most individuals to stop their use of tobacco, opportunities for intervention with tobacco use and addiction are vastly neglected. Reduction and cessation are critical steps for improving the health of individuals who use or are addicted to tobacco products.

REFERENCES

1   World Health Organization. WHO report on the global tobacco epidemic, 2008: The MPOWER package. Geneva: Author; 2008.

2   Centers for Disease Control and Prevention. Cigarette smoking-attributable morbidity—United States, 2000. Morbidity and mortality weekly report; 2003 [accessed 2012 Jan 24]. Available from: http://www.cdc.gov/mmwr/preview/mmwrhtml/mm5235a4.htm.

3   Mackay J, Eriksen M, Shafey O. The tobacco atlas, 2nd ed. Atlanta: American Cancer Society; 2006.

4   Proctor RN. Golden holocaust: origins of the cigarette catastrophe and the case for abolition. Berkeley CA: University of California Press; 2011.

5   Irvin JE, Hendricks PS, Brandon TH. The increasing recalcitrance of smokers in clinical trials: pharmacotherapy trials. Nicotine Tob Res. 2003; 5:27-35.

6   Jha P, Ranson MK, Nguyen SN, Yach D. Estimates of global and regional smoking prevalence in 1995 by age and sex. Am J Public Health. 2002;92(6):1002-6.

7   World Health Organization. The framework convention on tobacco control; 2003 [accessed 2012 May 5]. Available from: http://www.who.int/fctc/en/.

8   McLellan A, Lewis D, O'Brien C, Kleber H. Drug dependence, a chronic medical illness: implications for treatment, insurance, and outcomes evaluation. JAMA. 2007;284:1689-95.

9   Levy DT, Mabry PL, Graham AL, et al. Reaching healthy people 2010 by 2013—a SimSmoke simulation. Am J Prev Med. 2010;38:S373-81.

10   US Department of Health and Human Services. The health consequences of smoking: a report of the Surgeon General. Atlanta: US Department of Health and Human Services, Centers for Disease Control and Prevention, National Center for Chronic Disease Prevention and Health Promotion, Office on Smoking and Health; 2004 [accessed 2012 May 30]. Available from: http://www.cdc.gov/tobacco/data_statistics/sgr/2004/complete_report/index.htm.

11   American Psychiatric Association. Diagnostic and statistical manual of mental disorders, text revision, 4th ed. Washington DC: Author; 2000.

12   World Health Organization. ICD-10: International statistical classification of diseases and related health problems, tenth revision. Geneva: Author; 2007.

13   West R. Theory of addiction. Alcohol Alcohol. 2006;42(2):161-3.

14   Heather N. A conceptual framework for explaining drug addiction. J Psychopharmacol.1998; 12:3-7.

15   Benowitz N. Pharmacology of nicotine: addiction, smoking-induced disease, and therapeutics. Annu Rev Pharmacol Toxicol. 2009;49:57-71.

16   Walsh H, Govind AP, Mastro R, et al. Upregulation of nicotinic receptors by nicotine varies with receptor subtype. J Biol Chem. 2008;10:6022-32.

17   World Health Organization. Constitution of the World Health Organization [accessed 2012 May 30]. Available from: http://www.who.int/governance/eb/constitution/en/.

18   CAN-ADAPTT. Canadian smoking cessation clinical practice guideline. Toronto: Canadian Action Network for the Advancement, Dissemination and Adoption of Practice-informed Tobacco Treatment, Centre for Addiction and Mental Health; 2011 [accessed 2012 May 30]. Available from: https://www.nicotinedependenceclinic.com/English/CANADAPTT/Pages/Home.aspx.

19   Kroenke K, Spitzer RL, Williams JB. The Patient Health Questionnaire-2: validity of a 2-item depression screener. Med Care. 2003; 41:1289-92.

20   Leatherdale S, Shields M. Smoking cessation: intentions, attempts and techniques. Statistics Canada: Health Reports. Catalogue no. 82-003-XPE. Ottawa: Statistics Canada; 2009.

21   World Health Organization.The Ottawa Charter for Health Promotion. November 1986. http://www.who.int/healthpromotion/conferences/previous/ottawa/en

22   Wilkins K, Campbell NRC, Joffres MR, et al. Blood pressure in Canadian adults. Statistics Canada: Health Reports. Catalogue no. 82-003-X. Ottawa: Statistics Canada; 2010.

23   Woolacott NF, Jones L, Forbes CA, et al. The clinical effectiveness and cost-effectiveness of bupropion and nicotine replacement therapy for smoking cessation: a systematic review and economic evaluation. Health Technol Assess. 2002;6:1-256.

24   Woolf SH. The need for perspective in evidence-based medicine. JAMA. 1999; 24:2358-65.

25   Aveyard P, Raw M. (2012). Improving smoking cessation approaches at the individual level. Tob Control. 2012;21:252-7.

26   Reda AA, Kaper J, Fikretler H, et al. Healthcare financing systems for increasing the use of tobacco dependence treatment. Cochrane Database Syst Rev. 2009;2:CD004305.

27   Woolacott NF, Jones L, Forbes CA, et al. The clinical effectiveness and cost-effectiveness of bupropion and nicotine replacement therapy for smoking cessation: a systematic review and economic evaluation. Health Technol Assess. 2002;6:1-256.

28   Bobak M, Jha P, Nguyen S, Jarvis M. Poverty and smoking. Tobacco Control in Developing Countries. P Jha, F Chaloupka Eds. 2000. Oxford:Oxford Medical Publications.

29   Anderson JM, Rodney P, Reimer-Kirkham S, Browne AJ, Khan KB, Lynam MJ. Inequities in health and healthcare viewed through the ethical lens of critical social justice: contextual knowledge for the global priorities ahead. ANS Adv Nurs Sci. 2009;32(4):282-94.

30   Gollust SE, Schroeder SA, Warner KE. Helping smokers quit: understanding the barriers to utilization of smoking cessation services. Millbank Q. 2008;86(4):601-27.

31   Docherty G, McNeill, A. The hardening hypothesis: does it matter? Tob Control. 2012;21;267-8.

2

Legal Duty to Treat Tobacco Use and Addiction

PATRICK HLAVAC-WINSOR, CHARL ELS, DAVID SWEANOR AND
DIANE KUNYK

THE LAW IS ONE OF A NUMBER OF FORCES THAT MAY HELP HEALTHCARE PROFESSION-als to ameliorate the scope of the tobacco epidemic. The following chapter examines the physician's legal duty to his/her patients to treat tobacco use and addiction. It is beyond this chapter's scope to delve into an in-depth comment on all aspects of the legal implications concerning the treatment of mental illness and other addictions, but it is useful to carry out a cursory overview of the tort law framework under which a negligence claim could be made for the failure to identify and treat the effects of tobacco addiction.

Both the *DSM* and the *ICD* recognize tobacco addiction as a bona fide, chronic relapsing medical condition, and evidence-based treatment guidelines exist for its safe and effective treatment. Given the high prevalence rates of smoking, its addictive properties and its proven hazardous effects on human health, it is surprising that there is a lack of concrete jurisprudence in Canada regarding a physician's duty of care for the treatment of tobacco addiction. Not simply an academic debate on tort law, this is a relevant issue for public policy, evidence-based treatment, and an illustration of the unrealized public health gains that could flow from the use of current tort law in Canada. Although focused on physicians, this discussion may be of relevance to other healthcare practitioners.

In proving medical malpractice, a plaintiff must establish all four elements of the tort of negligence:

1. A duty of care existed or was owed.
2. The duty of care was breached, suggesting the treatment provider failed to conform to the relevant standard care.
3. The damage(s) resulted, and needs to be proven
4. The breach was a proximate cause of damages/injury.

The issue of injury and negligence permeates all aspects of the physician–patient relationship, which gives rise to a duty of care. The fact that there is a relationship and a fiduciary duty by the physician toward the patient speaks to several aspects that make up the tort claim framework. The physician–patient relationship is informed with a certain standard of care within its context, and any tort claim rests on the fact that damages have been incurred due to the breach of the standard of care owed to the patient—this reflects the causation aspect of a tort claim.

Once a relationship is established between a physician and a patient, the physician owes the patient a duty of care centred on a duty to treat the patient's illnesses. The duty to treat continues until the physician severs the relationship. Along with a duty to treat, the physician owes the patient a duty to disclose the risks of treatment. This duty to disclose is a continuing one when the condition requires long-term treatment.[1] Similarly, a physician has a duty to inform the patient of the effects of declining treatment.[2] The extent of this duty is highlighted in the case of *Hollis v. Birch*, where the court stated that "every individual has the right to know what risks are involved in undergoing or foregoing medical treatment and a concomitant right to make meaningful decisions based on a full understanding of those risks."[3]

The duty of care established by the physician's relationship with the patient is governed by the standard of care measured by whether the physician meets the standard of the "normal, prudent practitioner" in an objective way.[4] As pointed out by Picard and Robertson, the medical practitioner is therefore measured "objectively against a reasonable medical person who possesses and exercises the skill, knowledge and judgment of the normal, prudent practitioner of his or her special group."[2 (p.227)] Based on this standard, a specialist would be held to a higher standard based in his or her particular field. Additionally, the standard of care is influenced by the risk of the treatment, correspondingly increasing to coincide with increased risk.[5 (pp.285–88),6] Lastly, the standard must be judged "in light of the knowledge that ought to have been reasonably possessed at the time of the alleged negligence."[2 (p.240)] This means that the standard of care must be looked at in the context of knowledge at the time of treatment. Knowledge in this case must be at the level recognized by professional certification boards and overseeing bodies.

Following the establishment of a duty of care to the patient, along with a breach of the standard of care and resulting damages, the plaintiff patient would still need to establish causality of the injury by the deviation from the standard of care. This means that the plaintiff must show that but for the deviation from the established standard of care, the injury would not have happened. Within the context above, the courts have spoken specifically about individual duties comprising treatment and standards of treatment, and these will now be discussed.

DUTY TO DIAGNOSE

Picard and Robertson noted: "A thorough history, proper examination, appropriate tests, and consultations with colleagues and specialists where necessary, are clearly basic to a proper diagnosis. A reasonable [physician] should also heed a patient's complaints during treatment for they may be harbingers of change in condition. A [physician's] role in diagnosis cannot be just a passive one. Within reason, if appropriate tests are indicated they should be carried out and their results carefully reviewed, and if certain symptoms could be critical they should be canvassed with the patient."[2 (pp.302–5)]

DUTY TO REFER

In certain circumstances the Supreme Court of Canada has stated that there is a duty to refer in cases such as where the physician is unable to diagnose a condition, in cases of unresponsiveness to treatment, or in cases where "treatment is required which the [physician] is not competent to give."[2 (pp.312–14),7]

DUTY TO INSTRUCT THE PATIENT

In determining whether the patient can take on the responsibility for following instruction regarding their treatment, a physician must take into account the patient's ability to follow treatment. In this sense, the [physician] must take cognitive impairment or the effects of the very illness which is being treated … into account in assessing the extent to which the patient will be able to understand and carry out instruction. When the [physician] delegates to the patient the performance of some part of the treatment, there is a duty on the [physician] to explain clearly what is expected of the patient and to give a warning as may be required by the circumstances.[2] The Supreme Court of Canada stated in *Neutzen v. Korn*: "It is generally accepted that when a doctor acts in accordance with a recognized and respectable practice of the profession, he or she will not be found to be negligent."[8] In cases where a patient does not follow instructions, such as following up on appointments, they may be held to have contributory negligence. In *Patmore v. Weatherston* the court stated that the physician was not "obliged to 'chase' or 'hunt down' a patient who fails to return at the appropriate interval where there is nothing unusual about her condition."[9] Contributory negligence may result in a reduction of the damages awarded to the plaintiff if the other aspects of the negligence claim are made.

CAUSATION

In order to make out a claim for damages under torts, the plaintiff must show causation of the breach of the physician's standard leading to the damages. According to current case law interpreting the *Reibl* test, there is both "a subjective and objective requirement" in some cases, while other cases specifically continue to view the objective test only "what a reasonable person would have done."[2] [(p.190),10] The foregoing is however informed by the Supreme Court's ruling in *Arndt v. Smith* where the court stated the test involves "reasonable beliefs, fears, desires and expectations … in deciding what a reasonable person in the patient's circumstances would have done if properly informed."[2 (p.197),11] Academics have noted that the dicta in *Reibl v. Hughes* suggests that "the court must be satisfied that a reasonable person in the plaintiff's position would have declined the treatment at the particular time … this seems to imply that a decision to postpone treatment is sufficient to establish causation."[2 (pp.201–7)]

In essence, the courts have settled the fact that a physician has a duty to disclose possible treatments and their corresponding risks, including the implications of not having treatment. With this in mind, if the patient does not receive the broad disclosure about treatment options and is able to make an informed decision about treatment, the potential claim for an injury stems from the causation of delayed treatment or incomplete treatment.[2 (pp. 201–7)]

When dealing with the issue of treatment or the lack thereof, the traditional approach in torts is to illustrate elements of medical negligence. In broad strokes, negligence is proven if the defendant owed the plaintiff a legal duty of care; that the defendant breached that duty; that the plaintiff suffered damages; and that the damages were caused as a result of the defendant's breach of duty of care.[12] Within this framework, physicians are subjected to accepted standards regarding treatment as well as the notion that a patient should receive treatment in the first place.

The issue of tobacco use and addiction (and its resulting diseases) is unique in that it does not offer a clear-cut approach from the medical establishment. On the one hand, if tobacco addiction is seen as a voluntary activity and not as a medical condition, it may itself not warrant treatment but may be a factor in the treatment of another illness. If on the other hand, tobacco use is diagnosed as an illness (mental or otherwise), a physician may very well be required to offer treatment for the condition itself, or at least viable ways to reduce risk such as long term substitution of less hazardous nicotine delivery products. In either case, the physician faces the risk of not addressing the use of tobacco and therefore failing to honour a duty of care to the patient or to treat the patient to an adequate standard of care.

In the traditional sense of tort proceedings, one would need to prove, on a balance of probabilities, that an individual was detrimentally affected by a physician's failure to provide/establish treatment of tobacco use and addiction or amelioration of its harm. By the very nature of the relationship between the patient and the doctor, the doctor would have a duty to treat. This is, however, only the first step in the tort debate over negligence. Under certain circumstances, such as a physician's inability to offer adequate treatment, the duty of care may only extend as far as finding a qualified specialist capable of treating the condition, or to interventions that fall short of effective cessation but still significantly reduce risk.

A successful claim for negligence must show that the standard of care was below accepted norms. While jurisprudence has shown some willingness of the courts to recognize the changing nature of treatments, it has opened up the debate on whether there are differing community standards with regard to the level of treatment received. Even though this is a nuance in the standard of care debate, the pith of the matter rests on whether a physician treated the patient in the standard accepted by the medical establishment or a respected minority opinion of that establishment. In the case of tobacco use, case law illustrates that an acceptable standard to which a physician is held takes into account the effect of tobacco use on other conditions. For example, when dealing with a heart condition, a physician may be found to have breached the standard of care if he did not take into account a prolonged use of tobacco over the patient's lifetime. While not directly dealing with the issue of tobacco use, the standard of care to which the physician was held takes into account the detrimental impact of tobacco use on the treatment of a heart condition. In other medical negligence cases, it was often the lack of notice of other factors beyond the immediate symptoms of illness, which led to a court's finding that the standard of care fell below acceptable norms.

In several cases, the courts viewed the loss of opportunity for treatment and reduced resulting lifespan as damages.[5 (pp.405–22),13] One must remember that every case is judged on its facts and the evidence in support of a patient's claim of damages. Jurisprudence refers to statistics on the probability of successful treatment of various conditions when addressing the issue of damages. It may not be evident whether an individual could be successfully treated; however, the loss of opportunity for treatment may in some instances mean the difference between life and death. Not addressing an underlying condition such as the potential effect tobacco use may in fact carry with it the risk of treatment that is not adequately aggressive or that comes too late. As such the patients' claim of damages rests on the ability to show a statistical difference in outcome between treatment provided and the treatment that should have been provided given the circumstances.

Lastly, a patient must show that the resulting damages claimed stem from the breach of the physician's duty and standard of care. Due to the aggregate effects and prolonged exposure required to see a difference in the patient's health, the balance of probabilities required for successful claim is difficult to achieve given the countless factors affecting the patient's health over the same period of time. While recent case law states that a physician must investigate factors such as tobacco use when making a diagnosis and then following up on a referral to a specialist (or alternative provider) to deal with the treatment if unable to provide same themselves, long periods of time required to manifest illness (i.e. the insult-to-consequence latency period) make it difficult to show how the lack of treatment of tobacco use and addiction contributes to the patient's health. It is precisely because of this last step (but for test) that tort law can present a challenge in adequately addressing tobacco use and addiction treatment.[5 (pp.376–86)]

In recent academic discourse, tort law was described as having the fundamental purpose of providing a tool to remedy those injured by the willful or negligent conduct of others. While traditional tort law is able to cope with certain situations, others have pointed out it is "increasingly incapable of effectively dealing with some of the most grievous cases of harm by willful and negligent conduct on a modern society."[14] As such, this evolving aspect of tort law may need to take into account the growing scientific body of evidence showing harm and causation.

It is precisely along these lines that challenges to failure to adhere to standards of care for evidence-based treatment may fill in the gaps of traditional tort law. While traditional tort law would rely on the evidence presented—while based on long-standing legal principles—evidence-based treatment offers scientific methodology acquired over long periods of time and with large datasets. As such, evidence-based treatment serves as an impartial mechanism by which physicians have a base of decision-making about individual patients.[15] This evidence-based care helps to alleviate the subjective element when dealing with traditional tort matters. In the case of tobacco use and addiction, evidence-based treatment introduces a broad scientific body of knowledge with regard to tobacco effects. This body of knowledge, in turn, helps to clarify the need for a physician to address tobacco use or exposure and may, in fact, suggest that the standard of care required for its treatment has become more stringent. Departing from the medical standard of treatment and diagnosis may furthermore be shown to constitute negligence, given the body of empirical evidence connecting the use of tobacco and ill health effects. Additionally, given the increasing volume of knowledge demonstrating that tobacco use induces tobacco addiction, and given that addiction is recognized as a mental illness, a physician is more likely to have a duty of care for the treatment of this condition or the referral and proper follow-up to a specialist capable of treating the condition.

The evidence-based approach to these issues shifts the focus from the individual to the needs of society. Given the amount of time required to show symptoms of conditions like tobacco addiction, an evidence-based approach uses aggregated data to address large and costly medical issues. This approach not only impacts the traditional realm of tort law, it is a fundamental shift recognizing the high cost of care and social needs rather than an individualistic approach to treatment.[16] The impact of this approach is pronounced in all the factors showing negligence (be it from recognizing certain conditions as illness, understanding that effective treatment involves a certain standard of care for the condition, and that data supports the notion that prolonged exposure to tobacco products causes harm and if statistically significant in impacting the treatment or quality of life of a patient).

Apart from the potential risk for a successful tort case, whereby a physician has displayed negligence in the failure to treat tobacco addiction in a person under his/her care, there is the possibility of facing regulatory scrutiny. The provincial Colleges of Physicians and Surgeons have the mandate to guide the profession and to protect the public. From this perspective, if a patient can, based on a complaint filed to a specific College, demonstrate that a physician did not meet standards of care, the physician may be at risk of disciplinary action.

- Tobacco (nicotine) addiction is recognized as a bona fide chronic, relapsing medical condition.
- Country-specific clinical practice guidelines are available for the safe and effective treatment of this condition.
- In the context of a therapeutic relationship, where a duty to care exists, the failure to address tobacco addiction may potentially be viewed as a failure to meet standards of care, and as negligence under certain circumstances.

CONCLUSION

Tort law is a relevant framework for the issue of tobacco use and addiction treatment. Several aspects of the duty to treat and standard of care look to the medical establishment for guidance on acceptable standards. The courts are not experts and therefore look to governing medical bodies to establish the standard of treatment for tobacco use and addiction. The changing standards may make it more likely that a negligence claim can be made out if a physician did not actively comply with the accepted body of knowledge for tobacco treatment. While the tort framework may not immediately seem to apply to a duty to treat tobacco use and addiction, the reference to accepted treatment by governing medical bodies might serve a patient in making a negligence claim.

Given the high prevalence rates of tobacco use and addiction, the devastating health effects of tobacco consumption, and existence of Canadian practice guidelines for the treatment of tobacco use and addiction, it is the authors' belief that the likelihood of a successful tort case for damages sustained as a result of failure to provide treatment, is not only possible, but even likely under certain circumstances. Physicians' knowledge of the potential legal and regulatory risk associated with not providing treatment for tobacco use and addiction may increase their motivation to treat patients under their care. It is the duty of each physician to familiarize him/herself with the existing standards of care for the treatment of tobacco use and addiction based on Canadian guidelines, and to ensure that he/she has the necessary knowledge and skills to satisfy legal duties in terms of the management of the public health disaster: tobacco use and addiction.

REFERENCES

1   Peppin P. Informed consent. In: Downie J, Caulfield T, Flood C, editors. Canadian health law and policy. 3rd ed. Markham ON: LexisNexis Canada Inc; 2007. p.202.

2   Picard E, Robertson G. Legal liability of doctors and hospitals in Canada. 4th ed. Toronto: Thomson Carswell; 2007.

3   Hollis v. Birch, 129 D.L.R. (4th) 609 (S.C.C.) at 620 (1995).

4   Glass KC, Waring D. The physician/investigator's obligation to patients participating in research: the case of placebo controlled trials. J Law Med Ethics. 2005;33(3):575-85.

5   Jones M. Medical negligence. London UK: Sweet & Maxwell; 2003.

6   Lindahl v. Olsen, ABQB 639 (2004).

7   Rendek v. Dufresne, A.J. No. 1167 (2006).

8   Neuzen v. Korn, 3 S.C.R. 674 at 16 (1995).

9   Patmore (Guardian at litem of) v. Weatherston, B.C.J. No. 650 at 14 (1999).

10   Finch v. Carpenter, B.C.J. No. 1918 (S.C.) (1993).

11   Arndt v. Smith, 2 S.C.R. 539 (1997).

12   Restatement of the Law (2d) of Torts, 281, American Law Institute (1965).

13   Dickens B. Medical negligence. In: Downie J, Caulfield T, Flood C, editors. Canadian health law and policy. 3rd ed. Markham ON: LexisNexis Canada Inc; 2007. p.124.

14   McLachlin B. Negligence law – proving the connection. In: Mullany NJ, Linden AM, editors. Torts tomorrow: a tribute to John Fleming. Sydney: LBC Information Services; 1998:16 at 34.

15   Wilson K. Risk, causation and precaution: understanding policy-making regarding public health risks. In: Bailey T, Caulfield T, Ries N, editors. Public health law and policy in Canada, 2nd ed. Markham: LexisNexis Canada Inc; 2008. pp. 61-89.

16   Nixon S, Upshur RE, Robertson A, Benatar SR, Thompson A, Daar A. Public health ethics. In: Bailey T, Caulfield T, Ries N, editors. Public health law and policy in Canada, 2nd ed. Markham: LexisNexis Canada Inc; 2008. pp. 47-58.

3

Health Effects of Tobacco and Secondhand Smoke

ROBERTA FERRENCE, SARAH MUIR AND JACLYN KAYE

FOR AT LEAST 5 CENTURIES, TOBACCO HAS BEEN VIEWED AS A HARMFUL PRODUCT. IN 1604, King James I of England quite accurately pronounced it "a custome loth-some to the eye, hatefull to the Nose, harmefull to the braine, dangerous to the Lungs, and in the blacke stinking fume thereof, neerest resembling the horrible Stigian smoke of the pit that is bottomelesse." In the 19th century, Dr. Joel Shew of England attributed heart disease, cancer, impotency, insanity, and receding gums to the effects of smoking and chewing tobacco. Even Henry Ford published on the topic. Although some felt it had benefits, such as protection from the plague, tobacco use continued its relentless spread around the world, followed by its legacy of death and disease.

Preceded by a reference in 1916 to a "careful study of six Canadian insur-ance companies that found the mortality rate of non-smokers to be 59 and that of moderate smokers 93," the first formal research studies showed a link between smoking and lung cancer as early as 1939. By the early 1950s, large-scale epi-demiological studies confirmed this link, supported by laboratory research that found tumours in mice painted with cigarette tar. Heart disease was soon added to the list, and a dose–response relationship for amount and duration of smoking was found between smoking and lung cancer.

In 1964, the publication of the landmark Report of the US Surgeon Gen-eral on Smoking and Health marked the beginning of the decline in cigarette use in North America. The report concluded that cigarette smoking caused lung and laryngeal cancer in men, probably in women, and was the most impor-tant cause of chronic bronchitis in both sexes. Subsequent reports established tobacco use as a cause of most types of cancer, a range of cardiovascular and respiratory diseases, and several other conditions. The 1988 Report on Nicotine Addiction confirmed that tobacco products are addicting, that nicotine is the drug that causes addiction, and that the processes involved in nicotine addiction are similar to those that determine addiction to heroin and cocaine. Canada produced its own report on nicotine addiction in 1989, confirming the addictive properties of nicotine.

MECHANISMS FOR HEALTH EFFECTS

Tobacco smoke contains more than 7,000 chemicals, many of which are poisonous. Hundreds are toxic; at least 70 can cause cancer. These poisons, including toxic metals, poisonous gases and cancer-causing chemicals, reach not only the lungs but also every organ of the body through the bloodstream. Repeated inhalation of smoke leads to inflammation and damage and causes continuous stress to the immune system.

SMOKING

Active smoking has major effects throughout the body and consequently is a major or minor cause of most diseases that afflict us. Cigarette smoking is associated with at least 14 types of cancer. In some cases, such as kidney and bladder cancer, about half of all cases are caused by smoking. Breast cancer is now associated with active smoking in women of all ages. Carcinogens in cigarette smoke cause cancer-causing chemicals to bind to DNA. Several pathogenic processes (exposure to tobacco carcinogens, DNA damage and mutations) lead to lung cancer, and quitting smoking is the only proven way to reduce the risk of disease.

Cigarette smoking causes cardiovascular disease, including coronary heart disease, stroke, and other related conditions, including abdominal aortic aneurism. It also produces insulin resistance, which can lead to diabetes, vascular complications, and nerve damage. Smoking is associated with higher serum levels of cholesterol, lower levels of high-density lipoprotein (HDL), the good cholesterol, and other cardiovascular disease-related risk factors.

Smoking dose-dependently increases the risk of impaired glucose intolerance, type-2 diabetes, and abdominal-type obesity. Persons with diabetes who also smoke have an increased risk of complications and death. Although smokers on average have a lower body weight than non-smokers, they tend to accumulate more abdominal fat, which is associated with a greater risk of developing health problems.

FIGURE 1: The health consequences associated with smoking and exposure to secondhand smoke

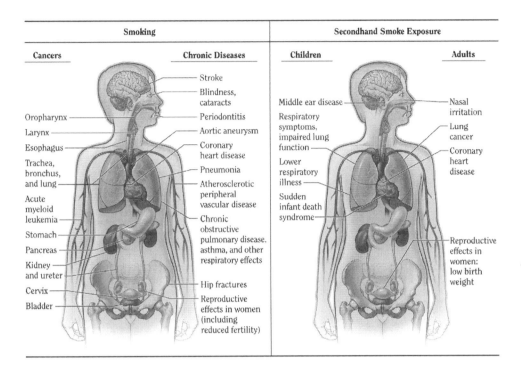

Source: US Department of Health and Human Services. How Tobacco Smoke Causes Disease – The Biology and Behavioral Basis for Smoking-Attributable Disease. A Report of the Surgeon General. Atlanta: US Department of Health and Human Services, Centers for Disease Control and Prevention, National Center for Chronic Disease Prevention and Health Promotion, Office on Smoking and Health; 2010. Used with permission.

It is well known that cigarette smoking causes chronic obstructive lung/ pulmonary diseases (COLD/COPD), which include emphysema, chronic bronchitis, and other disorders. Smoking produces oxidative stress, which can result in disease after several years.

There are a number of serious reproductive and developmental effects from smoking. These include chromosome changes and DNA damage in sperm cells, which affect male fertility and anomalies in offspring, such as cleft palate. Maternal smoking is linked to placental problems and can lead to fetal loss, preterm delivery, and low birth weight. Carbon monoxide exposure leads to low birth weight and may play a role in neurological deficits. Maternal smoking causes disease-related changes in the fetus, particularly brain and lung tissues.

A number of other conditions have been linked to cigarette smoking, including hip fracture, peptic ulcer, cataracts, and gum disease. Recent research implicates smoking in multiple sclerosis, rheumatoid arthritis, and other serious health conditions.

There is limited literature on the health effects of light and intermittent smoking, since most studies examine daily smokers. However, we do know that light smoking carries substantial health risks. Light and intermittent smokers may go undetected because they often don't see themselves as smokers or they deny their smoking.

Changes in cigarette design (filters, low-tar, or 'light' variations) have not reduced the overall risk of tobacco-related diseases among smokers and may have, in some cases, increased risk. The design characteristics of cigarettes (e.g. ventilation features, filters, paper porosity) can actually increase levels of toxic and carcinogenic chemicals in the inhaled smoke. With increased ventilation in 'light' cigarettes, smokers may inhale more deeply and cover ventilation holes with their fingers to get more nicotine and actually increase toxic exposures to the lung.

SMOKELESS TOBACCO

Use of smokeless tobacco may result in leukoplakia, oral cancer—especially squamous cell carcinoma—transient hypertension, cardiovascular disease, and nicotine dependence, as well as a reduction in the acuity of taste and smell. Smokeless tobacco use is associated with an increased risk of fatal myocardial infarction and stroke. A review of worldwide epidemiological data found that the risk of cancer for smokeless tobacco users is probably lower than that for smokers but higher than that of non-tobacco users. However, results from a study comparing carcinogen biomarkers in the urine of smokers and smokeless tobacco users show similar exposures to the potent tobacco-specific carcinogen NNK (Nicotine-derived nitrosamine ketone (NNK), or 4-(methylnitrosamino)- 1-(3-pyridyl)-1-butanone) in smokeless tobacco users and smokers, which does not support the use of smokeless tobacco as a safe substitute for smoking. The carcinogenic potential of smokeless tobacco is affected by the fermentation process, type of storage (refrigerated or not), and length of storage. While Swedish *snus* or snuff has been promoted as a reduced-risk product compared with traditional smokeless, its use is associated with a twofold increase in the risk of pancreatic cancer and a decrease in diastolic heart function in the left and right ventricles. Smokeless tobacco also appears to increase the prevalence of type-2 diabetes, particularly with high daily doses.

OTHER TOBACCO PRODUCTS

The tobacco industry has also developed newer smokeless tobacco products such as lozenges, tablets, tabs, strips, and sticks. These would present lower risk to individuals than cigarette smoking but may encourage nicotine addiction among youth, deter would-be cigarette quitters, and normalize the regular use of nicotine in society at large.

E-CIGARETTES

E-cigarettes or 'electronic nicotine delivery systems' (ENDS, the term used by the World Health Organization) deliver nicotine and other chemicals in vapour form. The e-cigarettes available in Canada do not contain nicotine. Potential hazards of inhalation of the complex mixture of chemicals found in e-cigarette vapours are not yet well documented, although early research shows some immediate adverse changes in pulmonary function. The effects of long-term use are unknown at this point. There is no evidence that e-cigarettes are effective treatment for nicotine addiction, and they are not approved as smoking cessation devices.

E-cigarettes are widely marketed on the Internet with added flavourings that appeal to youth, despite the fact that they are not approved for sale in Canada. Starter kits for e-cigarettes and e-hookah are now available in convenience stores as well as online. Early use of nicotine can quickly lead to nicotine addiction and ultimately uptake of cigarettes or other tobacco products. Many users of e-cigarettes (or "vapers" as some call themselves) may continue to use cigarettes in addition to their electronic ones. There are concerns that these electronic products are being used to undermine smoking bans, which could lead to increased use of all tobacco products. A recent case in which an e-cigarette exploded also suggests the difficulty with unregulated products.

SECONDHAND SMOKE

Exposure to secondhand smoke is known to cause lung cancer and nasal sinus cancer. There is strong evidence that it causes an increased risk of breast cancer among younger, mainly premenopausal, women. When the cells in the body are repeatedly exposed to the toxins in secondhand smoke, it causes irritation and inflammation, and ultimately DNA damage to the cells. This DNA damage causes out-of-control cell growth and can produce cancerous tumours.

There is no risk-free level of exposure to tobacco smoke. Tobacco smoke affects every organ in the body and can cause premature death and disease among smokers and non-smokers. Twenty years ago, secondhand smoke was classified as a 'Class A' carcinogen, which means it is a confirmed cause of cancer. The major adverse health outcomes caused by tobacco smoke occur via DNA damage, inflammation, and oxidative stress: cancers (respiratory and non-respiratory), cardiovascular disease, and pulmonary disease. There is also increasing evidence for a causal association between secondhand smoke and an increased risk of stroke.

There are many chemicals in secondhand tobacco smoke that can cause adverse health effects. Carbon monoxide in tobacco smoke decreases the availability of oxygen in the blood, which in turn increases the risk of heart attack. Other chemicals and toxins in secondhand smoke can cause formation of plaques, which can narrow and block the arteries.

The adverse health effects of secondhand smoke for children and infants can be more severe since their bodies are smaller, they have higher respiration rates than adults, and their bodies and lungs are still developing. Evidence shows that when fetuses and children are exposed to secondhand smoke, it can cause fetal growth impairment, low birth weight (due to maternal smoking or exposure to secondhand smoke), sudden infant death syndrome (SIDS), respiratory diseases and infections, worsening of asthma, and an increase in middle-ear infections.

The risk and severity of many adverse health effects (both acute and chronic) are directly related to duration and amount of exposure to tobacco smoke. However, even low levels of exposure to tobacco smoke can cause acute cardiovascular events and thrombosis. Many jurisdictions around the world have introduced smoking bans in workplaces and public places and have seen a substantial decrease in the rate of hospitalizations for heart attacks and a decrease in asthma and other respiratory symptoms.

Humans aren't the only ones affected: family pets are also seriously harmed by secondhand smoke. Animals inhale smoke as people do, but develop cancers and other diseases in a much shorter period of time and usually die from their smoking-related diseases. Dogs are particularly subject to lung cancer and nasal sinus cancer. Cats develop oral cancer and lymphoma. Lung cancer also afflicts pet birds.

There is good evidence now that outdoor exposure to tobacco smoke can be as high as indoors within 2 metres of a lit cigarette, with lower levels occurring up to and beyond 9 metres away. Even with indoor bans on smoking in most jurisdictions in North America, wait staff of restaurants and bars, as well as patrons, are still exposed for lengthy periods to hazardous amounts of second-hand smoke on outdoor patios that permit smoking.

Another consideration often ignored is the notion of social exposure to both cigarettes and secondhand smoke. Social exposure includes the visual and sensory cues associated with cigarette smoking. Young people in particular are influenced to smoke when those around them are smoking. By eliminating visibility of smoking and exposure to secondhand smoke, we are likely to see reduced relapse among smokers who have already quit, reduced initiation among never smokers, and an increase in smokers who quit.

THIRDHAND SMOKE

Thirdhand smoke has increasingly garnered attention as a potential health hazard related to smoking. Even though it is found in the research literature of the 1950s (remember those mice painted with 'tar'), it was not identified as a separate substance until the past decade. While secondhand smoke is a mixture of side-stream smoke (smoke emitted from a burning cigarette) and mainstream smoke (smoke exhaled by the smoker), thirdhand smoke is the residual tobacco smoke that persists as fine particles in dust that is found on surfaces such as clothing, hair, skin, walls, furniture, carpets, and inside cars, after the cigarette is extinguished. It contains nicotine, cancer-causing agents such as formaldehyde and tobacco-specific nitrosamines (TSNAs), and heavy metals such as lead, cadmium, and arsenic. When nicotine from thirdhand smoke on indoor surfaces combines and reacts with nitrous acid in indoor air, it forms new carcinogens; these new secondary pollutants are in addition to those found in freshly emitted tobacco smoke. The presence of nitrous acid from unventilated combustible appliances makes the home a major source of exposure to thirdhand smoke.

TABLE 1: Confirmed and suspected diseases caused by smoking and secondhand smoke exposure

Disease		Active Smoking		Passive Smoking				
		Confirmed	Suspected	Confirmed			Suspected	
				Adults	Children	Pets	Adults	Children
Cancers	Lung	✓		✓		✓ (Dogs, Birds)		
	Oropharynx	✓						
	Lip and Oral Cavity	✓						
	Nasal Cavity & Paranasal Sinus	✓		✓		✓ (Dogs)		
	Esophagus	✓						
	Trachea	✓						
	Bronchus	✓						
	Acute Myeloid Leukemia (Bone Marrow)	✓						
	Stomach	✓						
	Pancreas	✓						
	Kidney	✓						
	Uterine Cervix	✓					✓	
	Ureter	✓						
	Bladder	✓						
	Breast	✓		✓ (Pre-menopausal Women)				
	Colorectal		✓					
	Liver		✓					
	Oral Cancer					✓ (Cats)		
	Lymphoma					✓ (Cats)		
Cardiovascular Disease	Stroke	✓					✓	
	Aortic Aneurysm	✓						
	Coronary Heart Disease	✓		✓				
	Peripheral Vascular Disease	✓						
Respiratory Diseases	Chronic Obstructive Pulmonary Disease (COPD)	✓						
	Pneumonia	✓						
	Asthma	✓ (Worsening)			✓ (Worsening)			✓ (Induction)
	Coughing, phlegm, wheezing	✓			✓			
	Impaired Lung Function	✓			✓*			
	Lower respiratory illness				✓			
Reproductive Effects	Reduced Fertility in Mother and Offspring	✓			✓*			
	Sudden Infant Death Syndrome (SIDS)	✓			✓			
	Low Birth Weight	✓			✓*			
	Stillbirths and Fetal Death	✓						
	Pregnancy Complications	✓						
	Ectopic Pregnancy		✓					
	Miscarriage						✓	
	Fetal Growth Impairment				✓*			
Other Effects (Adults)	Hip fractures	✓						
	Low Bone Density	✓						
	Cataracts, Blindness	✓						
	Post-Surgical Healing Complications	✓						
	Peptic Ulcer Disease if *Helicobacter Pylori* positive	✓						
	Gum Disease	✓						
	Dental Caries		✓					
	Erectile Dysfunction		✓					
	Age-related Macular Degeneration (AMD)		✓					
	Multiple Sclerosis		✓					
	Absenteeism	✓		✓	✓			
Other Effects (Children)	Middle Ear Disease				✓			
	Oral Clefts in Infants		✓*					
	Adverse Impact of Cognition and Behaviour							✓
	Worsening of Cystic Fibrosis							✓

*In utero exposure

Thirdhand smoke has also been found on the interior surfaces of cars. The nicotine that is emitted during smoking can persist on indoor surfaces for weeks, months, or years, and when smoking occurs regularly in the same indoor location, layers of the toxins and carcinogens continually accumulate on these surfaces. Exposure to thirdhand smoke can occur via different routes such as: 1) skin contact with indoor surfaces (skin, hair, clothing, furniture, carpets, walls) that have accumulated the toxins, 2) ingestion of toxins from the indoor surfaces that have accumulated these toxins (e.g. infants crawling and playing with toys on the floor or carpet), or 3) inhalation of toxins that are found in dust particles on indoor surfaces. Though all ages are at risk of exposure to thirdhand smoke from indoor surfaces, children and infants are particularly at risk since they have regular contact with the floor, frequently put their fingers and objects in their mouths and have a higher respiration rate and lower body weight than adults. Additionally, outdoor-only smoking policies do not fully protect children and non-smokers in the home since thirdhand smoke particles can travel on the smoker's skin, hair, and clothing to indoor surfaces and the skin of others, particularly infants.

Family pets also spend much of their time indoors in home settings. Dogs and cats are exposed when they sit or lie on carpets, furniture, and other surfaces, and cats ingest toxic substances while grooming themselves.

While we cannot draw firm conclusions about the health hazards and negative health effects of exposure to thirdhand tobacco smoke, some of the toxins found in thirdhand smoke are known carcinogens, in particular, NNK, a lung carcinogen. If levels of this carcinogen accumulate over time on indoor surfaces, this exposure could contribute to lung cancer among both smokers and non-smokers exposed to secondhand and thirdhand smoke.

A growing concern is the thirdhand smoke that persists in homes previously occupied by smokers, even after smokers move out and the home is cleaned and left vacant for up to 2 months. New non-smoking residents will be exposed to thirdhand smoke particles and dust left on the indoor surfaces. Research shows that while the nicotine levels in the home declined with the new non-smoking residents, overall nicotine levels were still higher compared with homes of non-smokers.

While the emerging evidence about thirdhand smoke is not conclusive at this point, there are strong reasons to protect non-smokers and children from the potential health effects of thirdhand smoke exposure. Since higher levels of secondhand smoke are found in the homes of families of lower socioeconomic status, who are more likely to live in multi-unit social housing, there are important equity issues to be considered in providing protection.

WATERPIPE (HOOKAH, SHISHA OR NARGHILE) SMOKING

Research evidence on the harmful effects of waterpipe smoking, both tobacco and non-tobacco or herbal, has grown substantially in the past decade. We can now say with certainty that all waterpipe smoke is harmful to users and to those in the immediate environment. There are several areas of concern: high levels of exposure to carbon monoxide (CO), far greater than those for cigarette smoking; substantial exposure to the other products of combustion, including several carcinogens, the threat of infectious disease from sharing of mouthpieces, the lack of any kind of regulation of these products or where they can be used, and the widespread misperception that waterpipe is safer than cigarette smoking and that herbal waterpipe products are non-toxic.

Waterpipe smoking produces high levels of exposure to CO. There is research evidence for hospital admissions for CO poisoning at levels (20–30 ppm) that are commonly experienced in waterpipe smoking sessions. Waterpipe smoking significantly reduces lung function compared with non-smokers, but not compared with cigarette smokers.

Waterpipe tobacco smoking is associated with a more than twofold risk of respiratory illness, low birth-weight, cardiovascular disease, and lung cancer. Periodontal disease risks are 3–5 times higher. Disease types and rates for cigarette smokers have been established over the past 70 years, and longer follow-up will be required to establish these for waterpipe smoking. However, since the resulting smoke is the same, we can expect similar or even higher rates of both chronic and acute disease. Of particular concern is the fact that young women who smoke or are exposed to tobacco smoke before first pregnancy are at greatly increased risk of breast cancer, because young people are the major users of waterpipe.

Infectious diseases, such as tuberculosis, hepatitis, meningitis, and respiratory infections, can be transmitted by the use of shared mouthpieces. Some waterpipe cafes avoid cleaning mouthpieces and hoses to retain the flavour for the next user. Risks may actually be higher with longer follow-up periods, since research in this area is relatively new.

Addiction is a serious effect of waterpipe tobacco smoking, and, given the likelihood that nicotine may be added, of non-tobacco waterpipe smoking as well. Anecdotal evidence from tobacco enforcement inspectors suggests that herbal products are routinely spiked with 'e-juice' (pure nicotine used in e-cigarettes), which would also lead to addiction and potentially other damage. Since waterpipe is often used at a young age, it could serve as a gateway drug to cigarette smoking.

Puff topography research indicates that waterpipe users take 18 times as many puffs as cigarette smokers, with a resulting puff volume that is 12 times as high and a duration that is twice as long with half the interval between puffs. A meta-analysis of studies examining nicotine absorption among waterpipe users found levels comparable to smoking 10 cigarettes daily.

In a laboratory study, compared with pre-smoking levels, CO emissions from waterpipe smoking increased 20-fold during a 45-minute session compared with a less than three-fold increase after smoking a single cigarette. Peak nicotine levels were similar for both groups but waterpipe users experienced much higher levels of smoke exposure. Waterpipe tobacco smoking also increases heart rate and nicotine concentration, due to the presence of nicotine.

New laboratory research shows no significant differences between waterpipe tobacco and waterpipe herbal preparations in exposure to toxicants that are products of combustion. These include a variety of carcinogens and other substances that cause smoking-related cancers and cardiovascular disease. Specifically, when the researchers compared levels of carbon monoxide, nitric oxide, volatile aldehydes, nicotine, tar, and polycyclic aromatic hydrocarbons in both tobacco and herbal waterpipe products, only the level of nicotine was different.

Waterpipe use has become an issue of worldwide concern in recent years, particularly with regard to young people. While all other forms of tobacco smoking are banned in indoor public places across Canada, waterpipe use has been tolerated, mainly because federal and provincial legislation cover tobacco products rather than all smoked products, and waterpipe smoking may use tobacco, herbal product, or a mixture of both. This has led to an inability in many jurisdictions to control exposure to waterpipe smoke because most legislation applies only to tobacco products. This means expensive and time-consuming testing is usually required to prove that the product contains tobacco.

Since hookah, a type of waterpipe, smoking occurs in a group and tends to involve several smokers for long periods of time, it is reasonable to conclude that outdoor hookah smoking will also cause serious health effects. Even 30 minutes of exposure to cigarette smoke can cause cardiovascular harm. This is also a serious workplace issue as wait staff are not accorded normal occupational health safeguards and can be exposed to high levels of waterpipe smoke for full eight-hour shifts both indoors and outdoors.

NICOTINE

Nicotine is a chemical compound found in tobacco that causes and sustains powerful addicting effects of tobacco. It has long been recognized as the main factor in continued smoking, although other factors may be involved. Inherited variations of genes (e.g. CYP2A6) that affect the speed at which nicotine is metabolized contribute to different patterns of smoking behaviour and smoking cessation. Slow metabolizers on average consume fewer cigarettes and may find it easier to quit. Although it is well known that nicotine is very addictive for its consumers, it has additional health effects that are not widely known. Nicotine can have significant cardiovascular effects, depending on the speed at which it is administered—very quickly with inhalation but slowly with nicotine patch or gum. Nicotine also causes new growth of blood vessels, which can promote the growth of tumors or arterial plaque. The effects of nicotine are further detailed in Chapter 5.

Nicotine replacement therapy (NRT) is widely used as an adjunct to quitting. The nicotine used in the gum and patch is released slowly into the bloodstream, and is unlikely to cause significant cardiovascular or other effects. The effects of long-term use are not confirmed, although they would be favourable compared with continued smoking. Chapter 9 explores NRT in further depth.

Nicotine use in pregnancy poses a dilemma. Prenatal exposure to nicotine can cause significant damage to the fetal pancreas and raise the risk of metabolic disorders such as diabetes and obesity in childhood and adulthood. Nicotine exposure can also reduce fertility in daughters by 50% to 75%, and cause stillbirths, cardiovascular disease, and possibly attention deficit hyperactivity disorder and other disorders. In animal studies, it alters lung function and airway geometry, acting through nicotinic receptors. Yet continued smoking would cause greater harm to the fetus than nicotine alone. Quitting during pregnancy is more difficult because increased body water requires more nicotine to maintain the same blood level for the smoker. Thus, ideally, quitting should occur well before pregnancy begins.

BENEFITS AND RISKS OF QUITTING

Quitting smoking has both long-term and short-term benefits. Smoking cessation at all ages reduces the risk of premature death. It reduces the risk of developing many types of cancer, cardiovascular disease, and chronic lung disease. Women who quit during their reproductive years reduce their risk of infertility. The risk of having a low-birth-weight baby decreases for women who stop smoking before they are pregnant or during the first 3–4 months of pregnancy. Quitting at any time in pregnancy is considered to be beneficial. Quitting is also beneficial for both men and women to halt bone mineral density loss at hip sites.

Short-term benefits of cessation accrue in part because of increased oxygen to the body. Thus, smokers are strongly advised to quit smoking, even temporarily, before surgery for at least three to four weeks to reduce the risk of complications, including wound healing and pulmonary complications. Each additional week of smoking cessation has a significant impact on reducing post-operative complications. A meta-analysis of several clinical trials and observational studies showed a relative risk reduction of 41% for the prevention of post-operative complications with cessation.

Quitting reduces the risk of amputation after peripheral arterial surgery. It reduces the risk of developing gastric ulcers and the risk of recurrence due to failure to heal. It also improves pulmonary function by 5% and reduces respiratory symptoms within a few months of quitting. Based on numerous epidemiological studies, quitting smoking before the age of 35 decreases the risk of tobacco-related disease or death by nearly 100% compared with that for never-smokers. On average, cigarette smokers die 10 years younger than non-smokers. Stopping at age 60, 50, 40, or 30 gains about 3, 6, 9, and 10 years of life, respectively. Risk of dying has a much stronger relationship with duration of smoking than with number of cigarettes smoked, in part because number of cigarettes is not a very good measure of actual exposure to toxicants. A major review in 2008 showed that smoking cessation could lead to a 36% reduction in the relative risk of all-cause mortality for patients with coronary heart disease regardless of age, gender, index cardiac event, and country of residence.

Complete cessation following short-term use of NRT is theoretically safer than is long-term NRT use to maintain abstinence, but if the smoker is at a high risk of relapse, long-term NRT use is better than returning to smoking.

The long-term impact of reducing the number of cigarettes smoked without quitting is still unclear. Some research among long-term smokers shows that even halving the number of cigarettes does not significantly reduce fatal outcomes. However, other studies have shown some reduction in risk. At this point it would be inappropriate to present reduced smoking as a long-term option for smokers, particularly because smokers frequently compensate for reduced intake by taking more puffs, puffing harder, and covering ventilation holes. In effect, they may get the same amount of nicotine (and products of combustion) as they did before reducing their consumption.

CONCLUSION

Seventy years of research have produced a wealth of incontrovertible evidence for the major health effects of various forms of tobacco use and exposure. Despite major advances in tobacco control, this deadly product continues to be available day and night, on nearly every corner, with little control on use. Evidence produced over the past 2 decades has confirmed the very serious effects of secondhand smoke, leading to a more comprehensive view of smoking as a societal problem rather than one restricted to individuals. Although many strategies can reduce harm among individuals, it is critical to determine the overall risk/benefit to society when making recommendations to reduce harm. For example, the substitution of smokeless tobacco for cigarettes would likely reduce harm among individual smokers, but it might have a net harmful effect on society if it normalizes tobacco use and keeps people addicted to tobacco products. In fact, tobacco companies have used new forms of tobacco to expand upon their existing brands.

The health effects of tobacco products must not be viewed in isolation as strictly a medical issue. They have major implications for mental as well as physical health, and their social as well as physical effects need to be recognized. Social exposure to smoking can be just as harmful as physical exposure for children and young adults. We need to expand our perspective to embrace the social and interpersonal aspects of the smoking epidemic if we are to fully galvanize 'social treatments' in addition to medical approaches.

It will be many more decades before we have a full understanding of all the health impacts of tobacco and nicotine use. However, the strength of the current evidence is sufficient at this point to invoke the precautionary principle and develop a plan to eliminate tobacco products from our societies.

REFERENCES

1 American Cancer Society. Guide to quitting smoking: when smokers quit – what are the benefits over time? [cited 2012 Jan 30]. Available from: http://www.cancer.org/Healthy/StayAwayfromTobacco/GuidetoQuittingSmoking/guide-to-quitting-smoking-benefits.

2 Akl EA, Gaddam S, Gunukula SK, Honeine R, Jaoude PA, Irani J. The effects of waterpipe tobacco smoking on health outcomes: a systematic review. Int J Epidemiol. 2010;39:834-57.

3 Boffetta P, Hecht SS, Gray NJ, Gupta PC, Straif K. Smokeless tobacco and cancer. Lancet Oncology. 2008 Jul;9(7):667-75.

4 Boffetta P, Straif K. Use of smokeless tobacco and risk of myocardial infarction and stroke: systematic review with meta-analysis. BMJ. 2009 Aug 18;339:b3060.

5 Burton A. Does the smoke ever really clear? thirdhand smoke exposure raises new concerns. Environ Health Perspect. 2011;119:a70-a74. http://dx.doi.org/10.1289/ehp.119-a70.

6 Cameron M, Brennan E, Durkin S, Borland R, Travers MJ, Hyland A, et al. Secondhand smoke exposure (PM2.5) in outdoor dining areas and its correlates. Tob Control. 2010;19(1):19-23.

7   Chan A, Murin S. Up in smoke: the fallacy of the harmless hookah. Chest. 2011 Apr;139(4):737-8.

8   Chan WC, Leatherdale ST, Burkhalter R, Ahmed R. Bidi and hookah use among Canadian youth: an examination of data from the 2006 Canadian Youth Smoking Survey. J Adolesc Health. 2011 Jul;49(1):102-4. Epub 2011 Mar 12.

9   Cobb C, Ward KD, Maziak W, Shihadeh AL, Eissenberg T. Waterpipe tobacco smoking: an emerging health crisis in the United States. Am J Health Behav. 2010;34(3):275-85.

10   Collishaw N (chair). Canadian Expert Panel on Tobacco Smoke and Breast Cancer Risk. Ontario Tobacco Research Unit Special Report, Toronto, April 2009.

11   Doll R, Peto R, Boreham J, Sutherland I. Mortality in relation to smoking: 50 years' observations on male British doctors. BMJ. 2004;328:1519.

12   Dreyfuss JH. Thirdhand smoke identified as potent, enduring carcinogen. CA Cancer J Clin. 2010 Jul-Aug;60(4):203-4. Epub 2010 Jun 8.

13   Dugas E, Tremblay M, Low NCP, Cournoyer D, O'Loughlin J. Water pipe smoking among North American youths. Pediatrics. 2010;125:1184-9.

14   Eissenberg, T, Shihadeh A. Waterpipe tobacco and cigarette smoking: direct comparison of toxicant exposure. Am J Prev Med. 2009;37(6):518-23.

15   Health Canada. Smoking and mortality. 2011 [cited 2012 Jan 31]. Available from: http://www.hc-sc.gc.ca/hc-ps/tobac-tabac/legislation/label-etiquette/mortal-eng.php#note3.

16   Ivan B. Smoking-induced metabolic disorders: a review. Diabete Metab. 2008;34(4, Part 1):307-14.

17   Kalant H (Chairman), Clarke P, Corrigall W, Ferrence RG, Kozlowski LT. Report on nicotine dependence commissioned by the Royal Society of Canada, Ottawa, Canada, for the Health Protection Branch, Health and Welfare Canada, 1990.

18   Klepeis N, Ott WR, Switzer P. Real-time measurement of outdoor tobacco smoke particles. J Air Waste Manag Assoc. 2007;57:322-34.

19   Kuehn BM. FDA: Electronic cigarettes may be risky. JAMA. 2009 Sep 2;302(9):937.

20   Luo J, Ye W, Zendehdel K, Adami J, Adami HO, Boffetta P, Nyrén O. Oral use of Swedish moist snuff (snus) and risk for cancer of the mouth, lung, and pancreas in male construction workers: a retrospective cohort study. Lancet. 2007 Jun 16;369(9578):2015-20.

21   Matt AU, Quintana GE, Zakarian PJE, Fortmann JM, Chatfield AL, Hoh DA, et al. When smokers move out and non-smokers move in: residential thirdhand smoke pollution and exposure. Tob Control. 2011 Jan;20(1):e1. Epub 2010 Oct 30.

22   Maziak W. The global epidemic of waterpipe smoking. Addictive Behaviors. 2011;36(1-2):1-5.

23   Mills E, Eyawo O, Lockhart I, Kelly S, Wu P, Ebbert JO. Smoking cessation reduces postoperative complications: a systematic review and meta-analysis. Am J Med. 2011;124(2):144-54.e8.

24   National Cancer Institute at the National Institutes of Health. Harms of smoking and health, benefits of quitting [cited 2012 Jan 30]. Available from: http://www.cancer.gov/cancertopics/factsheet/Tobacco/cessation.

25   Oberg M, Jaakkola MS, Woodward A, Peruga A, Pruss-Ustun A. Worldwide burden of disease from exposure to second-hand smoke: a retrospective analysis of data from 192 countries. Lancet. 2011 Jan 8;377(9760):139-46.

26   Schick S. Thirdhand smoke: here to stay. Tob Control. 2011;20:13.

27   Shihadeh A, Salman R, Jaroudi E, Saliba N, Sepetdjian E, Blank MD, Cobb CO, Eissenberg T. Does switching from tobacco-based to herbal waterpipe products reduce toxicant intake? a crossover study comparing CO, NO, PAH, volatile aldehydes, "tar" and nicotine yields. Food Chem Toxicol. 2012 Mar 1;50(5):1494-98.

28   Statistics Canada. Health: less exposure to second-hand smoke; 2010 [cited 2012 Jan 31]. Available from: http://www41.statcan.ca/2007/2966/ceb2966_001-eng.htm.

29   US Centers for Disease Control and Prevention. Adult cigarette smoking in the United States: current estimate. Atlanta: US Centers for Disease Control and Prevention; 2009 [cited 2012 Mar 31]. Available from: http://www.cdc.gov/tobacco/data_statistics/fact_sheets/adult_data/cig_smoking/index.htm.

30   US Department of Health and Human Services.The health benefits of smoking cessation: a report of the Surgeon General. Atlanta: US Department of Health and Human Services, Public Health Service, Centers for Disease Control, Center for Chronic Disease Prevention and Health Promotion, Office on Smoking and Health; 1990.

31   US Department of Health and Human Services. The health consequences of smoking: a report of the Surgeon General. Atlanta: US Department of Health and Human Services, Centers for Disease Control and Prevention, National Center for Chronic Disease Prevention and Health Promotion, Office on Smoking and Health; 2004.

32   US Department of Health and Human Services.The health consequences of involuntary exposure to tobacco smoke: a report of the surgeon general. Rockville (MD): US Department of Health and Human Services, Centers for Disease Control and Prevention, Coordinating Center for Health Promotion, National Center for Chronic Disease Prevention and Health Promotion, Office on Smoking and Health; 2006.

33   US Department of Health and Human Services. How tobacco smoke causes disease: the biology and behavioral basis for smoking-attributable disease: a report of the Surgeon General. Atlanta: US Department of Health and Human Services, Centers for Disease Control and Prevention, National Center for Chronic Disease Prevention and Health Promotion, Office on Smoking and Health; 2010.

34   World Health Organization. Study group on tobacco product regulation. Waterpipe tobacco smoking: health effects, research needs and recommended actions by regulator. Geneva: Author; 2005.

4

Evidence for Developing and Implementing Cessation Services

ROBERT SCHWARTZ, JOLENE DUBRAY, ANNE PHILIPNERI,
MICHAEL CHAITON AND SHAWN O'CONNOR

THE DATA SPEAK FOR THEMSELVES. THEY TELL A VIVID AND CHILLING STORY OF THE dire and urgent need to encourage individuals who smoke to stop and to support them in their quit attempts. Very large numbers of Canadians and people across the world smoke regularly, resulting in morbidity, mortality, increased healthcare costs, and productivity losses of enormous proportions. The burden of tobacco use, however, falls unevenly on sub-populations who suffer in different proportions and numbers from the tobacco epidemic. This chapter presents data by sub-populations to help guide policy and practice decisions about where to focus cessation efforts. Data about the relationship of cigarette smoking to other chronic disease risk factors show readers the importance of addressing unhealthy behaviours. Finally, the chapter describes the current state of quitting behaviours across Canada. Data from standard cessation indicators (quit intentions, quit attempts, quit rates, consumption, and dependence) demonstrate the need for greater efforts to promote quitting and to support individuals until they have successfully stopped using tobacco.

GLOBAL TRENDS IN TOBACCO USE AND CESSATION

One billion men and 250 million women in the world are daily smokers. In high-resource countries, 35% of men and 22% of women smoke cigarettes. In middle- and low-resource countries, 50% of men and 9% of women smoke cigarettes.

Male smoking rates are slowly declining. Female smoking rates are also declining in most high-resource countries but are stable or increasing elsewhere.[1] Globally, smoking is recognized as the leading preventable causes of death and disease.[2,3] Tobacco use results in some 6 million deaths each year, a number that will grow to 8 million by the year 2030 if current trends continue, with most deaths occurring in low- and middle-income countries.[4]

The WHO Framework Convention on Tobacco Control (FCTC) specifies 3 categories of cessation support: cessation advice in health care, quitlines, and pharmacological therapy. Only a few of the 173 countries that are parties to the treaty provide and cover costs for all 3 of these services—14% of high-income, 5% of middle-income and 0% of low-income countries. A further 26% of high-income, 36% of middle-income and 5% of low-income countries cover the costs of some cessation services.[4] In 2010 only 14% of the world population had coverage for cessation programs.[4]

International Tobacco Control Policy Evaluation Project (ITC) research in 15 countries shows considerable variation in the proportion of individuals who make quit smoking attempts and who seek cessation support.[5] More than half of smokers in each country—and over 80% in others—have tried to quit at least once. Between 30% and 70% of smokers had visited a health professional in the past year, and there was a similar variation across countries in the proportion who received advice to quit: 20% in the Netherlands and over 66% in Thailand, Malaysia and the US. The proportion of smokers who used quitline services ranged from less than 4% to 12% in New Zealand. Smoking cessation medications were used by over 40% of smokers who made quit attempts in the past year in Australia, Canada, the UK and the US. Use of medications was much less common in middle-income countries.

DATA SOURCES

To aid the reader, figures and tables depicting survey data are accompanied by a detailed title, which typically provides information on the survey question, population of interest, age, and survey year. Figures and tables also have data sources listed in figure and table notes.

CANADIAN TOBACCO USE MONITORING SURVEY (CTUMS)

This Health Canada survey is an ongoing cross-sectional nationwide, tobacco-specific, random telephone survey, conducted every year since 1999. Annual data are based on two cycles, the first collected from February to June, and the second from July to December. The sample design is a 2-stage stratified random sample of telephone numbers. To ensure that the sample is representative of Canada, each province is divided into strata or geographic areas (Prince Edward Island had only one stratum). As part of the two-stage design, households are selected first and then, based on household composition, one, two, or no respondents are selected. The purpose of this design is, in part, to over-sample individuals 15–24 years of age. In general, CTUMS samples the Canadian population aged 15 and older (excluding residents of the Yukon, Northwest Territories, Nunavut, and full-time residents of institutions). The annual sample for CTUMS in 2010 was 19,822. All survey estimates were weighted, and variance estimates were calculated using bootstrap weights.

CANADIAN COMMUNITY HEALTH SURVEY (CCHS)

This is an ongoing cross-sectional population survey that collects information related to health status, healthcare utilization and health determinants. Initiated in 2000, it operated on a 2-year collection cycle but changed to annual data collection in 2007. The CCHS samples respondents living in private dwellings in the ten provinces and the three territories, covering approximately 98% of the Canadian population aged 12 or older. People living on reserves or Crown lands, residents of institutions, full-time members of the Canadian Forces and residents of certain remote regions are excluded from the survey. The CCHS uses the same sampling frame as the Canadian Labour Force Survey, which is a multistage stratified cluster design, where the dwelling is the final sampling unit. The annual targeted sample size for 2009/10 was 124,188. The CCHS is designed to provide reliable estimates at the health region level. All survey estimates were weighted, and variance estimates were calculated using bootstrap weights.

DEFINITIONS

Unless otherwise noted, current smoking is defined as past 30-day use and 100 cigarettes in lifetime. All tobacco use (and alternative tobacco products) is based on past 30-day use only.

SMOKING RELATED MORTALITY AND MORBIDITY IN CANADA

Mortality   The most recent estimate for the death toll in Canada due to smoking comes from 2002, when 37,209 deaths were attributable to smoking, representing 16.6% of all deaths.[6,7] These estimates are based on mortality and morbidity data from the Canadian Institute of Health Information; smoking-attributable fractions and numbers were calculated based on relative risk estimates from comprehensive meta-analyses. The number of deaths was also associated with significant premature mortality, accounting for approximately 515,608 years of life lost.[7] Failure to reduce the prevalence of smoking will lead to approximately one million deaths in Canada over the next 20 years.[8]

Nearly 90% of lung cancers and 15% of heart disease and stroke deaths in Canada are attributable to smoking.[7] In 2002, this translated into 17,427 deaths due to malignant neoplasms; 10,276 deaths due to cardiovascular disease; and 8,282 deaths due to respiratory disease. The diseases which caused the most deaths due to smoking were lung cancer (13,401) and chronic obstructive pulmonary disease (7,533).[6]

These mortality and morbidity estimates are similar to those from 1992[9] but are lower than those reported in a study using 1998 data.[8] Baliunas and colleagues suggest that the difference may be methodological (i.e. using meta-analyses to derive smoking attributable fraction) or may be due in part to improved heart disease survival.[6] These estimates are also consistent with estimates from other comparable countries: in the UK, smoking was estimated to have caused over 100,000 deaths per year over the past 10 years.[10]

Morbidity   Baliunas and colleagues estimated that in 2002 in Canada 339,179 hospital diagnoses were smoking-attributable, for a total of 2,210,155 (10.3%) acute care hospital days.[11] The estimate using 2002 data was 34% lower than that using 1992 data. Heart disease was the single largest contributor to smoking-attributable hospital days (21.0%; 463,625 hospital days). The overall average age for a smoking-attributable hospital diagnosis was 61.9 years for men and 62.8 years for women.

Sex differences   Smoking-attributable mortality is significantly higher among men than women: 21% vs. 12.2%. The Canadian Cancer Society projects that males will continue to have higher cancer incidence and mortality rates than females in 2011 (incidence: 65 vs. 51 per 100,000; mortality: 56 vs. 39 per 100,000); however, there is a difference in male and female lung cancer trends, which reflects the decline in smoking among males that began in the mid-1960s while the decline among females began in the mid-1980s.[12]

Secondhand smoke   There is growing evidence for a causal link between secondhand smoke and death; early studies found a causal relationship between secondhand smoke and lung disease, and secondhand smoke and heart disease.[7] However, the burden of disease attributable to secondhand smoke has increased and will continue to do so: globally, 603,000 deaths in 2004 could be attributed to secondhand smoke, or about 1.0% of worldwide mortality.[13] This estimate included 379,000 deaths from heart disease, 165,000 from lower respiratory infections, 36,900 from asthma, and 21,400 from lung cancer.

TOBACCO USE IN CANADA

In 2009–2010, 19% (or 5.5 million) of Canadians (across all provinces and territories) aged 12 years and over identified as having smoked 100 cigarettes in their lifetime and smoked within the past 30 days (Figure 1). Since 2000–2001 the prevalence of current smoking has decreased significantly from 25% to 19%. In 2009–2010, the prevalence of current smoking was lowest in British Columbia (15%) and highest in Nunavut (57%). Use of other tobacco products among Canadians aged 15 years and over (across all provinces, data not shown) was low in 2010: <1% pipe, 1% cigars and 3% little cigars or cigarillos. Use of smokeless tobacco was not reportable.[14]

Daily and occasional smoking Of Canadians aged 12 and over, 15.6% smoked daily and 3.5% had smoked occasionally in the past month (Figure 2). The rate of daily smoking decreased significantly between 2007–2008 and 2009–2010 (17.3% vs. 15.6%). The rate of occasional smoking has remained unchanged in recent years.

GRAPH 1: Current smoking prevalence, by province, ages 12+, Canada, 2009–2010, %

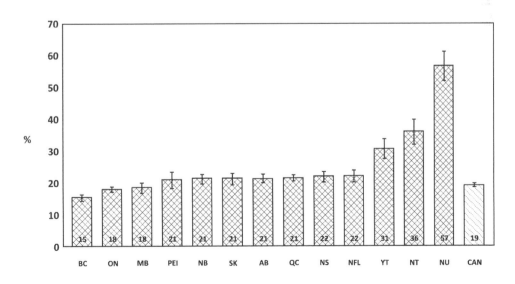

Note: All vertical lies represent 95% Confidence Intervals.
Source: Canadian Community Health Survey 2009–2010.

GRAPH 2: Daily and occasional smoking (past 30 days), by year, ages 12+, Canada

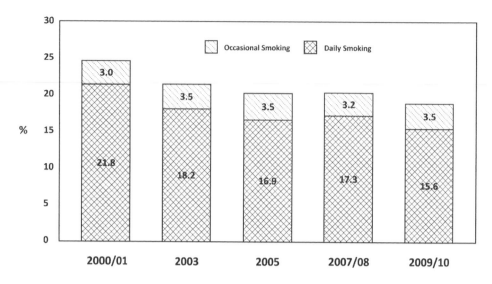

Source: Canadian Community Health Survey 2000–2001 to 2009–2010.

GENERAL ANALYSIS OF CURRENT SMOKING BY SUB-POPULATIONS

Smoking rates vary widely among sub-populations. Data from the Canadian Community Health Survey allow for the analysis of smoking prevalence across several groupings, including: socio-economic status, country of origin, occupation, immigration status, risk behaviours, and health status. Among the sub-populations analyzed, the prevalence of current smoking ranged from a high of 38.3% of individuals living in households with very low incomes ($5,000–$9,999) to a low of 5.8% of people born in India.

The 5 sub-populations with the highest prevalence of current smoking were: household income of $5,000–$9,999 (38.3%), Aboriginal peoples (35.9%), household income of $10,000–$14,999 (35.4%), individuals with a clinically diagnosed mood disorder (33.6%), and individuals who work in the trades (32.9%). While attention is often focused on sub-populations with high prevalence rates, it is important to note that the groups with the largest number of individuals smoking are not the same as those with the highest prevalence rates. The 5 sub-populations with the most current smoking rate were: individuals born in Canada (4.5 million), individuals who identified as being white (4.5 million), individuals who speak English at home (3.7 million), individuals who did not eat at least 5 servings of fruit or vegetables a day (3.6 million), and individuals who first learned to speak English (3.2 million).

Age and sex The prevalence of current smoking among Canadians (2009–2010) varied substantially by age and sex (Figure 3). The prevalence of current smoking was highest among males aged 25 to 29 years (30%), representing 334,300 of the 3.1 million male smokers aged 15 years or over in Canada (6% of all smokers). Males between the ages of 18 and 64 years had a significantly higher smoking prevalence than their female counterparts. The greatest number of current smokers among males was observed in the 45 to 49 year age group, representing 355,800 of the 3.1 million male smokers aged 15 years or over in Canada (7% of all smokers). The greatest number of current smokers among females was also observed in the 45 to 49 year age group, representing 300,300 of the 2.4 million female smokers aged 15 years and over in Canada (6% of all smokers).

GRAPH 3: Current smoking prevalence, by age and sex, ages 15+, Canada, 2009–2010, %

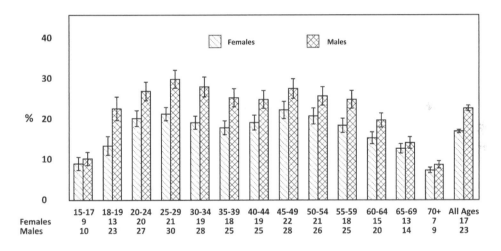

Note: All vertical lines represent 95% Confidence Intervals.
Source: Canadian Community Health Survey 2009–2010.

Education The prevalence of current smoking is significantly higher for Canadians with lower levels of education compared with those with higher levels of education. Canadians aged 18 years or over who had less than a high school education, completed high school, or completed some post-secondary education reported a higher prevalence of current smoking (29%, 24%, and 23%, respectively) than those who had completed post-secondary education (17%). Nevertheless, the greatest number of current smokers was observed among Canadians who had completed post-secondary education, representing 2.6 million of the 5.4 million smokers aged 18 years or over in Canada (or 49% of all smokers).

Occupation and unemployment status The prevalence of current smoking was highest among workers in the trades (33%) and manufacturing (26%), representing a combined total of 997,500 of the 5.4 million smokers in Canada aged 15 to 75 years (19% of all smokers). Individuals who worked in areas of health, science, culture, and social science reported significantly lower prevalence of current smoking (14%, 14%, 13%, and 12% respectively) (Figure 4). The category of sales reported the most current smokers, representing 941,400 of the 5.4 million smokers in Canada aged 15 to 75 years (18% of all smokers). Among unemployed Canadians aged 15 to 75 years, the prevalence of current smoking was 31%, representing 397,600 of the 5.4 million smokers in Canada aged 15 to 75 years (7% of all smokers).

GRAPH 4: Current smoking prevalence, by occupation, ages 15–75, Canada, 2009–2010, %

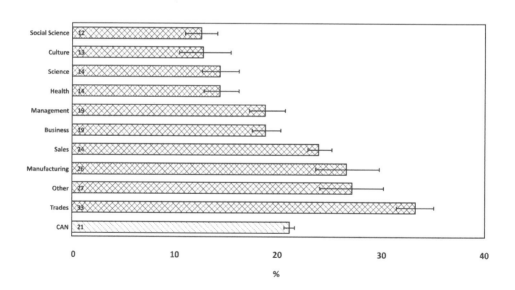

Note: All horizontal lines represent 95% Confidence Intervals.
Source: Canadian Community Health Survey 2009–2010.

Income The prevalence of current smoking is particularly high in very low-income households: 38% among Canadians (aged 18+) with household incomes ranging from $5,000 to $9,999 and 35% for those with household income of $10,000 to $14,999. The national rate for this age group is 20%. The largest number of smokers is in the $20,000 to $29,999 household income group - 483,200 of the 5.4 million smokers aged 18 years or over in Canada (9% of all smokers).

Immigration status and country of origin Perhaps contrary to some common preconceptions, the prevalence of current smoking is higher among non-immigrants (Canadian-born) (21%) than immigrants to Canada (13%). Of the 5.5 million smokers in Canada, 4.5 million are Canadian-born (or 83% of smokers). The prevalence of current smoking among Canadian residents born in certain countries was much lower than the national average of 19%; these include the US (15%), UK (14%), Holland (11%), China (11%), Italy (11%), Philippines (9%), Jamaica (8%), Hong Kong (8%), and India (6%). The prevalence of current smoking among immigrants did not vary by the number of years since immigrating to Canada.

Ethnic background and language spoken at home The prevalence of current smoking was highest among residents who identified as Aboriginal (36%), representing 329,900 of the 5.5 million Canadian smokers (6% of all smokers in Canada). Canadian residents who identified as South East Asian (14%), Black (13%), Latin American (12%), Korean (12%), Filipino (9%), Chinese (9%), or South Asian (8%) reported a lower prevalence of current smoking compared with the national average (19%). Not surprisingly, the greatest number of current smokers was among Canadian residents who identified as white, representing 4.5 million of the 5.5 million smokers in Canada (or 81% of all smokers in Canada). The next biggest identifiable group was Aboriginal (6%).

Canadian residents who spoke French at home reported a slightly higher prevalence of current smoking compared with the national average (22% vs. 19%, respectively). Canadian residents who spoke neither English nor French at home reported a lower prevalence of current smoking compared with the national average (12% vs. 19%, respectively).

Other sub-populations Eleven percent of pregnant women aged 15–49 years in Canada were current smokers, representing 29,500 of the 1.5 million female smokers aged 15–49 years in Canada (or 2% of all smokers). Approximately one-quarter (23%) of Canadian residents aged 18–59 years who identified as being homosexual or bisexual were current smokers, representing 137,200 of the 4.6 million smokers aged 18–59 years in Canada (or 3%). In Ontario and Quebec the prevalence of current smoking amongst residents aged 18–59 years who identified as being homosexual or bisexual exceeded the provincial averages (31% vs. 22% and 37% vs. 26%, respectively).

GRAPH 5: Clustering of unhealthy eating, inactive living, and diagnosed mood disorder by smoking status, Canada, 2009–2010, %

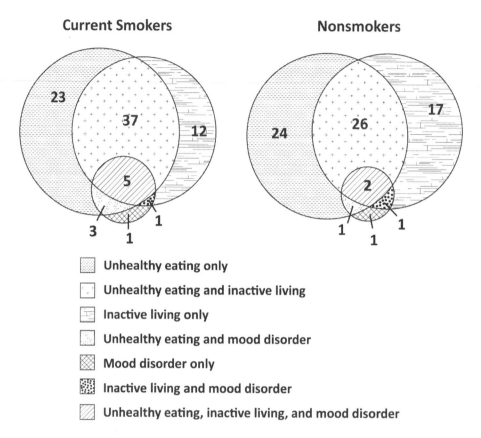

Current Smokers   Nonsmokers

- ☐ **Unhealthy eating only**
- ☐ **Unhealthy eating and inactive living**
- ☐ **Inactive living only**
- ☐ **Unhealthy eating and mood disorder**
- ☒ **Mood disorder only**
- ☐ **Inactive living and mood disorder**
- ☐ **Unhealthy eating, inactive living, and mood disorder**

Source: Canadian Community Health Survey 2009–2010. Area-proportional Venn diagrams obtained using the application by Chow et al.[15]

SMOKING AND OTHER CHRONIC DISEASE RISK FACTORS

Smokers are somewhat more likely than non-smokers to report most other chronic disease risk factors, yet because smokers represent only about one fifth of the population the number of non-smokers is larger than the number of smokers with each chronic disease risk factor. Compared with non-smokers, current smokers reported a higher prevalence of being clinically diagnosed with a mood disorder (11% vs. 5%), being inactive (55% vs. 46%), and eating fewer than 5 servings of fruits or vegetables (68% vs. 53%). The prevalence of being overweight/obese is similar for smokers and non-smokers (49% each). More smokers than non-smokers suffer from two or more other risk factors

(Figure 5). Eighty-three percent of current smokers are either inactive, unhealthy eaters, or diagnosed with a mood disorder, a much higher prevalence compared with non-smokers (72%) A significantly higher percentage of current smokers (5%) have all three conditions (unhealthy eating, inactive living, and diagnosed mood disorder) compared with non-smokers (2%). Unhealthy eating and inactivity are much higher among current smokers (42%) compared with non-smokers (28%).

Looking at the relationship between smoking cigarettes and other chronic disease risk factors in a different way, the prevalence of current smoking among Canadians reporting each chronic disease risk factor tends to be relatively high. Thus, Canadian residents who reported having a diagnosed mood disorder had the highest prevalence of current smoking (34%) even though they represent only 621,100 of the 5.5 million Canadian smokers (or 11% or all smokers; Figure 6). The prevalence of current smoking for overweight/obese people did not differ from the national average of 19%. However, the prevalence of current smoking among overweight/obese people was significantly higher than the provincial average in all provinces and territories except Nunavut. Canadian residents who reported being inactive or who ate fewer than 5 servings of fruits or vegetables a day had a significantly higher prevalence of current smoking compared with the national average (23% and 23%, respectively vs. 19%).

GRAPH 6: Current smoking prevalence, among those with other chronic disease risk factors, ages 12+, Canada, 2009–2010, %

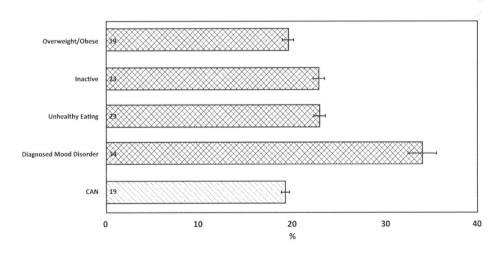

Note: All horizontal lines represent 95% Confidence Intervals.
Source: Canadian Community Health Survey 2009–2010.

SMOKING CESSATION IN CANADA

The ultimate objective of cessation strategies is to increase the proportion of those who have quit smoking.[16] In working toward this goal, desired outcomes include: increasing the proportion of smokers intending to quit, increasing the actual number of quit attempts, decreasing cigarette consumption, and decreasing tobacco dependence.

In 2010, 58% of current smokers, aged 15 years and older, intended to quit smoking in the next 6 months, representing 2.5 million Canadians. One-fourth of current smokers in 2010 wanted to quit smoking in the next 30 days. In recent years, there has been no significant change in the percentage of current smokers who intend to quit smoking in the next 6 months or in the next 30 days (Figure 7). Six-month quit intentions were lowest in Saskatchewan (53%) and highest in Newfoundland and Labrador (67%). Thirty-day quit intentions were lowest in Saskatchewan (21%) and highest in Newfoundland and Labrador (32%).

GRAPH 7: Intention to quit smoking within next 30 days and next 6 months, current smokers, ages 15+, Canada, 2004–2010, %

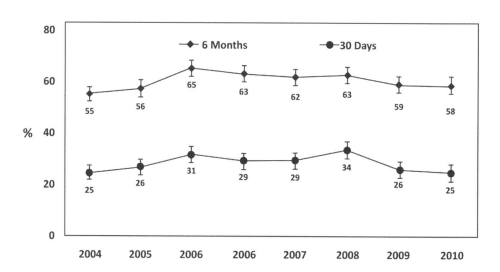

Note: All vertical lines represent 95% Confidence Intervals.
Source: Canadian Tobacco Use Monitoring Survey 2010.

Intention to quit smoking in the next 6 months was highest among youth smokers (15–19 year olds: 65%) and lowest among the oldest age group of smokers (45 years and older: 58%). Thirty-day quit intention was lowest among young adult smokers, aged 20–24 years (22%) (Figure 8). Six-month quit intentions were lowest among smokers with less than secondary education (43%) and that rate was significantly different from that of smokers who had only completed secondary education (64%). Smokers with less than secondary education reported the lowest rate of 30-day quit intention (20%). Similar rates of 30-day and 6-month quit intentions have been reported by male and female smokers since 2004.

GRAPH 8: Intention to quit smoking within next 30 days and next 6 months by age, current smokers, Canada, 2010, %

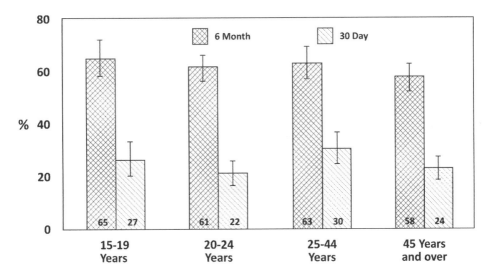

Note: All vertical lines represent 95% Confidence Intervals.
Source: Canadian Tobacco Use Monitoring Survey 2010.

Quit attempts In 2010, 47% of all smokers in Canada tried to stop smoking for at least 24 hours; 16% of smokers made only one quit attempt in the past year. Similar quit attempt rates have been reported since 2005 (Figure 9), and similar quit attempt rates were reported by males and females, across occupational groups and across educational groups (data not shown). Youth (15–19 year olds) (64%) and young adults (20–24 year olds) (57%) reported a higher percentage of quit attempts compared with older smokers (25–44 year olds: 43%; 45+ year olds: 40%) (Figure 10). A higher percentage of multiple quit attempts was reported by youth (44%) and young adults (40%) compared with older smokers (25–44 year olds: 27%; 45+ year olds: 24%).

GRAPH 9: Past year quit attempts, current smokers, ages 15+, Canada, 2005–2010, %

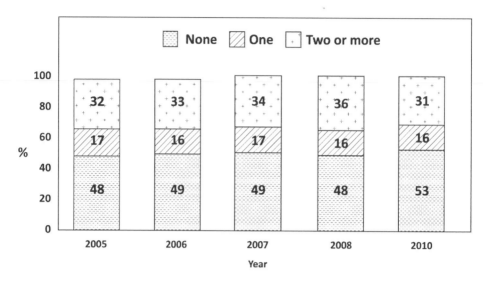

Source: Canadian Tobacco Use Monitoring Survey 2010.

GRAPH 10: Past year quit attempts by age, current smokers, Canada, 2005–2010, %

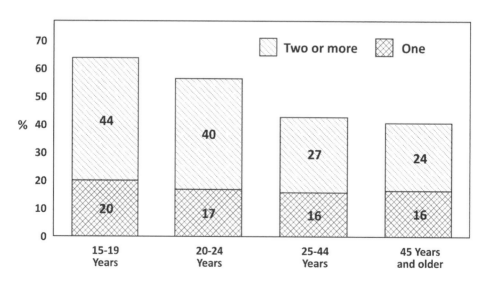

Source: Canadian Tobacco Use Monitoring Survey 2010.

Quits   In 2010, 6 in 10 Canadians who had ever smoked in their lifetime had quit for at least 30 days (Table 1). Among ex-smokers, 4.6% reported quitting for at least 30 days in the past year in 2010, representing 339,000 Canadians. In recent years there has been no significant change in lifetime or past year quit rates. Based on the estimates from the Ontario Tobacco Survey, 83% of past year quitters will relapse in the next year, meaning only 0.8% of quitters will remain abstinent throughout the following year.

Lifetime quit rate was lowest among youth (15–19 year olds) and young adults (20–24 year olds) compared with older ever-smokers. Lifetime quit rate was significantly lower among blue-collar workers (47%) and sales and service workers (49%) compared with white-collar workers (67%).

TABLE 1: Quit rate, 2005–2010, Canada, %

Year	Lifetime Quit Rate (%)	Past Year Quit Rate (%)	Adjusted Past Year Quit Rate (%)
2005	60.0 (58.3-61.8)	5.3 (4.3-6.3)	0.9
2006	60.0 (58.3-61.8)	5.3 (4.3-6.3)	0.9
2007	59.1 (57.3-60.9)	5.4 (4.2-6.5)	0.92
2008	62.2 (60.2-64.1)	5.3 (4.2-6.4)	0.9
2009	61.0 (59.1-63.0)	4.6 (3.7-5.6)	0.78
2010	62.3 (60.3-64.4)	4.6 (3.5-5.8)	0.78

CONSUMPTION

Change in the average number of cigarettes smoked (consumption) among those who continue to smoke is a commonly used indicator in tobacco control. In recent years, the mean number of cigarettes smoked among daily smokers has remained unchanged at about 15 cigarettes per day.

DEPENDENCE

The Heaviness of Smoking Index (HSI) combines the time to smoking the first cigarette each morning and the number of cigarettes smoked per day.[17] A score of 0–2 indicates low dependence; 3–4, moderate dependence; and 5–6, high dependence. In Canada, the proportion of highly dependent smokers significantly decreased between 2000 and 2009 (2.5% vs. 1.3%, $p<0.001$; see Figure 11), as has the proportion of all current smokers (10% in 2000 vs. 7% in 2009, $p=0.002$).

GRAPH 11: Heaviness of Smoking Index, by year, age 15+, Canada, %

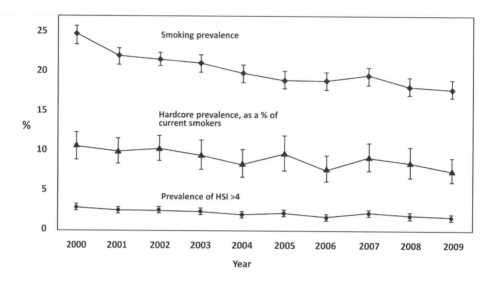

Source: Canadian Tobacco Use Monitoring Survey 1999–2010.

SUMMARY

It cannot be disputed that the data presented in this chapter indicate a need for concerted efforts to encourage and support smokers to quit. With some 5.5 million current smokers, Canada is paying a very high price in productivity losses, healthcare costs, morbidity, and mortality. While the prevalence of smoking is high or very high among low-income, low-education, Aboriginal, and other sub-populations, the bulk of smokers have post-secondary education, middle and high income, are white, and were born in Canada. Contrary to common belief, immigrants to Canada tend to have lower rates of smoking than native-born Canadians.

Canada has failed in recent years to increase the proportions of smokers who intend to quit, make quit attempts, successfully quit, or even decrease their daily consumption of cigarettes. While close to 60% of smokers intend to quit in the next 6 months and 40% attempt to quit, fewer than an estimated 1% successfully quit within a year. There is much work to be done.

REFERENCES

1   Shafey O, Eriksen M, Ross H, Mackay J. The tobacco atlas. 3rd ed. Atlanta: American Cancer Society; 2009 [cited 2012 Feb 29]. Available from: http://www.tobaccoatlas.org/.

2   Jha P. Avoidable global cancer deaths and total deaths from smoking. Nature Rev Cancer. 2009;9(9):655-64.

3   Murray CJL, Lopez AD. Alternative projections of mortality and disability by cause 1990–2020: global burden of disease study. Lancet .1997;349:1498-1504.

4   World Health Organization. WHO report on the global tobacco epidemic, 2011: warning about the dangers of tobacco. Geneva: Author; 2011 [cited 2012 Mar 8]. Available from: http://whqlibdoc.who.int/publications/2011/ 9789240687813_eng.pdf.

5   International Tobacco Control Policy Evaluation Project. Tobacco dependence and cessation: evidence from the ITC Project; 2010 Nov [cited 2012 Mar 8]. Available from: http://www.itcproject.org/documents/keyfindings/ itccessationreportpdf.

6   Baliunas D, Patra J, Rehm J, Popova S, Kaiserman M, Taylor B. Smoking-attributable mortality and expected years of life lost in Canada 2002: conclusions for prevention and policy. Chronic Dis Can. 2007;27(4):154-62.

7   Rehm J, Baliunas D, Brochu S, Fischer B, Gnam W, Patra J, et al. The costs of substance abuse in Canada 2002. Ottawa: Canadian Centre on Substance Abuse; 2006 [cited 2012 Mar 8]. Available from: http://www.ccsa.ca/2006%20CCSA%20 Documents/ccsa-011332-2006.pdf.

8   Makomaski Illing EM, Kaiserman MG. Mortality attributable to tobacco use in Canada and its regions 1998. Can J Public Health. 2004;95(1):38-44.

9   Single E, Robson L, Xie X, Rehm J. The costs of substance abuse in Canada. Ottawa: Canadian Centre on Substance Abuse; 1996.

10   Allender S, Balakrishnan R, Scarborough P, Webster P, Rayner M. The burden of smoking-related ill health in the UK. Tob Control. 2009 Aug;18(4):262-7.

11   Baliunas D, Patra J, Rehm J, Popova S, Taylor B. Smoking-attributable morbidity: acute care hospital diagnoses and days of treatment in Canada, 2002. BMC Public Health. 2007 Sep 18;7:247.

12   Canadian Cancer Society, Steering Committee on Cancer Statistics. Canadian cancer statistics 2011. Toronto: Author; 2011 [cited 2012 Feb 29]. Available from: http://www.cancer.ca/~/media/CCS/Canada%20wide/Files%20List/English%20files%20heading/PDF%20-%20 Policy%20-%20Canadian%20Cancer%20Statistics%20-%20English/Canadian%20Cancer%20 Statistics%202011%20-%20English.ashx.

13   Öberg M, Jaakkola MS, Woodward A, Peruga A, Prüss-Ustün A. Worldwide burden of disease from exposure to second-hand smoke: a retrospective analysis of data from 192 countries. Lancet. 2011;377(9760):139-46.

14   Health Canada. Canadian tobacco use monitoring survey 2010. Ottawa: Author; 2011 [cited 2012 Mar 8]. Available from: http://www.hc-sc.gc.ca/hc-ps/tobac-tabac/research-recherche/stat/ctums-esutc_2010-eng.php.

15   Chow S, Rodgers P. Extended abstract: constructing area-proportional Venn and Euler diagrams with three circles. Presented at Euler diagrams Workshop; 2005; Paris [cited 2012 Mar 9]. Available from: http://www.cs.kent.ac.uk/ people/staff/pjr/EulerVennCircles/EulerVennApplet.html

16   Copley TT, Lovato C, O'Connor S. Indicators for monitoring tobacco control: a resource for decision-makers, evaluators and researchers. On behalf of the National Advisory Group on Monitoring and Evaluation. Toronto: Canadian Tobacco Control Research Initiative; 2006 [cited 2012 Mar 9]. Available from: http://ctcri.ca/fr//index.php?option=com_docman&task=doc_download&gid=49.

17   Heatherton TF, Kozlowski L, Frecker RC, Rickert W, Robinson J. Measuring the heaviness of smoking: using self-reported time to the first cigarette of the day and number of cigarettes smoked per day. Brit J Addict. 1989;84:791-9.

5

Nicotine

HANS ROLLEMA

THIS CHAPTER REVIEWS KEY ASPECTS OF NICOTINE PHARMACOLOGY, WITH THE emphasis on the current understanding of nicotinic mechanisms that underlie tobacco dependence.

HISTORY

Nicotine is one of many alkaloids in plants and animals that act as natural repellants and insecticides and are toxic for the predator by interfering with the cholinergic system. Several of these alkaloids have been investigated for their pharmacological properties and as possible leads in drug discovery. Nicotine from tobacco leaves became the most used alkaloid after the worldwide popularization of smoking cigarettes as a form of self-administration of nicotine.

Tobacco smoking   Nicotine is an alkaloid in tobacco plants that grew indigenously in North and South America. It was used as a holy, healing herb in sacred ceremonies for many centuries. The *Nicotiana tabacum* plant, named after Jean Nicot de Villemain, who in the 16th century introduced tobacco from Brazil into Europe as a therapeutic herb for several diseases, became the main source for commercial production of cigarettes. Gaining popularity in England after tobacco was introduced to the English court, by the mid-17th century about half of the adult men in England used tobacco daily, mostly chewing or smoking pipes yet not all were enthusiastic about this "habit" and there warnings of its health risks.[1] Despite these warnings, smoking was generally thought to be beneficial and became increasingly popular. The possibility to mass-produce cigarettes, together with the highly effective advertising campaigns and market expansions in the 20th century, led to a steep rise in smoking cigarettes, resulting in the current worldwide nicotine dependence pandemic.[2] However, since the 1950s the serious health consequences of smoking became known, for a large part because of seminal studies by Sir Richard Doll and colleagues,[3] while in the US the Surgeon General started issuing reports on the dangerous health effects of smoking since 1964 and published the most recent, 29th report in 2010. In the meantime the search for a treatment of tobacco addiction had resulted in the concept of nicotine replacement therapy and the FDA approved nicotine gum in 1984 and nicotine patch in 1991, while bupropion and varenicline were approved as smoking cessation aids in 1997 and 2006, respectively.

Nicotine   Nicotine was isolated from tobacco leaves in 1828 and the first pharmacological studies were already performed as early as 1843, which was about 50 years before its chemical structure was elucidated in 1893 and 60 years before its laboratory synthesis in 1904. Nicotine constitutes between 0.6-3% of the dry weight of a tobacco plant and a typical cigarette contains about 6–11 mg nicotine, from which approximately 1–3 mg will be delivered systemically to a smoker upon smoking a whole cigarette. When burning the tobacco, part of the nicotine is vaporized and inhaled with the smoke as a gas, absorbed in the lungs and rapidly distributed in the body, including the brain, via the blood stream.

Since nicotine as a base is more volatile and more easily absorbed than as a salt, the 'nicotinic potency' of a cigarette can be enhanced when nicotine in the cigarette is in the base form, which will increase the amount of nicotine base in the smoke. Cigarette manufacturers achieve this with ammonia, usually added to the cigarette in the form of diammonium phosphate, a process that has been called 'freebasing,' in analogy of the conversion of cocaine into its free base, crack cocaine, to enhance potency.

The selective pharmacological actions of nicotine and muscarine, a natural product from the *Amanita muscaria* mushroom, observed during experiments performed in the early 1900's that led to the discovery of acetylcholine as a neurotransmitter by Dale and Loewi, were the basis for differentiating sympathetic and parasympathetic neurotransmission and later for defining acetylcholine receptors as nicotinic or muscarinic receptors. It was later discovered that these receptors represent different types of neurotransmission, the muscarinic receptors (M1-M5) being metabotropic or G-coupled receptors, and the nicotinic receptors (nAChR subtypes) belonging to the family of ionotropic or ligand-gated channels (see below: Nicotinic acetylcholine receptors).

CHEMISTRY, PHARMACOLOGY, AND PHARMACOKINETICS OF NICOTINE

Chemistry   Nicotine is 3-(1-methyl-2-pyrrolidinyl)-pyridine (Figure 1), with molecular formula $C_{10}H_{14}N_2$ and molecular mass 162.2. It has a chiral centre at C2 and the biologically active levorotatory enantiomer of nicotine, S-nicotine or (-)-nicotine, is selectively synthesized in tobacco plants. Pure nicotine is a liquid at room temperature and as a weak base (pKa=8.5) it can combine with acids to form salts that are usually solid and water-soluble. A salt form that is frequently used in pharmacological studies is nicotine bitartrate ($C_{10}H_{14}N_2 \cdot 2C_4H_6O_6$, molecular mass 462.4), which contains about 35% active nicotine. Nicotine bitartrate should therefore be given in 2.8 times higher doses than the intended dose of active nicotine. Although the active enantiomer of nicotine can be synthesized in the laboratory, the primary source of nicotine for nicotine replacement therapy formulations and pharmacological studies is the natural product that is extracted and purified from tobacco leaves.

FIGURE 1: Structures of (-)-nicotine and its primary metabolite (-)-cotinine

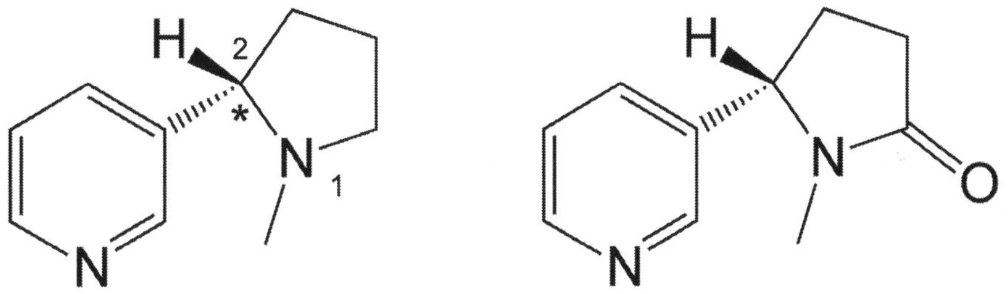

(-)-nicotine   (-)-cotinine

Pharmacology   Nicotine's pharmacological actions are primarily mediated via central and peripheral ganglionic nicotinic acetylcholine receptors (nAChRs) as it has very low affinity for the muscle type nAChR and poor binding affinity for other neurotransmitter receptors, ion channels, transporters, or enzymes. The pharmacology of nicotine is complex, since it can both activate and desensitize (i.e. inactivate) nAChRs depending on the concentration of nicotine and the duration of its exposure to the nAChR (see below: Nicotinic acetylcholine receptors: properties and function). The effects of nicotine are thus highly concentration-dependent and it is important to keep in mind that some of the pharmacological effects observed in preclinical in vitro and in vivo models using high nicotine concentrations do not occur in humans at the concentrations associated with cigarette smoking or the use of nicotine replacement therapy (NRT).

In the central nervous system nicotine acts as a stimulant and increases the release of neurotransmitters such as dopamine. Its effect on dopamine release in the reward circuitry of the midbrain is a key mechanism in initiating and maintaining nicotine addiction and will be discussed in detail below (see: Nicotine addiction). Nicotine also increases alertness, reduces anxiety, and causes muscle relaxation.

In the peripheral nervous system, the biphasic nature of nicotine's effects is illustrated by initial stimulation and subsequent depression of autonomic ganglia. Low doses of nicotine will directly stimulate and facilitate impulse neurotransmission, while high doses will initially stimulate and then block neurotransmission. A similar biphasic effect is observed in the adrenal medulla where at low doses, nicotine interacts with $\alpha 3\beta 4$ nAChRs and stimulates the release of norepinephrine, while high doses reduce the release of these catecholamines via activation of the splanchnic nerve. Nicotine increases heart rate and blood pressure, as well as blood glucose by stimulation of the sympathetic nervous system and increasing catecholamine release.

Nicotine is an emetic and can induce vomiting by a central mechanism via the chemo-emetic trigger zone in the area postrema, and by a peripheral mechanism via activation of the vagus nerve. Pure nicotine base has been used as an insecticide and it is easily absorbed through the skin with an LD_{50} of about 0.5 to 1 mg/kg. Toxic doses of nicotine cause parasympathetic stimulation with initial signs of nausea, salivation, vomiting, cold sweat, headache, drop in blood pressure, and subsequently tremors and convulsions via direct stimulation of nAChRs in the medulla oblongata; activation of the muscle type nAChR will result in contractions and fatal respiratory paralysis.

Pharmacokinetics   Smoking is an optimal nicotine delivery system to the brain that is under complete control by the smoker, who can regulate the nicotine dose via the number of cigarettes smoked, the number of puffs taken and how deep and often the smoke is inhaled. The pharmacokinetic properties and dispositional profile of nicotine have recently been reviewed by Benowitz and colleagues.[4]

Absorption and distribution   During smoking, a large portion of the nicotine in the tobacco is burnt but part is vapourized and inhaled with the cigarette smoke into the lungs from where nicotine is readily absorbed and distributed via the bloodstream throughout the body, including the brain. The absorption of nicotine is pH-dependent, since the base (the predominant form at pH>7) crosses membranes more readily than ionized nicotine (the main form at pH<6). Nicotine delivery via smoke is similar or higher than intravenous injection, in that high nicotine concentrations are rapidly achieved in the brain, which increase sharply with each puff, reaching a maximum level after each cigarette. Nicotine concentrations in arterial blood can be very high and levels close to 100 ng/mL (600 nM) have been reported, but the usual range is between 20 and 60 ng/mL (120–350 nM), while blood levels decline rapidly when not smoking anymore. Since nicotine has low protein binding of <5% and can readily cross the blood-brain-barrier, brain concentrations of unbound nicotine are estimated to be in the same range as unbound plasma levels. A recent PET study with ^{11}C-nicotine confirmed that these estimates were accurate and found that after a single puff the brain levels of nicotine were 40 nM and increased after smoking a single cigarette to 357 nM.[5] Nicotine replacement therapy (see chapter on NRT) uses transdermal patch, gum, or inhaler for a continuous delivery of nicotine that result in sustained blood levels of nicotine, which are usually 30–70% lower than from cigarette smoking, ranging from 5–20 ng/mL (30–120 nM).

Metabolism and excretion Nicotine is extensively metabolized in the liver by the cytochrome P450 enzymes CYP2A6 and CYP2B6 to six primary metabolites, with cotinine (Figure 1) as the main metabolite. About 75% of nicotine is converted to cotinine (not psychoactive) that has a half live of 16–20 hours, remains for a long time in the blood and is detectable for up to a week after the use of tobacco. Cotinine blood concentrations (250–300 ng/mL) are much higher and more stable than those of nicotine and are therefore used as a biomarker for nicotine exposure, which can be measured in plasma, saliva, urine, hair or nails, both in cigarette smokers and passive smokers who inhaled secondhand smoke.

Nicotine is excreted by glomerular filtration and tubular secretion and eliminated with a plasma half-life after cigarette smoking of about 2 hours in humans, which is much longer than the half-life in species used in pharmacological studies, i.e. 45 minutes in rats and 2 minutes in mice.[6] A 2-hour half-life implies that during a day of smoking, nicotine accumulates and will still be present in significant amounts after the last cigarette in the evening and during the night. Finally, the metabolism and excretion of nicotine metabolism are determined by genetic factors and strongly influenced among others by age, gender, race, kidney disease, smoking, and the presence of drugs that can inhibit or induce the activity of CYP2A6.

NICOTINIC ACETYLCHOLINE RECEPTORS: PROPERTIES AND FUNCTION

The interaction of nicotine with certain nicotinic acetylcholine receptor subtypes in mesolimbic regions of the brain underlies the addictive effects of nicotine. This section describes briefly the structure and function of these receptors.[7–10]

Nicotinic acetylcholine receptors Two types of receptors are activated by the neurotransmitter acetylcholine (ACh), muscarinic acetylcholine receptors (mAChR), belonging to the family of metabotropic G-protein coupled receptors that use second messengers, and nicotinic acetylcholine receptors (nAChR), which are ionotropic receptors that are directly linked to an ion channel. The nAChRs result from the assembly of five proteins or subunits (Figure 2) that form both the ligand binding site and a small ionic pore in the center and are located on the postsynaptic side of the neuromuscular junction and in the plasma membranes of certain neurons. The muscle nAChRs are formed by α1, β1, δ, and γ (embryonic) or ε (adult) subunits, the neuronal nAChRs are either composed of 5 identical subunits (e.g. α7) or various combinations of the subunits α2-α10, β2, β3 and β4 (e.g. α4β2, α3β4, α4β2α6, α9α10). The combination of several subunits allows the assembly of a large number of different nAChRs (Figure 2).

FIGURE 2: Structure of a nAChR in the plasma membrane (on the left) showing two α4 and three β2 subunits. On the right, cross sections of the muscle nAChR and two different central nAChR subtypes. The black dots between the subunits indicate the ligand binding sites.

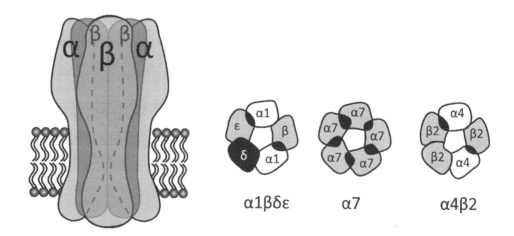

Modified after Rollema H, Bertrand D, Hurst RS, Nicotinic agonists and antagonists, in Encyclopedia of Psychopharmacology, ed. IA Stolerman, Berlin: Springer-Verlag; 2010, p. 888. Reproduced with permission of Springer Science+Business Media.

Activation, desensitization and upregulation Depending on the concentration and duration of exposure at the receptor, nicotine can activate, desensitize and upregulate central nAChRs, pharmacological events that are thought to play a role in nicotine addiction. The nAChRs have ligand binding sites between adjacent subunits and the binding of an agonist causes subtle changes in the conformation of the trans-membrane subunits that form the ion channel. As a result, the diameter of the central pore increases and allows the influx of sodium ions and efflux of potassium ions, causing depolarization of the plasma membrane and excitatory postsynaptic potentials in the neuron. Some nAChRs also allow calcium ions to enter the cell, which modulates the release of neurotransmitters. When activated by brief exposures to an agonist, the channel opens and closes as soon as the agonist dissociates from the binding site, in a matter or milliseconds, so that the nAChR is deactivated and can be activated again by another short pulse of the agonist. However, upon prolonged or repeated exposure to an agonist, the nAChR can transition to a state that cannot be activated, but is desensitized. This desensitized state represents a high affinity, non-conducting agonist-bound state that has high ligand affinity. It is thought that the binding affinities (K_i) of nAChR ligands represent binding to the desensitized receptor. Only when the agonist dissociates from the binding site the receptor will transition to the deactivated closed state and is ready to be activated again by an agonist (Figure 3).

FIGURE 3: Simplified schemes of the equilibrium between the closed (deactivated), open (activated) and desensitized (inactivated) states of a nAChR. Short exposure to a full agonist (left panel) activates the channel and favors the open state more compared to the binding of a partial agonist (right panel), which allows fewer ions to cross the cell membrane. Upon prolonged exposure to agonists the equilibrium is shifted to the desensitized state.

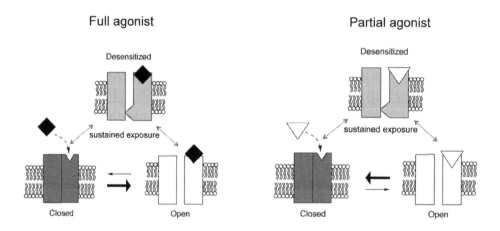

Modified after Rollema H, Coe JW, Chambers LK, Hurst RS, Stahl SM, Williams KE. Rationale, pharmacology and clinical efficacy of partial agonists of alpha4beta2 nACh receptors for smoking cessation. Trends Pharmacol Sci. 2007;28(7):316–25. Reproduced with permission of Elsevier Ltd.

A critical feature of nicotine pharmacology is that chronic nicotine will cause an increased density of nAChRs, which was termed receptor up-regulation. While most other cell surface receptors will down-regulate in response to sustained exposure to an exogenous or endogenous agonist, repeated exposure to nicotine and other nAChR ligands causes an increase in surface nAChRs. The increase in the number of nAChRs in smokers compared to non-smokers has been known for a long time and nicotine-induced nAChR increases were later demonstrated to occur in vitro and in laboratory animals. While the molecular mechanisms underlying receptor upregulation are not yet fully understood, it is likely a response to receptor desensitization and can be brought about by e.g. decreased receptor turnover, by increased synthesis of new proteins, and/or by increased receptor assembly and subsequent trafficking to the cell surface that can be enhanced by nicotine acting as a chemical 'chaperone.'[11] Besides the direct actions of nicotine that are mediated by nAChRs, nicotine-induced upregulation of nAChRs is an additional mechanism that is thought to play an important role in addiction. Moreover, upregulation may also have therapeutic benefits, since drug-induced increases in nAChR density may 'restore' deficits or malfunctioning of nAChRs in certain disorders.

Agonists, partial agonists, and antagonists Full agonists bind to and activate the nAChR and cause the channel to transition with 100% probability to the open state (Figure 3). A partial agonist binds to the same site and also shifts the equilibrium to the open state, but with less probability, while increasing the partial agonist concentration will not result in a larger response. Thus at a given level of receptor occupancy, partial agonists enable fewer ions to cross the cell membrane, resulting in a smaller excitatory signal and at maximal concentrations partial agonists evoke thus less than the maximal effect, i.e. have lower intrinsic activity, than a full agonist (Figure 4).

GRAPH 1: Theoretical concentration-response curves for the effects of a full agonist (ACh or nicotine) and a partial agonist (e.g. varenicline or cytisine) at a4β2 nAChR. In this example the partial agonist has lower intrinsic efficacy (~35% of the efficacy of the full agonist), but is more potent (lower EC_{50}, i.e. the concentration causing half maximal activation) than the full agonist.

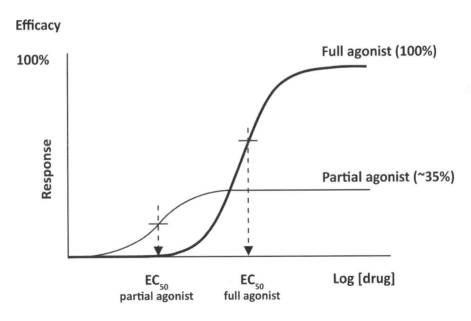

Modified after Rollema H, Bertrand D, Hurst RS, Nicotinic agonists and antagonists, in Encyclopedia of Psychopharmacology, ed. IA Stolerman, Berlin: Springer-Verlag; 2010, p. 889. Reproduced with permission of Springer Science+Business Media.

Since a partial agonist occupies the same binding site as a full agonist, it will competitively inhibit receptor activation by a full agonist, such as endogenous ACh or nicotine from smoking, a principle that was the basis for developing a4β2 nAChR partial agonists as smoking cessation aids (see chapter 9 on varenicline). While ACh is a full agonist at all nAChR subtypes, exogenous compounds can be partial agonists at certain nAChRs relative to the full agonist ACh, and full agonists or antagonists at other subtypes. This is actually the case for nicotine, which is a full agonist at a4β2 nAChRs (K_i=16 nM), a 75% partial agonist at a7 (K_i=2.1 μM), a high efficacy 85% agonist at α3b4 (K_i=520 nM), and a 60% partial agonist at the a4a6β2 subtype (K_i=270 nM).

Interestingly, agonists are usually much more potent in desensitizing than activating most nAChRs, as exemplified by a typical concentration-dependent inactivation and activation profile for a full agonist in Figure 5. The potency to inactivate nAChRs, expressed as the concentration needed to desensitize the receptor by 50% (IC_{50}, in the nM range), is often at least an order of magnitude higher than the activation potency, expressed as the concentration that produces half maximal activation of the nAChR (EC_{50}, in the μM range).

This has important implications, since nicotine and drugs like varenicline are exposed to the receptor for sustained periods, in contrast to the endogenous neurotransmitter ACh, which is immediately broken down by the enzyme acetyl-cholinesterase after being released. Therefore, short exposures to ACh will activate nAChRs, but nicotine and (partial) agonists will mainly cause receptor desensitization, which is a key mechanism in the addictive actions of nicotine and likely of the therapeutic effects of drugs (see below: Nicotine addiction).

GRAPH 2: Hypothetical concentration-dependent activation and inactivation (desensitization) curves for a full nAChR agonist. The activation and desensitization potencies are indicated by EC_{50} and IC_{50} values, respectively.

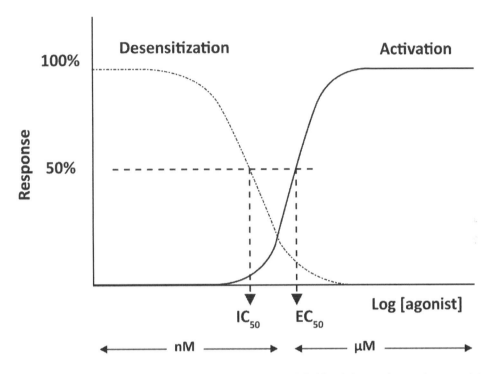

Modified after Rollema H, Bertrand D, Hurst RS, Nicotinic agonists and antagonists, in Encyclopedia of Psychopharmacology, ed. IA Stolerman, Berlin: Springer-Verlag; 2010, p. 889. Reproduced with permission of Springer Science+Business Media.

Antagonists are compounds that bind to the receptor, either at the binding site (competitive antagonists) or elsewhere on the nAChR (non-competitive antagonists), but have no effect and will prevent agonists to interact with the nAChR. Many naturally occurring toxins that act as repellants in plants or animals[12] are non-competitive nAChR antagonists, while some of the few natural products that are competitive antagonists have become important pharmacological tools for the identification and characterization of nAChR subtypes, e.g. methyllycaconitine (a7 antagonist), β-dihydroerythroidine a4β2 antagonist) and a-bungarotoxin (α1 and a7 antagonist). Mecamylamine is an antagonist of nicotinic acetylcholine receptors.

NICOTINE ADDICTION

Effects on mesolimbic dopamine release   Inhalation of tobacco smoke rapidly delivers nicotine to the brain where it can interact with different nAChR subtypes, which trigger the release of a variety of neurotransmitters, including dopamine that mediates the reinforcing effects of nicotine and other drugs of abuse. Nicotine has higher affinity for a4β2 nAChRs (K_i=16 nM) than for other subtypes (K_i> 250 nM) and will thus preferentially bind to this subtype. There is convincing evidence that the interaction of nicotine with a4β2 containing nAChRs in the mesolimbic pathway, which has cell bodies in the ventral tegmental area (VTA) and terminals in the nucleus accumbens and prefrontal cortex (Figure 6), mediates the addictive effects of nicotine.

FIGURE 4: Schematic of inhaled nicotine-induced dopamine release in the nucleus accumbens mediated by its interaction with α4β2 nAChR (insert) in the ventral tegmental area

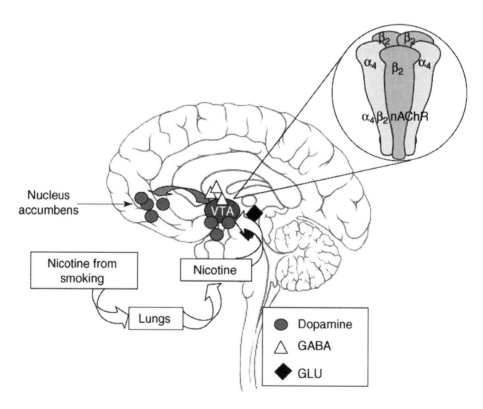

Modified after Rollema H, Coe JW, Chambers LK, Hurst RS, Stahl SM, Williams KE. Rationale, pharmacology and clinical efficacy of partial agonists of alpha4beta2 nACh receptors for smoking cessation. Trends Pharmacol Sci. 2007;28(7): 316–25. Reproduced with permission of Elsevier Ltd.

For instance, in transgenic mice the elimination of either the a4 or β2 subunit attenuates the pharmacological and behavioural effects of nicotine,[13,14] and the targeted expression of β2 subunits in the VTA of β2-knockout mice reinstates nicotine-seeking behaviour and nicotine-induced mesolimbic dopamine release,[15] while lesions of mesolimbic dopaminergic neurons abolish the reinforcing effects of nicotine. Clinical evidence that a selective partial agonist of a4β2 nAChRs, varenicline, is an efficacious smoking-cessation agent (see chapter 9 on varenicline) further supports the role of a4β2 containing nAChRs in tobacco dependence.

A comparison of nicotine concentrations that are predicted to be in the brain of an individual who smokes with nicotine's in vitro functional potency at different nAChR subtypes can indicate whether or not those concentrations can functionally interact with a nAChR subtype. This is shown for a4β2 nAChRs in Figure 7 and reveals that the predominant effect of nicotine from smoking or NRT is a4β2 nAChRs desensitization, with only a tiny fraction of receptors being activated by nicotine concentrations in people who smoke.[16]

FIGURE 5: Nicotine concentrations in the brain of a smoker (grey bar) superimposed over its activation and desensitization curves at human a4β2 nAChRs, show that the predominant effect of these nicotine concentrations is desensitization with minimal activation of the a4β2 nAChR.

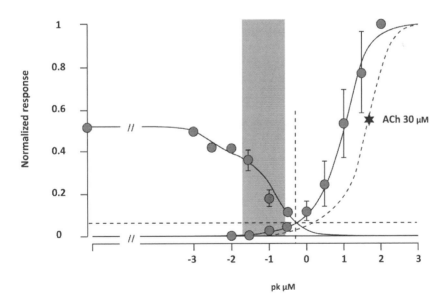

Modified after Rollema H, Shrikhande A, Ward KM, Tingley FD, Coe JW, O'Neill BT, et al. Pre-clinical properties of the alpha4beta2 nicotinic acetylcholinic receptor partial agonists varenicline, cytisine, and dianicline translate to clinical efficacy for nicotine dependence. Br J Pharmacol. 2010;160:334–45. Reproduced with permission of Nature Publishing Group.

Such extensive desensitization seems at odds with the fact that nicotine stimulates dopamine release, but nicotine interacts with a4β2 nAChRs located on different neurons that can have opposing effects on dopamine release. While desensitization of a4β2 nAChRs on dopaminergic neurons is likely to *decrease* dopamine release, concurrent desensitization of a4β2 nAChRs located on GABAergic neurons will have the opposite effect, since attenuation of the GABA-mediated inhibitory drive will *increase* dopamine release. Activation of a4β2 nAChRs on these different neurons will obviously have the opposite effect on terminal dopamine release, while nicotine also interacts with nAChRs on glutamate neurons, which in turn regulate the activity of dopaminergic and GABAergic neurons in the VTA. In addition, over time the number of a4β2 nAChRs will increase via up-regulation that adds to the complexity of these processes. The net result of these differential effects is enhanced dopamine release in the nucleus accumbens.

Finally, recent studies on nAChR subtypes that mediate nicotine-evoked effects, including dopamine release, revealed that nicotine also interacts with a6 containing subtypes, e.g. a4a6β2 or a4a6β3 nAChRs, which play a key role in mediating dopamine release.[17] Moreover, it was recently shown that the a6 containing subtypes are not extensively desensitized by brain concentrations of nicotine, which explains that nicotine can stimulate dopamine release via activation of a subtype that is not readily desensitized.[18]

Pharmacological mechanisms in nicotine addiction The nicotine-induced release of dopamine in the mesolimbic reward pathway initiates a physiological response that contributes to the reinforcing effects of nicotine.[19] Between cigarettes, brain nicotine levels gradually decrease, triggering several processes that contribute to the cycle of craving and urge to smoke that maintains nicotine dependence. It is believed that the rapidly recurring and transitory increases in mesolimbic DA levels following repeated exposure to, and withdrawal from, nicotine transmit salient reward and aversive signals to higher cortical centers, facilitating the learning and associations that lead to physical dependence, which is characterized by both somatic and psychoactive symptoms. These responses contribute to both the reinforcing effects of nicotine and the craving symptoms upon smoking cessation.

PET studies with a selective α4β2 radioligand found that after 1–2 puffs half of the brain α4β2 nAChRs were occupied by nicotine and that smoking only 1 cigarette delivered sufficient nicotine to the brain for almost complete occupancy of central α4β2 nAChRs for several hours.[20] Since the α4β2 nAChRs will be in the desensitized state, it has been proposed that smokers smoke a next cigarette to maintain all α4β2 nAChRs desensitized. In this scenario craving and withdrawal symptoms will be experienced when desensitized α4β2 nAChRs transition to the deactivated state during abstinence and are responsive to nicotine again. It should however be mentioned that recent studies have shown that withdrawal symptoms may be mediated by other neuronal connections, including the medial habenula and the interpeduncular nucleus, which express β4 and α5 containing nAChR subunits, indicating that different nAChR subtypes play a role in addiction and withdrawal symptoms associated with tobacco use.[21]

NICOTINE AND NACHR LIGANDS AS THERAPEUTICS

Since smoking improves mood and concentration, and reduces stress and anxiety, nicotine also has beneficial properties and it has been suggested that smoking cigarettes is a form of self-medication, e.g. to attenuate symptoms of depressed mood, of schizophrenia or cognitive deficits. As nicotine lacks good drug-like properties, compounds with an improved pharmacokinetic profile and more selectivity for a certain nAChR subtype are being designed as potential novel therapeutics for several disorders.

Nicotine addiction As discussed, α6 containing receptors play an important role in mediating nicotine-induced dopamine release and discovery efforts are focused on the design and development of ligands that selectively interact with α6 containing nAChRs,[22] but so far no clinical data have been disclosed. Another nAChR subtype that may have a role in addiction and withdrawal is the α3b4 nAChR, and antagonists are studied as potential smoking cessation agents.[23]

A completely different approach is vaccination, an immunotherapy with the potential to treat addictions to nicotine and other drugs of abuse with relatively few or mild adverse events (also see Chapter 9).[24] A nicotine vaccine will raise nicotine-specific antibodies in the blood that bind to nicotine. As the nicotine-antibody complex cannot enter the brain, nicotine does not have central effects and the smoker will thus not experience reinforcement from smoking.[25] Several companies are developing nicotine vaccines and initial results showed that high antibody levels were associated with higher quit rates at 1 year than lower tiers. However, one of the vaccines, NicVax, failed to meet the primary endpoint in two large phase 3 clinical trials, having the same 11% abstinence rate at 1 year as placebo treatment.[26] It is possible that vaccines prepared with different carriers and adjuvants may improve the immune response.

Depression Interest in the antidepressant potential of nicotine and nAChR ligands was stimulated by the finding that these compounds display antidepressant-like activity in preclinical rodent models and by clinical studies on the antidepressant activity of the non-selective nAChR antagonist mecamylamine. It was hypothesized that antagonists and partial agonists of a4β2, a7 or α3b4 nAChRs will reduce the hyperactivity of the cholinergic system, which is thought to cause depressive symptoms. Treatment with either a nAChR antagonist that blocks the receptor, or with a nAChR partial agonist that reduces cholinergic tone or desensitizes the receptor, should result in decreased nAChR signalling.[27-29] While nicotine and several nAChR ligands have shown preclinical activity in the forced swim test, results from phase-2 and -3 trials with nAChR ligands in combination with classical antidepressants in treatment-resistant patients have been mixed. Positive outcomes were reported for mecamylamine and its S-(+)-enantiomer, TC-5214, in double-blind studies and for the a4β2 selective partial agonist varenicline in a small open-label study. However, four large phase-3 studies with TC-5214 in treatment resistant depressed patients did not meet primary endpoints, while interim results from a phase-2 trial with the a4β2 selective partial agonist, CP-601927 were also negative. Results from further trials have to be awaited before conclusions can be drawn about the potential of nAChR antagonists or partial agonists as adjunct therapy for depression.

Cognitive deficits   Nicotine and nicotinic agonists improve information processing, attention, and memory in animal cognition models and in human clinical studies, indicating that the central cholinergic system plays an important role in cognition.[30] and a4β2 and a7 subtypes are drug targets to improve cognitive deficits associated with schizophrenia, Alzheimer's disease, and attention deficit hyperactivity disorder.[31]

Cognitive impairment is one of the hallmarks of schizophrenia, and there is preclinical evidence that selective a7 or α4β2 nAChR ligands can enhance cognitive performance. Several a7 and α4β2 nAChR compounds are now being investigated for cognitive impairment associated with schizophrenia, but while initial trials showed positive results, larger trials have thus far had mainly negative outcomes.

Deterioration of memory and cognitive function is also a key feature in Alzheimer's disease (AD), characterized by declining cholinergic transmission due to the loss of mAChRs and nAChRs. A small number of α7 and α4β2 nAChR partial or full agonists have been advanced into clinical studies in AD patients. While some studies have shown significant improvements in measures of attention and memory, in several trials compounds failed to meet their primary endpoint.

Attention deficit hyperactivity disorder (ADHD) patients are known to use tobacco products at a much higher rate than the general population, and nicotine, mostly administered as a transdermal patch, has therefore been evaluated in a number of trials as a treatment of ADHD, which had promising results. Nicotine improved some measures of symptom severity, while selective a4β2 nAChR agonists (e.g. ispronicline, sofinicline, and ABT-089) significantly improved ADHD rating-scale scores in adults.

Parkinson's disease Epidemiological studies have shown that long-term smoking is associated with a decreased incidence of Parkinson's disease (PD) and it is believed that nicotine provides protection against neurodegeneration of dopaminergic neurons. Nicotine-evoked dopamine release in striatum is mediated via a4β2 and a6* nAChRs and the number of these subtypes decline with disease progression.[32,33] It was recently found that concentrations of nicotine in the smoker's brain can activate a6* nAChRs,[18] and compounds that target a6 containing nAChRs thus have potential in treating Parkinson's. An alternative explanation for the protective effect of nicotine is that nicotine causes upregulation of nAChRs, which may to some extent restore the receptor deficit in the substantia nigra of PD patients.[34,35] This suggests that the impaired dopaminergic function in PD can be improved by nicotine and nicotinics via a6* and/or a4β2 nAChRs. While small clinical studies have shown that nicotine from smoking or NRT gum did not produce robust improvements in motor symptoms, better results were reported for nicotine given for 3.5 months in an oral capsule (NP002) that showed a trend to reduce dyskinesias due to L-dopa therapy in PD patients. Several studies are now in progress with selective a4β2 partial or full agonists in animal PD models, but initial results with the a4β2 partial agonist altinicline showed that 1-week treatment with this compound did not have anti-parkinsonian effects in humans and further studies are thus needed.

Pain It has long been known that nicotine and nicotinic natural products have analgesic effects, but the discovery of the remarkable analgesic potency of the a4β2 agonist epibatidine, a frog alkaloid, prompted extensive research on nicotinic compounds as novel pain treatments.[36] Unfortunately, the development of most compounds that showed potent analgesic activity (e.g. ABT-594 or tebanicline, sofinicline) has been discontinued, mostly because of a lack of tolerability.

In conclusion, the mixed results of clinical trials with nAChR ligands for several indications illustrate the challenges of developing nicotinic compounds as novel therapeutics. Despite decades of research, so far only one novel nAChR ligand has been discovered and approved for marketing, the smoking cessation aid varenicline, more than 50 years after the nAChR antagonist mecamylamine was introduced in the 1950's to treat hypertension. The main reason for discontinuing a compound has been a narrow therapeutic index, either due to insufficient efficacy or to a high incidence of adverse events, which are often gastrointestinal and central nervous system side effects. Clearly, more selective compounds with optimal functional potency at the appropriate target nAChR subtype that will reach adequate free brain concentrations are needed to increase the success rate of nicotinic drug development.

SUMMARY

This chapter reviews aspects of nicotine, a plant alkaloid that acts as a natural repellant against predators. Brief descriptions of the history of nicotine and cigarette smoking, and of the structure and function of nAChRs, precede more detailed discussions of the pharmacology and pharmacokinetics of nicotine. Acting almost exclusively on different subtypes of nAChRs that can be activated and desensitized by nicotine, it has complex and dose-dependent effects on the peripheral and central nervous systems. Nicotine has a relatively short half live of 2 hours in humans and is rapidly metabolized with cotinine as a primary metabolite. It is well established that the addictive effect of nicotine, which makes it so difficult for smokers to quit, is mediated via a4β2 nAChRs and that increased dopamine release in the mesolimbic system plays a key role in initiating and maintaining the addiction. However, a6 containing nAChRs have also been implicated in the effects of nicotine on dopamine release, while recent studies suggest that other subtypes, e.g. α3b4 containing nAChRs, may be involved in nicotine withdrawal. The chapter concludes with an overview of nicotinic ligands as potential treatments for nicotine addiction, depression, cognitive deficits in schizophrenia or Alzheimers' disease, ADHD, Parkinson's disease, and pain.

REFERENCES

1   James I. A counterblaste to tobacco; 1604/1905 [cited 2012 May 11]. Available from: http://www.laits.utexas.edu/poltheory/james/blaste/blaste.html.

2   Brandt AM. The cigarette century: the rise, fall and deadly persistence of the product that defined America. New York: Basic Books; 2007.

3   Doll R et al. Mortality in relationship to smoking: 20 years' observations on male British doctors. Brit Med J. 2004;6:1451-5.

4   Benowitz NL, Hukkanen J, Jacob P. Nicotine chemistry, metabolism, kinetics and biomarkers. Handb Exp Pharmacol. 2009;(192):29-60.

5   Rose JE, Mukhin AG, Lokitz SJ, Turkington TG, Herskovic J, Behm FM et al. Kinetics of brain nicotine accumulation in dependent and nondependent smokers assessed with PET and cigarettes containing ^{11}C-nicotine. Proc Natl Acad Sci USA. 2011;107:5190-5.

6   Matta SG, Balfour DJ, Benowitz NL, Boyd T, Buccafusco JJ, Caggiula AR, et al. Guidelines on nicotine dose selection for in vivo research. Psychopharmacol. 2007;190:269-319.

7   Albuquerque EX, Pereira EF, Alkondon M, Rogers SW. Mammalian nicotinic acetylcholine receptors: from structure to function. Physiol Rev. 2009;89:73-120.

8   Taly A, Corringer PJ, Guedin D, Lestage P, Changeux JP. Nicotinic receptors: allosteric transitions and therapeutic targets in the nervous system. Nat Rev Drug Discov. 2009;8:733-50.

9   Changeux JP. Nicotine addiction and nicotinic receptors: lessons from genetically modified mice. Nat Rev Neursci. 2010;11(6):389-401.

10   Hurst RS, Rollema H, Bertrand D. Neuronal nicotinic acetylcholine receptors: from basic science to therapeutics. Pharmacol Ther. 2012 (forthcoming).

11   Govind AP, Vezina P, Green WN. Nicotine-induced upregulation of nicotinic receptors: underlying mechanisms and relevance to nicotine addiction. Biochem Pharmacol. 2009;78:756-65.

12   Daly JW. Nicotinic agonists, antagonists, and modulators from natural sources. Cell Mol Neurobiol. 2005;25(3-4):513-52.

13   Picciotto MR, Zoli M, Rimondini R, Léna C, Marubio LM, Pich EM, Fuxe K, Changeux JP. Acetylcholine receptors containing the beta2 subunit are involved in the reinforcing properties of nicotine. Nature. 1998;391(6663):173-7.

14   Tapper AR, McKinney SL, Nashmi R, Schwarz J, Deshpande P, Cesar Labarca et al. Nicotine activation of alpha4* receptors: sufficient for reward, tolerance, and sensitization. Science. 2004;306(5698):1029-32.

15   Maskos U, Molles BE, Pons S, Besson M, Guiard et al. Nicotine reinforcement and cognition restored by targeted expression of nicotinic receptors. Nature. 2005;436:103-7.

16   Rollema H, Shrikhande A, Ward KM, Tingley FD 3rd, Coe JW, O'Neill BT et al. Pre-clinical properties of the alpha4beta2 nicotinic acetylcholine receptor partial agonists varenicline, cytisine and dianicline translate to clinical efficacy for nicotine dependence. Br J Pharmacol. 2010;160:334-45.

17   Drenan RM, Grady SR, Steele AD, McKinney S, Patzlaff NE, McIntosh JM et al. Cholinergic modulation of locomotion and striatal dopamine release is mediated by alpha6alpha4* nicotinic acetylcholine receptors. J Neurosci. 2010;30(29):9877-89.

18   Valera S, Bertrand B, Rollema H, Hurst RS, Bertrand S. Effects of nicotine and varenicline at alpha6 containing nAChRs: relevance for nicotine dependence. Soc Neurosci. 2010. Poster# 476.12/NN6.

19   Laviolette SR, Van der Kooy KD. The neurobiology of nicotine addiction: bridging the gap from molecules to behaviour. Nat Rev Neurosci. 2004;5:55-65.

20   Brody AL, Mandelkern MA, London ED et al. Cigarette smoking saturates brain alpha-4beta2 nicotinic acetylcholine receptors. Arch Gen Psychiatry. 2006;63:907-15.

21   De Biasi M, Dani JA. Reward, addiction, withdrawal to nicotine. Ann Rev Neurosci. 2011;34:105-30.

22   Marks MJ, Wageman CR, Grady SR, Gopalakrishnan M, Briggs CA. Selectivity of ABT-089 for alpha4beta2* and alpha6beta2* nicotinic acetylcholine receptors in brain. Biochem Pharmacol. 2009;78(7):795-802.

23   Zaveri N, Jiang F, Olsen C, Polgar W, Toll L. Novel alpha3beta4 nicotinic acetylcholine receptor-selective ligands. Discovery, structure-activity studies, and pharmacological evaluation. J Med Chem. 2010;53(22):8187-91.

24   Shen XY, Orson FM, Kosten TR. Vaccines against drug abuse. Clin Pharmacol Ther. 2012;91(1):60-70.

25   Ottney AR. Nicotine conjugate vaccine as a novel approach to smoking cessation. Pharmacotherapy. 2011;31(7):703-13.

26   Fahim RE, Kessler PD, Fuller SA, Kalnik MW. Nicotine vaccines. CNS Neurol Disord Drug Targets. 2012 Jan 10. [Epub ahead of print] PMID: 22229310.

27   Shytle RD, Silver AA, Lukas RJ, Newman MB, Sheehan DV, Sanberg PR. Nicotinic acetylcholine receptors as targets for antidepressants. Mol Psychiatry. 2002;7:525-35.

28   Philip NS, Carpenter LL, Tyrka AR, Price LH. Nicotinic acetylcholine receptors and depression: a review of the preclinical and clinical literature. Psychopharmacol. 2010;212:1-12.

29   Mineur YS, Picciotto MR. Nicotine receptors and depression: revisiting and revising the cholinergic hypothesis. Trends Pharmacol Sci. 2010;31:580-6.

30   Poorthuis RB, Goriounova NA, Couey JJ, Mansvelder HD. Nicotinic actions on neuronal networks for cognition: general principles and long-term consequences. Biochem Pharmacol. 2009;78:668-76.

31   Wallace TL, Ballard TM, Pouzet B, Riedel WJ, Wettstein JG. Drug targets for cognitive enhancement in neuropsychiatric disorders. Pharmacol Biochem Behav. 2011;99(2):130-45.

32   Quik M, O'Leary K, Tanner CM. Nicotine and Parkinson's disease: implications for therapy. Mov Disord. 2008;23:1641-52.

33   Chen H, Huang X, Guo X, Mailman RB, Park Y, Kamel F, Umbach DM et al. Smoking duration, intensity, and risk of Parkinson disease. Neurology. 2010;74:878-84.

34   Srinivasan R, Pantoja R, Moss FJ, Mackey ED, Son CD, Miwa J, Lester HA. Nicotine up-regulates alpha4beta2 nicotinic receptors and ER exit sites via stoichiometry-dependent chaperoning. J Gen Physiol. 2011;137:59-79.

35   Xiao C, Nashmi R, McKinney S, Cai H, McIntosh JM, Lester HA. Chronic nicotine selectively enhances alpha4beta2* nicotinic acetylcholinic receptors in the nigrostriatal dopamine pathway. J Neurosci. 29(40):12428-12439.

36   Gao B, Hierl M, Clarkin K, Juan T, Nguyen H, Valk M, Deng H, Guo W et al. Pharmacological effects of nonselective and subtype-selective nicotinic acetylcholine receptor agonists in animal models of persistent pain. Pain. 2010;149:33-49.

6

Assessing Tobacco Use in Clinical Practice: A Step-Wise Approach

MILAN KHARA, AMIT ROTEM AND ALLISON VAN DRIESUM

This chapter has been adapted from the original article: Els C & Selby P. A step-wise approach to assessment: informing about cessation and optimizing outcomes. Smoking Cessation Rounds. 2009; 2(7): The Minto Prevention and Rehabilitation Centre, University of Ottawa Heart Institute and the Addiction Medicine Service, Centre for Addiction and Mental Health, University of Toronto, used with permission.

AS NO TWO INDIVIDUALS ARE THE SAME, IT FOLLOWS THAT ASSESSMENT AND TREATment of tobacco use and addiction must be tailored in order to take into account the dynamic circumstances and changing needs of the individual over time. Assessment aims not only to identify tobacco use and detect addiction but also to inform treatment decisions and measure outcomes over time. It requires the identification and exploration of factors that could potentially impact outcomes. These include the patient's level of motivation, intention to quit, levels of self-efficacy, level of nicotine dependence, social supports, stress, and outcome expectancy.[1–3]

Tobacco use and addiction is often a precursor to other chronic health conditions or may co-occur with physical or mental (including addictive) disorders. Individuals with comorbid psychiatric conditions (especially severe and persistent mental illness) and substance-related disorders (e.g. cocaine, opioid, and alcohol dependence) also want to quit smoking but, when neglected, these conditions are among the most important factors negatively impacting on smoking cessation outcomes. To optimize cessation outcomes, it is fundamentally important to include the identification of other health conditions in the assessment for the purposes of guiding treatment.

Adequate assessment of tobacco use and addiction can be brief, concrete, and practical. It almost universally requires an iterative assessment approach to assessment to reflect experimentation, readiness to cut down or quit, response to treatment and relapses. This chapter recommends a brief and pragmatic approach to comprehensive assessment. Proper assessment guides treatment and lays the foundation for safe and effective therapy; it is fundamental to optimized outcomes.

ASSESSMENT PROTOCOL

The following model serves as a generic template for assessment. This step-wise approach to assessment involves three steps totalling five tasks: Step 1: Screening, Diagnosis, Step 2: Triage, Treatment planning, and Step 3: Outcome monitoring.

STEP 1: IDENTIFICATION OF TOBACCO USERS

Most Guidelines recommend the institutionalization of tobacco screening and documentation of tobacco use. These recommendations suggest that all patients be asked about their use of tobacco and that this status be documented on a regular basis. The single question: "Do you currently use any tobacco products?" is designed to yield, with sufficient sensitivity, an accurate identification of most current tobacco users. Such screening for current (or past) tobacco use will result in four possible responses:

- Currently using tobacco and willing to make a quit attempt at this time (or in the near future).
- Currently using tobacco but not willing to make a quit attempt at this time.
- Formerly used tobacco.
- Never regularly used tobacco.

Individuals identified as currently using tobacco should be subject to more in-depth assessment, while former or never-smokers may be counselled in a fashion to reinforce their respective nonsmoking status. This forms part of the systematic implementation of the complete '5-A' approach (Ask, Advise, Assess, Assist, and Arrange) for brief interventions (a full description of this intervention approach can be found in Chapter 8).

STATEMENT 1: Questions to assess the stage of change for quitting smoking

---

1. **Are you intending to quit smoking in the next six months?** If no, the patient is in precontemplation. If yes, please proceed to the next question.
2. **Are you intending to stop smoking in the next month?** If no, the smoker is in the contemplation stage. If yes, proceed to the next question.
3. **Did you try to quit smoking in the past year?** If no, the smoker is in the contemplation stage. If yes, the smoker is in the preparation stage.
4. (if the smoker has already quit) **How long ago did you stop smoking?** If <6 months ago, the patient is in the action stage. If >6 months, he/she is in the maintenance stage.

Source: Prochasa JO, Goldstein MG. Process of smoking cessation. Implications for Clinicians. Clin Chest Med. 1991;12(4):727-37. Copyright Elsevier 1991. Used with permission.

TOXICOLOGICAL TESTING TO VERIFY SMOKING STATUS

The primary clinical application of biochemical testing is verification of abstinence, as opposed to identification of tobacco users in clinical settings. Biochemical verification of smoking status can be conducted, but the clinical application in primary care treatment planning and follow-up monitoring remains limited. Testing for cotinine, the main metabolite of nicotine, will only be detectable in the body for a limited time after exposure to nicotine.

A positive **cotinine** level has limited value in diagnosing tobacco addiction, but it does confirm recent exposure to nicotine that may be due to secondhand smoke exposure or the use of any nicotine replacement therapy. Testing may have special applications in sub-populations where self-reports may be dubious or inaccuracy is suspected, possibly to avoid facing the consequences such as in adolescents, pregnant women or in patients on lung-transplant lists. The costs associated with conducting such testing are significant, and the clinical application of determining cotinine levels in primary-care settings for smoking cessation is limited.

Another test that also determines possible exposure to tobacco smoke involves **thiocyanate** (another metabolite of nicotine) and, similar to cotinine, tests can be conducted on a variety of bodily matrices (e.g. blood, sputum, urine, and hair). Sputum measurements are generally considered inferior to serum determinations as a testing matrix due to the inherent limitations in the saliva distribution of nicotine breakdown products. Although it is less invasive, the clinical applications remain limited; nevertheless, cost allowing, serum cotinine point-of-care testing is commercially available and may serve as a detector of possible relapse. Hair analysis for cotinine determination is expensive and has no clinical application in assessment for the purpose of treatment planning on a primary-care level.

Carbon monoxide (CO) measurement has a much larger clinical application in daily smoking cessation practice. It is usually measured in expired air, with the aid of a special device, which is commercially available and relatively inexpensive. A CO reading >10 parts per million (ppm) is usually indicative of the consumption of cigarettes or smoking, but this is not specific to tobacco. It does not detect the use of other nicotine-delivery systems, only the inhalation from a combustible tobacco-delivery system. Serial measurements of CO (e.g. every clinic visit) have a useful application in cessation settings for monitoring outcome. It is also a useful tool to further engage individuals in the ongoing process of stopping smoking and receiving treatment, by providing tangible evidence of progress. However, CO measurement may lead to a positive result when persons are exposed to inhaling secondhand smoke so results must be interpreted with caution.

STEP 2: TRIAGE

To conduct a more comprehensive assessment of tobacco use and addiction, the combination of an unstructured clinical interview and psychometric testing (i.e. using selected rating scales) is recommended. The minimum set of clinical data should be collected for treatment planning. Factors that are commonly assessed to be relevant in planning treatment include the duration of smoking (often expressed as pack-years as calculated by packs smoked per day × years as a smoker) and the use of other tobacco products e.g. smokeless tobacco (including *snus*). Assessment should include detection of potential withdrawal symptoms or mood changes associated with previous quit attempts, cravings, possible triggers and sources of secondhand smoke exposure (e.g. others smoking in the home or vehicle). Post-cessation weight gain is a commonly expressed concern;[5]

therefore, serial weight monitoring is necessary to allow the prevention of avoidable or significant changes in weight when quitting smoking. Useful and available questionnaires are available, for example to determine the reasons why an individual smokes (The "Why" Test)[6] and reasons for quitting.[7] Inquiry about daily caffeine consumption is relevant, since individuals may develop symptoms of caffeine intoxication due to a change in the pharmacokinetics of CYP1A2 substrates with tobacco reduction and cessation.

After smoking status has been determined, it is important to confirm the diagnosis of tobacco dependence through the use of either the *Diagnostic and Statistical Manual of Mental Disorders, Fourth Edition, Text Revision (DSM-IV-TR)*[8] criteria for the diagnosis of Nicotine Dependence (Table 1) or the International Classification of Diseases (ICD-10)[9] criteria. There are subtle differences between these classification systems and the use of either to confirm the diagnosis is considered feasible. Revisions are expected for the diagnostic entity of Nicotine Dependence, and the proposed designation is Tobacco Use Disorder.[10] The proposed changes better align the category of tobacco use disorder with other categories of substance addiction, and also reflect a maladaptive pattern of use, leading to clinically significant impairment or distress. The time period remains 12 months, and severity, course, and remission specifiers are added as well as specifiers of "with or without physiological dependence." The proposed revisions are detailed on the *DSM-5* development website hosted by the American Psychiatric Association.

TABLE 1. DSM IV-TR Criteria for Nicotine Dependence

A maladaptive pattern of substance use, leading to clinically significant impairment or distress, as manifested by three (or more) of the following, occurring at any time in the same 12-month period:

(1) Tolerance, as defined by either of the following:

> (a) A need for markedly increased amounts of the substance to achieve intoxication or desired effect   (b) markedly diminished effect with continued use of the same amount of the substance

(2) Withdrawal, as manifested by either of the following:

> (a) The characteristic withdrawal syndrome for the substance (refer to Criteria A and B of the criteria sets for Withdrawal from the specific substances) (b) the same (or a closely related) substance is taken to relieve or avoid withdrawal symptoms.

(3) The substance is often taken in larger amounts or over a longer period than was intended

(4) There is a persistent desire or unsuccessful efforts to cut down or control substance use

(5) A great deal of time is spent in activities necessary to obtain the substance (e.g., visiting multiple doctors or driving long distances), use the substance (e.g., chain-smoking), or recover from its effects

(6) Important social, occupational, or recreational activities are given up or reduced because of substance use

(7) The substance use is continued despite knowledge of having a persistent or recurrent physical or psychological problem that is likely to have been caused or exacerbated by the substance (e.g., current cocaine use despite recognition of cocaine-induced depression, or continued drinking despite recognition that an ulcer was made worse by alcohol consumption)

Specify if:

> **With Physiological Dependence:** evidence of tolerance or withdrawal (i.e., either Item 1 or 2 is present) **Without Physiological Dependence:** no evidence of tolerance or withdrawal (i.e., neither Item 1 nor 2 is present).

Reprinted with permission from the Diagnostic and Statistical Manual of Mental Disorders, Fourth Edition, Text Revision. Copyright 2000. American Psychiatric Association.

Assessment of motivation to change behaviour   The clinical practice guidelines underscore the necessity to assess readiness to quit (the third A of the 5-A Approach). For those who are not ready to quit, the use of the motivational 5-R's (Relevance, Risks, Rewards, Roadblocks, Repetition) is recommended, which then becomes part of the assessment in those unwilling to make a quit attempt. Scaling questions to assess readiness to quit assists in matching stage-appropriate motivational interventions to the level of readiness of the patient. Three questions are routinely posed:

- On a scale from 0–10, how important is it for you to quit at this time?
- On a scale from 0–10, how confident are you that you can quit smoking at this time?
- On a scale from 0–10, how ready are you to make this change?

In addition to these questions, asking whether the patient has set a quit date, and when it is planned, may also assist in determining the relative readiness to change.

THE FAGERSTRÖM TEST FOR NICOTINE DEPENDENCE

Nicotine dependence level is most commonly determined with the use of a self-report rating scale, the Fagerström test for nicotine dependence (FTND).[11] The six questions (Table 2) in this scale are scored individually and the total for all the questions is calculated, providing a cumulative score out of 10. Among these questions, the single factor most strongly associated with the degree of nicotine dependence is the time from waking up to the first cigarette (Question #2). The number of cigarettes per day is considered a less indicative measure for the level of addiction because there are large inter-individual variations in the efficiency with which people smoke. The FTND score provides an indication of the level of dependence, and is categorized as follows: 0–2 = very low level of dependence, 3-7 = moderate, and 8–10 = very high level of dependence. The FTND remains a gold standard in assessment of tobacco addiction.

THE HEAVINESS OF SMOKING INDEX is a subset of questions from the FTND for determining level of addiction to nicotine. It consists of FTND Item 1 and 4; using the same response scales and calculating the total score using the sum of the scores on those two items. Scoring: 0-2 =mild; 3-4=moderate; 5-6= severe dependence.

TABLE 2. The Fagerström test for nicotine dependence.

How many cigarettes per day do you usually smoke?	10 or less	0
	11-20	1
	21-30	2
	31 or more	3
How soon after you wake up do you smoke your first cigarette?	≤ 5 minutes	3
	6-30 minutes	2
	>30 minutes	1
Do you find it difficult to stop smoking in no-smoking areas?	No	0
	Yes	1
Which cigarette would you hate most to give up?	The first 1 of the morning	1
	Other	0
Do you smoke more frequently in the first hours after waking up than during the rest of the day?	No	0
	Yes	1
Does your smoking make you so ill that you are in bed most of the day?	No	0
	Yes	1

Source: Heatherington TF, et al. The Fagerström Test for Nicotine Dependence: a revision fo the Fagerström Tolerance Questionnaire. Br J Addict. 1991:86(9):1119-27.

Assessing medication use One of the key recommendations in the updated USDHHS clinical guidelines is for clinicians to encourage the use of pharmacotherapy by all patients attempting to quit smoking unless medically contraindicated or in specific populations where there is insufficient evidence of effectiveness (smokeless-tobacco users, pregnant women, youth, and light smokers). To guide current treatment recommendations in selecting medications, the previous use of cessation medication should be examined to determine which of any of the 7 first-line options (5 NRT options, bupropion, or varenicline) had worked in the past. Previous use may guide the next choice for pharmacotherapy as well as the exploration of any related side effects, and the dose, duration, and adequacy of previous medication use.

Clinical practice guidelines suggest that counselling and medication in combination are more effective than either option alone; therefore, it is useful to determine if any psychosocial interventions were used in the past. This will guide the selection of psychosocial interventions and counselling recommendations for the current cessation attempt. Past quit attempts and experience should be assessed as well for planning the next intervention. Thus clinicians should encourage all individuals to use both counselling and medication when attempting to stop smoking, and the selection of current interventions may be guided by previous successes and challenges.

Assessment to detect comorbid mental illness   Evaluation of the mental status and psychiatric history of a patient may be best achieved by conducting a standardized psychiatric interview. However, the most relevant questions in a smoking-cessation context would be to exclude any previous history of psychiatric illness (e.g. major depressive disorder, schizophrenia, anxiety disorders, bipolar disorder), previous hospitalizations or treatment for psychiatric reasons, previous suicide attempts, and a determination of any significant level of exacerbation in pre-existing psychopathology during the last quit attempt. Safety of patients is paramount; therefore, assessment in this context serves to exclude any imminent risk of harm to self or others.

In some individuals, mood exacerbations can occur up to 6 months after tobacco abstinence, with or without the use of pharmacotherapy; as a result, this aspect must be serially and diligently monitored. The proposed assessment also incorporates screening for possible mood disorders as well as quantifying any changes in mood over time during the reduction and cessation process. One example of a brief, appropriate screener is the Patient Health Questionnaire (PHQ-2) as it inquires about the frequency of depressed mood (feeling down, depressed or hopeless) and anhedonia (little interest or pleasure in doing things) over the past 2 weeks. The purpose of incorporating a screening tool is not to establish a final diagnosis or to monitor the severity of comorbid depression but rather to screen for depression only as a "first step" in a broader approach. Patients who screen positive on the PHQ-2 should be further evaluated with the PHQ-9 (or reasonable alternative), and to determine whether they meet criteria for a *DSM-IV-TR* Major Depressive Episode or Disorder. One example of integrating the mood screening in the usual 5-A treatment algorithm for tobacco addiction treatment, is the Safety-Sensitive Algorithm (Chapter 1).

The use of standardized and alternative rating scales supplement the interview, and the use of the Beck Depression Inventory or a Hamilton Depression Scale (HAMD-7) may offer useful mood-related information, if administered over time and serially. Changes in mood or the development of an imminent and substantial risk of harm (as a result of a psychiatric condition) warrant the attention of the primary-care provider or attending psychiatrist, and must be sufficiently addressed to ensure the patient's safety and optimal outcome. Ongoing mood monitoring is generally required and recommended for those with a history of major mood conditions or other neuropsychiatric conditions.

Assessment of possible drug interactions   The patient may be using certain psychotropic drugs that must be identified and may require special attention; among the most salient examples are the cytochrome P450 1A2 (CYP1A2) substrates, e.g. haloperidol, clozapine, olanzapine, and caffeine. Serial blood level determinations (of selected 1A2 metabolized psychotropic drugs, such as clozapine) may be required to monitor potential changes in blood levels of these drugs when patients quit smoking. Monitoring of caffeine reduction and consumption may prevent exacerbations of pre-existing anxiety conditions when patients stop smoking.

Assessment to detect substance-related disorders   Failure to identify and treat comorbid substance-use disorders in those quitting smoking may compromise outcomes and pose independent health risks. Alcohol and caffeine may be triggers. The detection of substance-related disorders is best done through a standard psychiatric interview, where direct inquiry about the use of alcohol, painkillers, street drugs, and caffeine is conducted.

The supplementation of the clinical interview with standardized rating scales may enhance the sensitivity of the interview and for the purposes of detecting substance related discorders including alcohol related disorders. The CAGE Questionnaire[12] (Ever felt like you need to *Cut* down on drinking? Ever felt *Annoyed* by criticism of drinking? Ever had *Guilty* feelings about drinking? Ever take a morning *Eye-opener* drink?) remains a sufficiently sensitive and specific screening tool. Obtaining collateral information and conducting laboratory testing (e.g. liver function testing) and toxicological testing can enhance the detection of drug use. Positive drug tests do not equate with either impairment or with addiction to drugs, but warrant further exploration and investigation.

STEP 3: MEASUREMENT OF OUTCOMES

Carbon monoxide measurement in expired air remains the standard outcome measurement in smoking cessation trials. Measurement of short-and long-term abstinence (LTA) rates is valuable for describing cessation outcomes, and the improvement in quality of life may be more sensitive in detecting subtle changes over the process of quitting. Assessing for the number of quit attempts may also be indicative of the impact of tobacco-control interventions, but key challenges remain in the methodology for accurate measurement.[13] Treatment retention and recidivism may also serve as predictors of outcome. Fundamentally, however, the measurement of outcome should not be based only on LTA rates, and this is especially the case in those persons with mental illness or addiction. Outcome measures should include some level of mood symptom monitoring irrespective of the selected medication by which cessation is achieved.

SUMMARY

A thorough assessment typically guides treatment decisions and profoundly impacts the course and prognosis of any medical condition. This chapter offered a pragmatic approach to the identification and assessment of tobacco use and addiction, with the purpose of informing treatment and measuring outcomes. This flexible model of assessment is applicable to all healthcare disciplines, across the spectrum of care, and sets the stage for the integration of smoking cessation interventions into busy daily practices.

An assessment minimally includes 3 steps: Identification (screening and diagnosis), Triage (and treatment planning), and outcome monitoring. Collecting the minimum amount of information is required to identify and confirmation of diagnosis develop an individualized evidence-based treatment plan. Ongoing monitoring of the progress and effectiveness of multimodal and guideline-driven treatment allows for a truly longitudinal approach required for successful chronic disease management.

An iterative process of assessment guides the appropriate level and intensity of treatment of tobacco use and addiction. The multi-domain assessment sets the stage for treatment decisions and greatly impacts on the course and prognosis of the condition. Ensuring the integration of safe and effective tobacco management into daily clinical practice hinges on the adoption of a thorough, frequent assessment process.

REFERENCES

1   Niaura R, Abrams DB. Smoking cessation: progress, priorities and prospectus. J Consult Clin Psychol. 2002;70(3):494-509.

2   Prochaska JO, Goldstein MG. Process of smoking cessation. Implications for clinicians. Clin Chest Med. 1991;12(4):727-35.

3   Abrams DB, Orleans CT, Niaura RS, Goldstein MG, Prochaska JO, Velicer W. Integrating individual and public health perspectives for treatment of tobacco dependence under managed health care: a combined stepped-care and matching model. Ann Behav Med. 1996;18(4):290-304.

4   United States Department of Health and Human Services; Public Health Service. Treating tobacco use and dependence: 2008 update [cited 2012 Feb 28]. Available from: http://www.ncbi.nlm.nih.gov/books/bv.fcgi?rid=hstat2.chapter.28163.

5   Simpson D. Smoking cessation and weight gain: a common problem and a unique opportunity. Smoking Cessation Rounds. 2008;2(4) [cited 2012 Feb]. Available from: http://www.smokingcessationrounds.ca/crus/smokingceseng_04_08.pdf.

6   American Academy of Family Physicians. The "Why"-Test. [2008; cited 2010 Nov]. Available from: http://family-doctor.org.

7   Downey L, Rosengren DB, Donovan DM. Sources of motivation for abstinence: a replication analysis of the reasons for quitting questionnaire. Addict Behav. 2001;26(1):79-89.

8   American Psychiatric Association. Diagnostic and statistical manual of mental disorders, 4th edition, text revision. Arlington VA: American Psychiatric Association; 2000.

9   World Health Organization. International statistical classification of diseases and related health problems, 10th revision; 2007 [cited 2012 Feb 28]. Available from http://www.who.int/classifications/icd/en/.

10   American Psychiatric Association. DSM-5 development, proposed revision R 09 Tobacco Use Disorder; 2012 [cited 2012 Feb]. Available from: http://www.dsm5.org/ProposedRevision/Pages/proposedrevision.aspx?rid=459.

11   Heatherington TF, Kozlowski LT, Frecker RC, Fagerström, KO. The Fagerström test for nicotine dependence: a revision of the Fagerström tolerance questionnaire. Br J Addiction. 1991;86(9):1119-27.

12   Mayfield D, McLeod G, and Hall P. The CAGE Questionnaire: Validation of a New Alcoholism Screening Instrument. Am J Psychiatry 1974;131:1121-1123

13   Cunningham JA, Selby PL. How you assess quit attempts for smoking makes a big difference to your results. Addiction. 2008;103(11):1761-2.

7

Unassisted Cessation

DIANE KUNYK AND CHARL ELS

THERE ARE MORE INDIVIDUALS WHO HAVE FORMERLY SMOKED AS COMPARED WITH those currently smoking in many developed countries—including Canada.[1] It has been estimated that between 2/3 and 3/4 of former smokers have quit on their own without formal evidence-based psychosocial and/or pharmacotherapy interventions.[2] For these individuals, abstinence was achieved either by gradually cutting down or by abruptly quitting, i.e. 'cold turkey.' Quitting without the formal assistance of tobacco reduction and cessation interventions is often referred to as unassisted cessation. High rates of natural recovery, where no professional help or pharmacotherapy is offered, are not uncommon within the field of addiction.[3,4]

As most individuals do not access more formal methods of treatment (i.e. evidence-based psychosocial and/or pharmacotherapy interventions), unassisted cessation has been described as the most successful method because of its reach.[2] West (2010) purports that the finding that more individuals quit smoking without formal assistance does not mean it is the most effective method. Rather they suggest that this reflects an access issue to evidence-based cessation interventions, with more attempting to stop without than those with assistance.[5] In order for individuals to seek out tobacco reduction and cessation treatments, it has been determined that there are two critical requirements. These are to know about their existence and to have access (their availability and affordability). The US Consumer Demand Roundtable has concluded that neither of these critical conditions has been attained, particularly for low-income and blue-collar populations where smoking rates remain the highest.[6]

The topic of unassisted tobacco cessation is one that has received high levels of interest and debate within in the tobacco control community, and given the strength of opposing forces, a resolution of these issues does not appear to be readily apparent. This chapter attempts to address the conflicting themes presented in the literature regarding unassisted cessation as it relates to tobacco cessation and treatment access.

UNASSISSTED AND ASSISTED TOBACCO REDUCTION AND CESSATION

Unassisted cessation is the method by which most individuals have achieved success with stopping smoking. Despite its relative success, it has been suggested that unassisted cessation is seldom emphasized by healthcare professionals when providing advice to their patients who express interest in quitting smoking.[7] Chapman (2010) has argued against this omission and asserts that the underlying message when formal cessation interventions are offered is that "you need help and you are unlikely to succeed alone." He suggests that this message erodes confidence in a process of stopping that has proven successful for many individuals and overstates the difficulty of quitting.[8 p.701] He also hypothesizes that this arguably misleading message of the need for formal assistance has coincided with the advent of cessation medications, and that this message requires a more balanced realignment to incorporate the most preferred and most successful method used by most former smokers.[8]

Britton (2011) notes that healthcare professionals need to be able to provide cessation support to the individuals they treat for tobacco use and addiction, and that many of these are desperate to quit and have repeatedly tried to quit cold turkey and failed.[9 p.704] Healthcare professionals are guided in their advice and interventions with their patients by best practice guidelines; these are formulated on critical reviews of existing and emerging evidence. Article 14 of the World Health Organization's Framework Convention on Tobacco Control (FCTC) suggests cessation should be part of every country's main armamentarium of tobacco control, and that country-specific clinical practice guidelines should be developed.[10] There is a large body of peer-reviewed research and literature reviews on the topic of smoking cessation interventions including empirical evidence reporting relapse curves of self-quitters or the efficacy of unassisted smoking cessation. In a review of tobacco dependence treatment guidelines in 31 countries, all recommended brief interventions, intensive behavioural supports, and nicotine replacement therapies, and most recommended bupropion (84%). Varenicline was not on the market in most of the countries surveyed at the time of the study.[11] The current approach of offering psychosocial and/or cessation medication for individuals who use and/or are addicted to tobacco is endorsed by the World Health Organization, the US Department of Health and Human Services Clinical Practice Guidelines, the US Centers for Disease Control and Prevention, the American National Academies of

Science Institute of Medicine, the Canadian Clinical Practice Guidelines (CAN-ADAPTT), and the Royal Australian College of General Practitioners (see Table 1). The latter's guidelines suggest that every individual who smokes and is willing to quit should be offered a medication option unless contraindicated. The Australian guideline further suggests: "Smokers who want to try unassisted quitting should be encouraged to do so. However, best results are achieved when medicines are used in combination with counselling and support."[12]

TABLE 1. Comparison of seven cessation-specific strategies

	MPOWER	FCTC	USDHHS	CDC	IOM	RACGP	CAN-ADAPTT
Advice	✔	✔	✔	✔	✔	✔	✔
Unassisted						✔	✔
Pharmacotherapy	✔	✔	✔	✔	✔	✔	✔
Counselling	✔	✔	✔	✔	✔	✔	✔

Legend: MPOWER: World Health Organization (WHO) initiative to denormalize and reduce tobacco use (see Chapter 12 for details); FCTC: WHO Framework Convention on Tobacco Control; USD-HHS: US Department of Health and Human Services; CDC: US Centers for Disease Control and Prevention; IOM: Institute of Medicine of the US National Academies of Science; RACGP: Royal Australian College of General Practitioners; CAN-ADAPTT: Canadian Action Network for the Advancement, Dissemination and Adoption of Practice-Informed Tobacco Treatment, Centre for Addiction and Mental Health.

There is skepticism among some critics regarding the evidence informing these guidelines as they pertain to cessation medications. It has been observed that pharmaceutical manufacturers of smoking cessation products are the funding source for many assisted cessation studies and this may be a source of bias. For example, a meta-analysis of randomized controlled trials of nicotine replacement therapies (NRT) determined that 51% of pharmaceutical-industry funded trials reported significant effects as compared with 22% of non-industry trials.[13] Chapman goes further with his argument that research on cessation is dominated by studies on interventions as opposed to unassisted cessation, that this is inversely proportional to how most individuals quit, and that this reflects influence by those whose careers depend on labour-intensive regimens and the pharmaceutical industry.[2] Opponents of the evidence-based guideline approach of offering psychosocial and cessation medications for every individual willing to attempt stopping tobacco use have also argued that these approaches deliberately over-medicalize the process of cessation.[2,7]

Most healthcare professionals endorse the disease concept of tobacco addiction as informed by both the World Health Organization's International Classification of Diseases and the American Psychiatric Association's *Diagnostic and Statistical Manual of Mental Disorders* (4th edition, text revision) recognition of tobacco addiction (nicotine dependence) as a chronic, relapsing disease.[14,15] The addictive qualities of the psychoactive compound nicotine as delivered by consuming tobacco and the brain neuro-adaptation resulting from chronic exposure to tobacco consumption are no longer disputed (Chapter 5). Yet despite the evidence and broad recognition of tobacco addiction as a medical disorder, its conceptualization varies between members of different professions with each focusing perhaps on a different aspect of the same medical condition. These differences inevitably inform viewpoints of what constitutes effective treatment and how resource allocation should be prioritized. Similar to other aspects of Western culture and pathology, the theories explaining tobacco addiction have evolved and will continue to do so. Yet despite this continuous evolution of knowledge, there is currently a remarkable degree of consensus within the healthcare professions on how to safely and effectively treat the medical condition of tobacco addiction.

Formal cessation assistance is considered clinically meaningful for tobacco use as well as for the disease of tobacco addiction. There are perhaps few diseases for which safe and effective therapies, including pharmacotherapies, are available where it may be considered justifiable to recommend unassisted self-management of the disease condition. It is recognized that individuals differ in the extent to which they use and/or are addicted as well as the ease with which they can quit tobacco.[5] In their study of 8,213 adults in the US, Donny and Dierker (2007) found that the greater the number of cigarettes smoked, the greater the odds were of meeting the diagnostic criteria for dependence. Under 50% of those who smoked 1–5 cigarettes were dependent, while >80% of those who smoked 30 cigarettes per day met the criteria. Further, more than 60% of (ever) daily smokers met the criteria for nicotine dependence.[16] Despite the limitations of using the categorical *DSM* criteria-based method to diagnose addiction, these findings do provide some mechanism to define the subset of individuals who use tobacco that may be addicted. The current evidence on interventions for tobacco use and cessation falls short of providing rigorous guidance on treatment matching for the needs and situations of individuals wanting to reduce or stop. As a result there appears to be a default to treating all individuals who use tobacco as heavily addicted and requiring the same intensity of treatment.

It has been suggested that it is harmful when individuals pay for cessation services and yet fail to quit.[8] It has been hypothesized that such experiences lower self-confidence even further than experiences with stopping unaided, and that the underlying message is, "So I got help, and I still failed. Perhaps I am now beyond help?"[8 p.35] The understanding of addiction as an often chronic, relapsing disease that may require repeated intervention and multiple attempts to quit[18] opens up an alternative hypothesis. Individuals with diabetes, for example, may not be able to manage their disease despite attendance at a specialized clinic, and require ongoing modifications in behavioural assistance, medical interventions, and monitoring over time. Although not the case for every tobacco user, individuals who are addicted to tobacco may also require intervention on such a longitudinal basis.

ACCESS TO TOBACCO REDUCTION AND CESSATION INTERVENTIONS

It has been argued that the economic costs associated with cessation interventions are a barrier, particularly to disadvantaged groups—and these are often groups with disproportional rates of smoking. This includes discussions of population level, as opposed to individual level, approaches to smoking cessation. It has been noted that the high cost of cessation medications have made these inaccessible to all but the wealthy in low-income countries.[8] As impoverished nations are limited in their resources, it has been asserted that cessation interventions are unlikely to achieve their population-wide cessation goals; therefore, diversion of limited tobacco control funding to individualized cessation approaches is inappropriate.[7]

Does this set up a false dichotomy between individual (clinical) interventions and other tobacco control strategies?[5] The FCTC guidelines include the adoption of clinical cessation programs within their tobacco control strategy including for those within low-income countries. Their implementation guidelines support the integration of cessation and treatment measures in conjunction with population-level interventions, purporting that these will have a synergistic effect and maximize their impact.[18] Bitton and Eyal observe that the line between clinical- and population-level cessation interventions are not always distinct with strategies such as telephone quitlines and cessation websites having the ability to reach broader populations. They argue that is it justified, and a moral obligation, to develop cessation programs in a stepwise manner alongside population-based programs.[19]

Noting that it makes most economic sense on a population level to offer the most inexpensive forms of intervention to support quitting, a treatment algorithm was developed within a population strategy to help Canadian tobacco users. The purpose of this algorithm was to triage treatment users to restrict the provision of intensive treatments on a population level. With this approach, individuals who had previously been unsuccessful (i.e. unassisted cessation) with lower-intensity interventions (i.e. self-help pamphlets) would be referred to progressively intensive interventions (psychosocial interventions and/or cessation medications).[20] Within this algorithm, the decision for the treatment intervention is not with the individual wanting to reduce or stop tobacco; it is based on failure to quit with a more inexpensive intervention.

One concern with this step-wise approach is that it does not address the urgency to stop using tobacco on the health of the individual. It has been demonstrated that the longer a person consumes tobacco, the greater is their risk of inducing a tobacco-related disease.[21] Consequently, tobacco reduction and cessation interventions are not only a treatment but also a preventative measure. This is arguably similar to individuals with elevated blood pressure (hypertension) or abnormal glucose levels (diabetes). There are some individuals with these conditions who are able reduce these risks through lifestyle changes such as diet change, weight loss, and increased exercise. It is considered appropriate for healthcare professionals to educate their patients on the menu and efficacy of options (behavioural change, psychosocial interventions, and available medications) to treat these conditions and prevent the expression of related diseases. The patient chooses what is best to suit his or her individual situation, and is encouraged to engage in follow-up on a longitudinal basis to monitor the efficacy of the chosen intervention, adjust as required, and monitor for the expression of related disease. There is no requirement for repeated failure or the expression of related disease before treatment is offered for the presenting condition. Is it appropriate for tobacco use and addiction to be managed differently for economic, or other, reasons?

SITUATING UNASSISSTED AND ASSISTED CESSATION

Will it be possible to resolve what appear to be differences of informed opinion? What does exist is a common goal to support individuals and populations to reduce and stop their tobacco use. Most individuals currently smoking want to quit and many have repeatedly failed in their efforts. It is critical that we learn how to best support cessation for their individual situations. There is much to be learned in this regard. There is also a growing body of evidence in the field of triaging tobacco use with intensities of treatment; it is also recognized that tobacco reduction and cessation interventions are most effective when in conjunction with population-level interventions.

It is generally agreed that everyone deserves the opportunity to obtain his or her own highest level of health. Tobacco use decisions (to start or not, to stop once started, or to resume once discontinued) are personal and individual. The decision of how best to manage one's own tobacco use and addiction is also personal and individual—and ought not to be determined by healthcare providers, health systems, tobacco control advocates or others. For those currently using tobacco, it is optimistic to learn that there are more ex-smokers than current smokers in many countries, and that stopping is an obtainable goal. Individuals who use and/or are addicted to tobacco have a right to be informed of their options so that they may make informed decisions, and these options are ideally available for their use. Healthcare professionals have a duty to continually inform their patients of the best evidence available to help reduce or stop their tobacco use so that their patients may make informed decisions around managing their own health. This includes the ability of some individuals to reduce and stop tobacco use without other forms of formal cessation interventions.

Most individuals who use and/or are addicted to tobacco want to reduce or stop their tobacco use, and many of these will succeed unassisted, i.e. without medication or professional help. Others will access and may potentially benefit from formal psychosocial or pharmaceutical supports, and there is some evidence to suggest that the use of assistance for cessation has increased over time.[22] Clearly a balance needs to be struck, and more research is required to determine which subset of tobacco users may benefit from formal help. The phenomenon of natural recovery from tobacco addiction requires attention from the tobacco control community as does potential conflict-of-interest from industries that may benefit from medicalizing tobacco use. The following chapters will explore these more formal tobacco reduction and cessation interventions in depth.

REFERENCES

1   Health Canada. Canadian tobacco use monitoring survey 2010. Ottawa: Author; 2011 [cited 2012 Mar 8]. Available from: http://www.hc-sc.gc.ca/hc-ps/tobac-tabac/research-recherche/stat/ctums-esutc_2010-eng.php.

2   Chapman S. The inverse impact law of smoking cessation. Lancet. 2009;9691;373-5.

3   Robins LN, Locke BZ, Regier DA. An overview of psychiatric disorders in America. In: Psychiatric disorders in America: the Epidemiologic Catchment Area Study. LN Robins, DA Regier, Eds. New York: The Free Press; 1991: p. 328-66.

4   Sluske WS. Natural recovery and treatment-seeking in pathological gambling: results of two US national surveys. Am J Psychiatry. 2006;193:297-302.

5   West R. Should smokers be offered assistance with stopping? Addiction. 2010;105:1867-9.

6   Husten C. A call for ACTTION: increasing access to tobacco-use treatment in our nation. Am J Prev Med. 2010;38(3S);S414-7.

7   Chapman S, MacKenzie R. The global research neglect of unassisted smoking cessation: causes and consequences. PLOS Medicine. 2010;7(2):e1000216.

8   Chapman S, MacKenzie R. Can it be ethical to apply limited resource to low-income countries to ineffective, low-reach smoking cessation strategies? A reply to Bitton and Eyal. Public Health Ethics. 2012;5(10):29-37.

9   Britton J. In defence of helping people to stop smoking. Lancet. 2009;373(9665):703-5.

10   World Health Organization. The framework convention on tobacco control; 2003 [accessed 2012 May 5]. Available from: http://www.who.int/fctc/en/.

11   Raw M, Regan S, Rigotti NA, McNeill A. A survey of tobacco dependence treatment guidelines in 31 countries. Addiction. 2009;104(7):1243-50.

12   Zwar N, Richmond R, Borland R, Peters M, Litt J, Bell J, Caldwell B, Ferretter I. Supporting smoking cessation: a guide for health professionals. Melbourne: The Royal Australian College of General Practitioners; 2011.

13   Etter JF, Burr M, Stapleton J. The impact of pharmaceutical company funding on results of randomized trials of nicotine replacement therapy for smoking cessation: a meta-analysis. Addiction. 2007;102:815-22.

14   American Psychiatric Association. Diagnostic and statistical manual of mental disorders, 4th edition, text revision. Arlington VA: American Psychiatric Association; 2000.

15   World Health Organization. International statistical classification of diseases and related health problems, 10th revision; 2007 [cited 2012 Feb 28]. Available from http://www.who.int/classifications/icd/en/.

16   Donny EC, Dierker LC. The absence of DSM-IV nicotine dependence in moderate-to-heavy daily smokers. Drug Alcohol Depend. 2007;89(1):93-6.

17   Fiore MC, Jaén CR, Baker TB, Bailey, WC, Benowitz, NL, Curry, SJ, et al. Treating tobacco use and dependence: 2008 update. Clinical practice guideline. Rockville MD: U.S. Department of Health and Human Services. Public Health Service; 2008 May [cited 2012 Mar 16]. Available from: http://www.surgeongeneral.gov/tobacco/treating_tobacco_use08.pdf.

18   World Health Organization. Guidelines for implementation of article 14 of the WHO Framework Convention on Tobacco Control. Geneva: Author; 2010.

19   Bitton A, Eyal N. Too poor to treat? The complex ethics of cost-effective tobacco policy in the developing world. Public Health Ethics. 2011;4(2);109-20.

20   McDonald P. A recommended population strategy to help Canadian tobacco users. Toronto: Ontario Tobacco research Unit, Special Report Series; Sept. 2003 [cited 2012 June 8]. Available from: http://www.otru.org/pdf/special/special_population_strategy.pdf.

21   Doll R, Peto R, Boreham J, Sutherland I. Mortality in relation to smoking: 50 years' observations on male British doctors. BMJ. 2004;328:1519.

22   Zhu S, Melcer T, Sun J, Rosbrook B, Pierce JP. Smoking cessation with and without assistance. Am J Prev Med. 2000;18:305-11.

TOBACCO CESSATION SELF-HELP BOOKS

Marilyn Herie

1. Riley, Gillian (2007). *How to Stop Smoking & Stay Stopped for Good:* **Ebury Publishing.**

This book provides a good overview of cognitive barriers to smoking cessation, as well as suggestions for how to address them. However, there is a great deal of current information about the neurobiology of addiction and nicotine & the brain that is not addressed, or is addressed in a way that minimizes this important dimension of tobacco addiction. There are many more up to date and credible smoking cessation resources available.

2. Carr, Allen (1995). *The Only Way to Stop Smoking Permanently:* **Penguin Books.**

This book is highly critical of the common research-based clinical practice approaches to smoking cessation. This book may appeal to those individuals looking for an alternative perspective to smoking cessation. The book is written in a highly motivating, engaging and humorous style.

3. Carr, Allen (2006) *Easy Way to Stop Smoking:* **Arcturus Canada.**

This is a well-written and persuasive book. It is easy to see why the author has been so successful at disseminating his ideas and method of quitting smoking. It is not based on any scientific evidence, and in fact dismisses well-validated smoking cessation approaches. Nonetheless, it may be useful for individuals who are unwilling to try nicotine replacement, or who have not found it helpful.

This book challenges mainstream smoking cessation approaches, but does so in a very empowering and person-centred fashion. Because the focus is on changing cognitive strategies around smoking behaviour, which has some demonstrated effectiveness in treating addictions, it may be very helpful for individuals who are ready to quit smoking. This might not be the best approach for thos individuals experiencing other problems, such as concurrent substance use or mental illness who are trying to quit smoking.

4. Prasad, Balasa L. (2005) *Stop Smoking for Good:* **Penguin Books.**

This book discusses the psychological factors leading to - and sustaining - nicotine dependence, but minimizes the neuro-biological impact of smoking on the brain. The author dismisses well-established and well-researched aids to quitting smoking, such as nicotine replacement, and promotes myths and misinformation about these approaches.

5. Rutter, Sandra (2006) *Quit Before You Know It:* **Hazelden.**

The book is based on relapse prevention strategies widely used in addiction treatment, but doesn't provide any information about alternative and complementary smoking cessation strategies, such as nicotine replacement. The book is published by a well-known treatment centre in the U.S. (Hazelden), and is endorsed by many medical and therapy practitioners. However, the bias of the approach (away from the well-supported use of nicotine replacement) undermines the credibility of this book.

6. Aldrich, Matthew (2006) *Stop Smoking:* **McGraw- Hill.**

This book summarizes the key cognitive distortions among people who continue to smoke, and does a good job of helping the reader to confront and debunk them. The section on risk situations and suggested coping strategies is also helpful. However, the book falls short of encouraging the reader to formulate a concrete plan for quitting smoking, and fails to note additional resources such as nicotine replacement and cessation counselling, that have been shown to be very effective. The book refers to the "harmful drug nicotine" – which is not accurate. Health risks relate to the other harmful chemicals in cigarettes, not to nicotine itself. This is a fairly major example of misinformation. Other information of the health risks of smoking and benefits of quitting are accurate. The book cover is well-designed and appealing, but the content does not deliver on this promise.

7. DeNelsky, Garland Y (2007) *Stop Smoking Now! The rewarding journey to a smoke-free life:* **Cleveland Clinic Press.**

This is an excellent, comprehensive resource. Includes practical and evidence based information about both behavioural and pharmacological approaches to quitting smoking. The information is enlivened by many case examples and also includes a brief but compelling chapter on the tobacco industry and the social/political context in the US. The resources and text is slanted towards the American context, but the information is presented in a very readable and practical form. Includes cutting-edge medications, such as Varenicline. This is an excellent resource for individuals who are considering quitting smoking as well as to health professionals new to the field of smoking cessation.

8. Ivings, Kristina (2006). *Free yourself from smoking: A three-point plan to kill nicotine addiction.* **London: Kyle Cathie Ltd.**

The inclusion of worksheets and exercises, accurate and up-to-date information (including detailed information on nicotine replacement), and guidelines for developing a plan for quitting make this an excellent resource. Although some of the language is geared to a U.K. audience, it does not detract from the overall readability and usefulness of the book.

9. Keelan, Brian (2004). *Free at last! Stop Smoking: How I did it, How you can do it too.* **Toronto: Hushion House.**

This is an engaging, inspiring and comprehensive book – well-written and presented, with clear, up-to-date information and a balanced perspective. Although written by a non-specialist (who quit smoking himself), the Canadian perspective and data, inclusion of useful websites, encouraging and motivational tone, and use of humour make this book an excellent complement to a formal cessation program, or a "standalone" self-help book.

8

Psychosocial Interventions

STEPHANIE COHEN, ROSA DRAGONETTI, MARILYN HERIE AND
MEGAN BARKER

THERE ARE INDIVIDUALS ABLE TO STOP USING TOBACCO INDEPENDENTLY WITHOUT treatment. Others that use or are addicted to tobacco may require formal assistance to achieve abstinence. For some, the process of quitting can be a complex process spanning months and/or years that requires support, medication, and multiple attempts. The optimal treatment design for tobacco use and addiction is one that is comprehensive and multi-pronged. According to the US Department of Health and Human Services Public Health Service best-practice guidelines for smoking cessation and the current Canadian guidelines (CAN-ADAPTT), a combined approach of medication and counselling is the most effective approach. It is recommended that both treatment components are available and offered to individuals consuming tobacco whenever possible.[1,2]

Through a bio-psychosocial lens, and within a harm reduction framework, this chapter will focus on the evidenced-based psychosocial interventions used for tobacco reduction and cessation. Counselling plays a critical role by increasing motivation to quit and providing support. It also addresses cognitive, affective, behavioural, and environmental barriers to quitting. Moreover, counselling provides both coping strategies and problem solving skills, and can boost the effects of pharmacotherapy treatment. Counselling and/or psycho-educational support sessions can provide opportunities to obtain instructions, information, and seek clarification around the use of pharmacotherapy in a tobacco treatment plan. Furthermore, counselling and psycho-educational support sessions can address cessation medications including unrealistic expectations about their use. Cessation medication can be very effective in helping to achieve tobacco abstinence; nonetheless, many would argue that the role of counselling is not equally important but actually more important.[3]

The psychosocial interventions and counselling approaches addressed in this chapter include brief intervention and the 5 A's, cognitive-behavioural therapy strategies, motivational interviewing, group treatment, telephone quit-lines, Web assisted tobacco interventions (WATI), and contingency management. Wherever applicable, this chapter will infuse the Canadian clinical practice guideline summary statements that have evolved out of the CAN-ADAPTT project. It is recognized that the optimal approach is a combination of medication and counselling.[4,5] Pharmacotherapy is discussed in Chapter 9.

CAN-ADAPTT SUMMARY STATEMENTS FOR COUNSELLING AND PSYCHOSOCIAL APPROACHES

1. ASK: Tobacco use status should be updated for all patients/clients, by all healthcare providers on a regular basis.
2. ADVISE: Healthcare providers should clearly advise patients/clients to quit.
3. Healthcare providers should assess the willingness of patients/clients to begin treatment to achieve abstinence (quitting).
4. ASSESS: All individuals working with Aboriginal peoples should seek appropriate training in providing evidence-based smoking cessation support.
5. ASSIST: Every tobacco use who expresses the willingness to being treatment to quit should be offered assistance.
   a. Minimal intervention, of 1-3 minutes, are effective and should be offered to every tobacco user. However, there is a strong dose-reponse relationship between the session length and successful treatment, and so intensive interventions should be used whenever possible.
   b. Counselling by a variety or combination of delivery formats (self-help, individual, group, helpline, web-based) is effective and should be used to assist patients/clients who express a willingness to quit.
   c. Because multiple counselling sessions increase the chances of prolonged abstinence, healthcare provid-

ers should provide four or more counselling sessions where possible.

d. Combining counselling and smoking cessation medication is more effective than either alone, therefore both should be provided to patients/clients trying to stop smoking where feasible.

e. Motivational interviewing is encouraged to support patients/clients willingness to engage in treatment now and in the future.

f. Two types of counselling and behavioural therapies yield significantly higher abstinence rates and should be included in smoking cessation treatment: 1) providing practical counselling on problem solving skills or skill training and 2) providing support as a part of treatment.

6. ARRANGE: Healthcare providers:

a. Should conduct regular follow-up to assess response, provide support and modify treatment as necessary.

b. Are encouraged to refer patients/clients to relevant resources as part of the provision of treatment, where appropriate.

Source: CAN-ADAPTT. Canadian smoking cessation clinical practice guideline. Toronto: Canadian Action Network for the Advancement, Dissemination and Adoption of Practice-informed Tobacco Treatment, Centre for Addiction and Mental Health; 2011. Available from: www.can-adaptt.net. Reprinted with permission.

BRIEF INTERVENTIONS[a]

Decades of accumulated evidence support the use of brief interventions to assist patients (or clients) with tobacco reduction and cessation.[1] Meta-analyses included in the Centers for Disease Control and Prevention (CDC) Guideline[1] demonstrated a dose–response relationship between session length and abstinence rates. An increase in abstinence rates with increasing "total amount of

---

[a]The content in this section was adapted from Herie M, Dragonetti R, Selby P. Assessment and brief interventions for alcohol and tobacco problems in primary health care. In: Khenti A, Sapag JC, Mohamoud S, Ravindran A, editors. Mental health and substance issues in primary care. Toronto: Centre for Addiction and Mental Health; 2012. Available from: www.camh.net. Used with permission.

contact time" up to a maximum of 90 minutes, and a dose–response relationship between number of sessions and treatment effectiveness was also determined. Slightly differing definitions of "brief intervention" exist; however, it is considered to be 1 to 4 counselling sessions of 5–15 minutes that include feedback on tobacco use, advice, goal setting, and follow-up appointments.[6,7]

TABLE 1: The 5A's for Treating Tobacco Use and Dependence

Ask about tobacco use (screening).   "How many cigarettes per day do you smoke?   Identify and document tobacco use status for every patient at every visit.
Advise all people who use tobacco to quit.
Assess "How ready is the patient to change?   Is the patient is willing to make a quit attempt at this time?
Assist all patients that use tobacco in making quit attempts.   *For the patient willing to make a change:* Offer medication and provide or refer for counseling or additional treatment to help the patient.   *For the patient presently unready to change:* Provide interventions designed to increase future change attempts.
Arrange follow-up and continue to support.   *For the patient willing to make a change:* Arrange for follow-up contacts beginning with the first week after the quit/change date.   *For the patient presently unwilling to change:* Address tobacco use and dependence and willingness to change at the next clinic visit.

Source: Fiore MC, Jaén CR, Baker TB, Bailey WC, Benowitz NL, Curry SJ et al. Treating tobacco use and dependence: 2008 update. U.S. Department of Health and Human Services. Public Health Service. 2008 May.

The 5 A's: Ask, Advise, Assess, Assist, and Arrange The USDHHS guidelines recommend the 5 A's model for treating tobacco use through brief interventions in primary care settings (Table 1).[1] The 5 A's are supported by the most current Canadian guidelines for tobacco screening and brief interventions.[2] Incorporating the FRAMES model into these 5 intervention steps can help enhance patients' motivation for change, as well as foster engagement and rapport. The acronym FRAMES is a helpful mnemonic for the components of brief motivational interventions:

- **Feedback**: Provide patients with personalized feedback regarding their individual status and risks.
- **Responsibility**: Emphasize personal responsibility for change and the individual's freedom of choice.
- **Advice**: Include a clear recommendation on the need for change, in a supportive rather than an authoritarian manner.
- **Menu**: Offer a menu of strategies for change, providing options from which the patient may choose.
- **Empathy**: Be empathic, reflective, warm, and supportive.
- **Self-efficacy**: Reinforce patients' expectation and optimism that change is possible.

***How to* Ask**   The first "A" requires the counsellor to *ask* the patient about tobacco use, which is essentially the screening component of the intervention. The counsellor explains that a standard series of health questions that are directed to all patients in order to improve their overall health. Questions that suggest a negative response are avoided. Once the patient responds negatively, it can be more difficult to explore the issue further:

- *Negative*: "You are not a smoker are you?"
- *Positive*: "Please tell me about your tobacco use."

In asking about tobacco use it is important to:

- Be nonjudgmental.
- Listen attentively to patient concerns and reflect what you hear and see.
- Refrain from negative comments or reactions that demean the patient. Be sensitive to broader issues such as poverty and social disadvantage.
- Make positive statements about progress at each visit however small.

***How to* Advise**   Advice to quit or reduce should be delivered in the same nonjudgmental and sensitive tone as in asking about tobacco use. Use positive statements to provide an accurate assessment of risks. Here are some examples of positive versus negative advice statements:

- *Negative*: "If you really loved your family, you wouldn't smoke inside your home or car."

- *Positive*: "The risk of secondhand smoke to your family has you concerned."

Note that advice is not admonition. It is a statement that reflects the patient's perceived risks or negative consequences related to tobacco use. If the patient does not have any concerns about use, or is not experiencing any consequences, advice can be premised by *asking for permission* to share concerns and information, as in the following examples:

- "Would it be OK if I shared the reasons for my concern about your tobacco use?"
- "I'd like to let you know about some of the risks in smoking that you might not already be aware of, but I want to emphasize that it is your choice alone to decide to make a change."
- "I really appreciate your honesty in telling me about your tobacco use. Would you like to hear about some steps that you can take to reduce your risk of future problems?"

In all cases, emphasizing the patient's autonomy (personal choice and control) can help to minimize resistance to talking about tobacco use, and communicates respect and affirmation of the patient's willingness to engage in talking about a potentially sensitive topic.

FIGURE 1. Readiness Ruler for Assessing Motivation to Change

A Antecedents	B Behaviour	C Consequences
Example: Alarm goes off, wakes up, goes to kitchen to make coffee, grabs cigarettes beside coffee maker, gets newspaper from front door...	*Example:* Drinks coffee and smokes 2 or 3 cigarettes at kitchen table while reading the paper...	*Example:* Positive — feels relief; needs coffee and cigarettes to wake up; enjoyable to have some time before kids wake up... Negative — doesn't eat proper breakfast; not so hungry after coffee and cigarettes; not healthy to skip breakfast; feels bad for smoking and especially in the house because of the kids...

How to **Assess**   In addition to offering brief advice, practitioners should *assess* patients' readiness to change. A helpful motivational tool to use in a consultation is the Readiness Ruler (Figure 1).[8] This asks patients to rate, on a scale from 0–10, the importance of making this change relative to other priorities in their life, as well as their confidence in their ability to change (self-efficacy) and overall readiness to make change. The practitioner may follow-up patients' self-ratings with these questions:

- "Why are you at __ and not zero?"
- "What would it take for you to go from __ to __?"
- "What is one small step that you could take in the next week?"

Practitioners can also calibrate their responses and suggested interventions to better fit the patient's motivation for change. For patients with low importance, confidence, and readiness, it is important to "keep the door open" for continued engagement and conversation.

Developing discrepancy can be especially helpful in making tobacco use more salient for the patient. This means contrasting the person's goals or values with their current behaviour. An example of developing discrepancy is:

- "You would like to avoid getting intubated for your cardio-obstructive lung disease (COLD); but you are clear in saying that you do not intend to make any changes to your smoking. I'm wondering how this fits?"

The above statement is offered in a spirit of collaborative curiosity, with no sarcasm or intent to "trap" the patient into acknowledging the need for change. The intention is to invite the patient to reflect on his or her inconsistencies in values/goals and behaviours, and to come to his or her own conclusions.

Patients who are not ready to change can benefit from exploring and resolving their ambivalence. Practitioners have an important role to play in raising doubt and concern in a supportive and nonjudgmental way. At an earlier stage in the patient's change process, "action-oriented" strategies on the part of the practitioner may be perceived as irrelevant (at best) or authoritarian and overbearing (at worst). The goal in assessing readiness to change is to ensure that our strategies are in line with the patient's motivation and priorities.

How to **Assist**   Once the patient has made a commitment to change, it is appropriate to *assist* by helping to develop a modified plan that includes recommending the use of medication. The modified plan should not include any contraindications with the medication. Practical counselling that will help the patient with problem solving and skills training may also be provided. Assisting should also include support and supplementary materials from the practitioner which may include information on specialist treatment programs, quitlines, self-help resources, or referral to another care-team member. The 5 R's model[1] provides a helpful framework in assisting patients to change, especially in the context of a brief intervention where time is limited. Each component is outlined below, with specific suggestions on what to say to the patient.

1. **Relevance**: Help patients to appreciate the relevance of the changes you are suggesting by personalizing your feedback so that it is salient to that individual. General exhortations to change are less effective than messaging that is targeted to the explicit concerns or presenting features of each unique patient. The examples below illustrate less and more relevant practitioner feedback:

Presenting Issue	Less Relevant Feedback	More Relevant Feedback
37-year-old male who reports daily smoking	"Smoking in the home is a big risk to your *and* your partner as well."	"I understand that you and your partner are hoping to start a family. I'm not sure if you already know about how men's tobacco use can affect the chances of getting pregnant and passing on dangerous chemicals to the fetus through sperm affected by tobacco smoke?"
14-year-old female who reports experimental alcohol and tobacco use	"You know that drinking and smoking are not good things to be doing."	"Why do you think that I might be concerned about your alcohol and tobacco use?"

2. **Rewards**: Understanding the benefits or rewards of using tobacco provide a picture of the role that tobacco plays in the person's life. To elicit the rewards, ask "I'd like to understand more about how tobacco fits into your life. What is good or helpful about smoking for you?"

3. **Risks**: Once you have explored rewards, the door is now open to explore the risks, or consequences, of tobacco use as perceived by the patient. To elicit the risks, ask "Now that we've looked at the good things, can we take a look at the other side? What is not-so-good about tobacco use for you?"

4. **Reflection**: Throughout the consultation, reflecting back your understanding of what the patient has said can enhance rapport and convey empathy and understanding. Reflective listening is a foundation skill in brief motivational interventions and is delivered in a nonjudgmental way. The following are some examples of reflective listening:

Patient Statement	Practitioners' Reflection	Follow up with...
"Yes, I am still smoking, and no, I don't want a lecture."	"You've been feeling pressured by me and probably others about your smoking."	"And what you do about your smoking is your choice. How could I be helpful to you in a way that wouldn't feel so pressuring?"
"I am a social smoker: just 2-3 cigarettes per day at the most."	"From your standpoint, you are smoking so little that it is not any cause for concern."	"Would you be interested to hear about risks associated with low levels of tobacco use?"
"My son is really on my case about my smoking."	"He is concerned about you, but it feels a bit like nagging."	"Can you tell me more about some of your son's concerns?"
"I have tried the patch before, and the cravings were just as bad as when I tried to quit cold turkey!"	"It's discouraging, and you're wondering whether there is an effective medication out there for you."	"Would you be interested to hear more about some new and different medication options that you can consider?"

5. **Roadblocks**: The final "R" is about exploring possible roadblocks to change. This facilitates problem-solving and invites the patient to mobilize his or her own best resources to support the change process. To invite an exploration of possible roadblocks, say: "What might stand in the way of this plan working for you?" "What else do you think you will need to support you in this plan for change?"

***How to* Arrange**   Finally, the brief intervention is completed by *arranging* a follow-up appointment either in-person or in the form of a phone call. Patients may be seen by a member of their healthcare team, or referred to community resources or specialist services, such as community-based cessation groups, tobacco quitlines, or addiction treatment. Follow-up can occur with any member or members of the care team, and can employ the variety of techniques and strategies outlined above. For example, many practitioners ask patients to complete a Readiness Ruler at each visit in order to continually assess motivation and self-efficacy. Agenda-setting is also an ongoing process as patients' priorities shift, emerging issues come to the forefront, and other concerns are resolved. The FRAMES acronym and the 5 R's provide helpful reminders of how to conduct follow-up consultations in a way that enhances motivation and increases the likelihood of change.

INTENSIVE COUNSELLING

There is a dose–response relationship between the intensity of counselling sessions provided and abstinence rates.[4,5] Brief interventions consisting of 1–3 minutes of counselling time, can increase 6-month abstinence rates by approximately 14%; still, if counselling contact is increased to 31–90 minutes this rate is increased to 27%.[4] It is important to note that these abstinence rates emerged from a meta-analysis of 35 randomized trials and that some of the studies incorporated medication across all counselling conditions.[4]

This section will discuss intensive counselling strategies that can help individuals address the cognitive, behavioural, and environmental factors that contribute to the maintenance of their tobacco use and addiction. Generally speaking, intensive treatment is defined as involving 4 or more counselling sessions that are a minimum duration of 10 minutes each.[5] It can be used to serve a variety of purposes: to increase motivation to reduce and/ or quit; to help establish a reduction and/or quit plan; to assist in the development of coping strategies; to troubleshoot and flag potential challenges during the quitting process; and to encourage the use of newly developed coping strategies.[4]

People most likely to benefit from intensive counselling interventions are essentially those people who have a more difficult time quitting including more heavily tobacco addicted people; people with alcohol and drug problems; people with mental health issues and/or concurrent disorders; people from deprived socio-economic groups; and those who live with others who smoke.[9] A cognitive-behavioural model provides many useful strategies that can be incorporated into an intensive counselling approach to meet the aforementioned objectives. Research suggests that both group and 1-to-1 counselling models can be effective formats for delivering cognitive behavioural strategies and psychosocial support; thus, the strategies discussed in this section can be incorporated into either treatment model.[3]

A history of multiple failed quit attempts does not predict future failure.[10] A factor correlated with smoking cessation success is a previous quit attempt where abstinence was achieved for 12 months or more and/or a recent attempt where the individual who smokes achieved abstinence anywhere from 6 to 14 days.[10] In other words, the more experience the individual has with achieving abstinence, the more practise of living without cigarettes and experiencing life as a former smoker.[10] Conversely, the less time that a tobacco addicted person has been abstinent the more likely he or she will benefit from an intensive intervention.

COGNITIVE-BEHAVIOURAL APPROACHES

Cognitive-behavioural therapy (CBT) focuses on changing the thoughts, feelings and behaviours that accompany tobacco use and addiction.[10] These approaches are strongly guided by the principles of social learning theory; as a result, this can be a very helpful approach for facilitating skill building, problem solving and relapse prevention strategies in tobacco addicted individuals. It is important to note that the counselling recommendations discussed in this section are directed towards individuals who are ready to make a quit attempt. Motivational interviewing strategies are recommended for those individuals who are unwilling to make a quit attempt and will be discussed later in this chapter.[4,5]

Quitting tobacco is not a linear event but a complex process. Thus, in order to increase the likelihood of a successful quit, people who use tobacco are strongly encouraged to devote some time to planning and preparation prior to embarking on a quit attempt.[3,5,10] Typically, the first few sessions of intensive counselling incorporate many or all of the following strategies: self-monitoring, increasing awareness of smoking triggers, developing coping strategies, increasing support, setting a quit date, and for some, initiation of pharmacotherapy.[4,10] The actual length of the planning phase is variable; it depends upon the program resources and the needs of the individual.[10]

Self-monitoring Many individuals describe their tobacco use as subconscious and automatic; it seems seamlessly interwoven into daily life. One of the first steps involved in changing this behavior is to help individuals increase awareness of their tobacco using behaviour through self-monitoring. Changes in behavior and thinking go hand-in-hand; therefore, one of the goals of self-monitoring is to help individuals identify the relationship between their feelings, thoughts, and their smoking behaviour.[3,10] It is recommended that individuals record every cigarette smoked while tracking their associated thoughts and feelings (Figure 2). For some, the very act of self-monitoring is a reduction strategy and through engaging in this process they decrease their use.[10] Still, in the initial phase of treatment, individuals are simply asked to observe their smoking behaviour and begin to identify patterns.

FIGURE 2. Daily Diary

What is your goal for this week? _____

	Did you smoke? If yes, how many cigarettes?	Describe the situation (e.g., were you alone or with others, at home or in a social setting, etc.)	Thoughts and feelings (what were you thinking and feeling in this situation?)
Monday			
Tuesday			
Wednesday			
Thursday			
Friday			
Saturday			
Sunday			

Triggers   The process of documenting thoughts, feelings, places, and events closely associated with tobacco enables the individual to analyze each episode in isolation and identify its antecedents. Thus, the term antecedent is synonymous with trigger as it refers to the places, people, feelings, thoughts, and essentially any other internal and/or external stimuli that the individual strongly associates with tobacco use. A functional analysis provides a tool with which individuals can gain a deeper understanding of the "function" of tobacco in their lives. Once this insight is gained, they can begin to develop and practise new strategies to deter smoking urges and disrupt the automatic tobacco-related behaviour chain of events.[3,10,11]

Tobacco functional analysis   Functional analysis, or the ABC model, is a helpful clinical tool for analyzing tobacco use episodes. It helps the individual to understand the function of their tobacco use and begin to develop ways to avoid future use. Functional analysis can be carried out during a group or individual counselling session, or assigned as homework. This simple format can help identify both triggers and consequences.

TABLE 2. ABC: Antecedents Behaviour Consequences

A Antecedents	B Behaviour	C Consequences
Example: Alarm goes off, wakes up, goes to kitchen to make coffee, grabs cigarettes beside coffee maker, gets newspaper from front door...	*Example:* Drinks coffee and smokes 2 or 3 cigarettes at kitchen table while reading the paper...	*Example:* Positive — feels relief; needs coffee and cigarettes to wake up; enjoyable to have some time before kids wake up... Negative — doesn't eat proper breakfast; not so hungry after coffee and cigarettes; not healthy to skip breakfast; feels bad for smoking and especially in the house because of the kids...

Setting a quit date and/or scheduled reduction date A strategy that is strongly encouraged with a CBT approach is setting a specific quit date. This provides patients with a clear target to work towards; at the same time, this date helps maintain the momentum of the quit process moving forward. The act of committing to a quit date or even the act of committing to a "trial" quit date provides the person who smokes with a clear window of time to mentally prepare for abstinence. Moreover, it provides an opportunity to practise and refine new skills and coping strategies that they will require to achieve abstinence.[3,10]

Although this strategy is recommended, it is important to remember that, in the field of tobacco use and addiction treatment, an effective one-size-fits-all model is not optimal. Some individuals may feel reluctant or even incapable to establish a quit date because a goal of abstinence feels unachievable. There are multiple ways to facilitate the goal-setting process in the planning phase of counselling. Target dates established around a "scheduled reduction" or a "trial quit day" may be more reasonable and feasible strategies for some tobacco addicted individuals. For those individuals who engage in counselling treatment with a goal of reduction rather than abstinence, it is more helpful to explore intermediate steps along the reduction and quitting continuum.[3] The most critical feature that underlies all phases of intensive counselling is the practitioner's ability to keep the patient engaged in the process.

Maintenance Patients may benefit from having a counselling session scheduled on the quit date and/or immediately after the quit date. This gives the practitioner an opportunity to offer support and encouragement and assist with optimizing the quit plan if needed. Research evidence validates the role of psychosocial support in successful cessation; furthermore, the individual's perceived amount of support plays a key role in enhancing treatment success.[10] The greater amount of support perceived by the individual making the quit attempt, the greater the chances of success.[10] Relapse rates are highest in the first 14 days post quit.[1,10]

The maintenance phase essentially involves the same ongoing process of trial and error around an individual's development and utilization of effective coping strategies as a means to maintaining abstinence. The practitioner's role in the maintenance phase of counselling continues to be both supportive and practical. The practitioner will continue to assist the individual to optimize his or her repertoire of coping skills while at the same time, providing positive reinforcement around healthy changes and gently encouraging the patient to continue on his or her quit journey.[10]

As the duration of abstinence increases, so does the patient's sense of self-efficacy.[10] In the initial phase of the reduction and/or quit process, patients are encouraged to employ avoidance as one of their main coping strategies. It is recommended that individuals remove tobacco from their home, car, and place of employment, harness the support of friends and family, and deliberately spend as much time as possible in environments that constrain smoking in order to increase chances of maintaining abstinence.[3,4] In addition to the avoidance strategy, which may or may not be a feasible long-term strategy with respect to all triggers, patients are encouraged to utilize a broader range of coping strategies and more active coping strategies such as physical exercise and/or healthy eating and/or relaxation during the maintenance phase.[3] Stress and weight gain are two of the most common challenges that people face during the quit process; as a result, people are encouraged to increase and/or engage in physical activity during the quit process as a means of coping with both potential barriers.[3,4] Similarly, individuals are encouraged to practice and utilize relaxation techniques as a means of coping with stress and/or cravings to smoke.[3] The more coping skills that a person is able to develop and employ during the quit process, the more likely treatment outcomes will be successful.[11]

Relapse Prevention Research informs us that most individuals will have to make multiple quit attempts before they are able to achieve long-term abstinence from tobacco.[1,9] It is critical that this information be shared with individuals, in advance of their quit attempts, so that any past experience of chronically quitting and/or attempting to quit can be normalized.[1] This information can also help normalize future struggles, as the quit process may not be easy. Due to the chronic and relapsing nature of tobacco addiction, it is anticipated that majority of people who smoke will experience difficulty in maintaining abstinence at some point.[3,9,10] Thus, the term relapse prevention is somewhat problematic in itself because research reveals that relapse prevention strategies have only modest effects at best.[3,9,11,12] It is therefore unrealistic to expect that relapse prevention strategies can completely prevent relapse. Consequently, from the onset of intensive counselling, the practitioner needs to build rapport and create a safe environment for the individual to talk openly and honestly. This sense of safety is most critical in counselling when quit plans do not unfold as anticipated. For example, when an individual has a relapse, rather than avoiding or withdrawing from treatment, he or she needs to feel safe enough to stay engaged in treatment or perhaps even seek additional treatment. Individuals should be encouraged to reframe their perceptions of "slips" and/or "relapses" early on in the counselling process; there are no failures in the quit process, only learning opportunities.[10] The key to quitting for all individuals is to not quit quitting.

MOTIVATIONAL INTERVIEWING

Some of the biggest challenges in the treatment of tobacco use and addiction can be regarded as problems related to motivation. Research suggests that nearly 3/4 of adults who smoke express interest in quitting, yet almost 80% have no intention to quit in the next month, and 30–45% have no plans to quit within 6 months.[10] This conflicting data suggests that the vast majority of individuals who smoke are highly ambivalent towards the quitting process. At the same time, research suggests that even individuals who are actively engaged in treatment, motivation levels can become problematic. A common problem in tobacco treatment is noncompliance with both medication and counselling plans.[4] Studies indicate that individuals seeking treatment often complete fewer than 50% of their scheduled counselling sessions; moreover, this lack of treatment adherence decreases one's chance of treatment success.[4] Thus, it appears that even in those groups of individuals motivated enough to seek treatment for tobacco dependence, motivation levels can change.

In a metaanalysis of 31 different studies examining the effectiveness of motivational interviewing (MI) in smoking cessation, the most promising results were found in those studies where MI was used with adolescents, people with medical conditions, people with low motivation, and people with low levels of tobacco dependence.[13] However, this meta-analysis also revealed that for some tobacco addicted individuals, motivational interviewing was found to have a smaller effect than expected.[13] In some studies, the results were only modest when compared to results seen with this approach used in the treatment of alcohol dependence and other substances.[13]

The core philosophy of MI is to work in a respectful and collaborative way with patients. It is a non-confrontational counselling approach that can be used to help people resolve their ambivalence around changing their tobacco use; at the same time, it can be used to strengthen their commitment to change.[14] Instead of advising the patient how to change, the counsellor evokes and elicits the patient's own reasons for change.[15] Research supports the use of MI as a method for improving practitioner–patient relationships; it also promotes behaviour change across a wide variety of healthcare issues including smoking cessation.[15] Motivational Interviewing practice is often described as a "way of being with people" versus a means of "tricking" people into doing something they do not really want to do.[16]

From an MI perspective, if the person seeking tobacco treatment is ambivalent, it is probably more helpful to ask *why* she or he would consider quitting. In contrast, a cognitive behavioural approach would focus on *how* the person can quit. Cognitive-behavioural strategies use learning processes and skill development to try to help people reduce or quit smoking. Motivational interviewing communicates that patients themselves hold the answers to change[10,15] Instead of teaching or training the patient to problem solve, MI recognizes that the patient has the expertise to change and the practitioner encourages the mobilization of the patient's own resources.[10,17]

Although these 2 approaches focus on different components of change, the models are compatible and can be combined.[17] For example, if a practitioner is working with a tobacco addicted person with low motivation and high ambivalence around the quit process, focusing on increasing motivation and strengthening commitment to treatment before developing coping skills would seem like a feasible and productive approach.[17] One example of a successfully integrated MI and CBT approach involved a randomized multi-site trial of personalized telephone counselling interventions with over 2,100 adolescent smokers. The studies found that this combined MI–CBT intervention increased successful 6-month abstinence rates.[18]

Similarly, motivational interviewing is compatible with a brief treatment approach to tobacco reduction and cessation. For example, with regards to the second of the 5 A's, *advise*, a simple motivational strategy that all practitioners can employ is the practice of asking patients for permission to give advice, rather than merely dispensing advice to patients.[19] For example, instead of simply handing a patient some pamphlets on smoking cessation medications, ask permission first. This small act of asking for permission may have a big impact on the practitioner's relationships with his or her patients and it can be used to strengthen rapport. It can be likened to the act of knocking on a door before entering; it conveys respect.[19]

Research reveals that the practitioner's style plays a significant role in predicting patient motivation and change.[10] For healthcare practitioners specifically, the traditional underlying principles of MI have been revised and reintroduced as the following concepts under the RULE acronym:[19]

- **Resist** the "righting reflex"
- **Understand** your patient's motivations
- **Listen** to your patient
- **Empower** your patient

The "righting reflex" refers to the widespread practice of healthcare professionals, across all healthcare disciplines "prescribing" change.[15] Furthermore, in a recent systematic review of 72 studies comparing an MI approach with a directive, advice-giving approach, the former was more effective in 80% of the studies.[15] The last guiding principle, empower the patient, highlights the person's autonomy in decision-making.[19] One of the hallmarks of MI is for the practitioner to explicitly acknowledge the fact that the decision to change ultimately rests in the hands of the patient. Practitioners cannot make people quit smoking and treatment is not about making people change. The following is an example of empowering the patient.

Patient: "Smoke free policies and nicotine patches are just another way your hospital picks on smokers and tries to force them to quit."

Practitioner: "Yet the reality is, no one can force you to quit. When you leave this building and hospital grounds, you can have a cigarette or as many cigarettes as you want to. Personally I do hope you decide to try quitting, for the sake of your health. Still you are absolutely correct: to smoke or to quit is your decision, no one else's."

GROUP TREATMENT

There remains a lack of evidence to determine which model of intervention is most effective with respect to both cost and treatment outcomes.[20] There is enough research to determine that groups are more effective than self-help and no treatment.[20] There is also limited evidence that group treatment enhances outcomes when combined with advice from a health professional or nicotine replacement therapy.[20] There is emerging evidence that some populations benefit from more intensive group counselling when it is combined with a more intensive pharmacotherapy component.[21] Not all people who use and are addicted to tobacco need a combination of intensive group and pharmacotherapy treatment, nor do all people need or want intensive group treatment in itself.

The decision to provide groups as a component of tobacco cessation treatment is affected by multiple factors: availability of resources, practitioner competency, and the needs and wants of the individual. Treatment planning should be a collaborative approach; the opinions and views of the individual should be solicited during this process.[10] It is important that the treatment plan be tailored to accommodate the individual's preferences for treatment whenever possible as their outcomes may improve.[10] This section provides a brief discussion of group models used in tobacco cessation. The evidence base around the effectiveness of group treatment compared to other forms of psychosocial support in tobacco cessation treatment is also discussed.

All of the psychosocial and/or counselling approaches can be delivered in a group format. Brief treatment typically occurs for those that do not have a focus of tobacco treatment (i.e. a parenting group or a psychiatric support group). Group programs that are not focused on tobacco treatment may choose to develop a module that addresses smoking and tobacco dependence in pre-existing group programs. An example of a group that lies somewhere between brief and more intensive group treatment is a 90-minute psycho-educational workshop; this provides people with an overview of a bio-psychosocial approach to quitting smoking, and discusses the different evidence-based treatment options. The cognitive-behavioural strategies can be delivered in an intensive group model. There is huge variation across the structure, size, group treatment goals, and participant composition of these intensive groups but, generally speaking, they are typically 4–8 sessions, and can range anywhere between 1 and 2 hours.[10] Motivational interviewing can also be delivered in a group format, but this approach is often less reliable when delivered in a group format and more challenging to deliver. For example, one challenge with MI groups is the fact that patients simply get less "air time" to talk about their own reasons for change in a group setting and research shows that outcomes are correlated with change talk. However, because MI does compliment the other treatment models such as CBT and brief treatment, a smoking cessation group may incorporate a blend of MI strategies and another treatment approach.

The group's design and participant composition is based on its purpose. The group's main objectives can be skill-based (i.e. helping to develop coping strategies and teaching relapse prevention skills) or support-based. Supportive groups provide the opportunity to interact and connect with others without a cigarette; a skill that is often underdeveloped in people who smoke, as cigarettes can be a social tool heavily relied upon. Whether the group is skill-based or not, people benefit by having additional social support during the quit process. Social support plays an important role in smoking cessation outcomes.[10] Moreover, perceived support in the individual's social environment is a key factor; the more support perceived the more likely the individual will succeed in his or her quit attempt.[10] As a result, groups may be especially beneficial for those individuals who indicate that they do not have a very large support system. People who indicate that they live with another person who smokes and/or have many friends who smoke may equally benefit from interacting with others actively engaged in the quitting process. Nevertheless, there are individuals who have nonsmoking friends and a nonsmoking home, but seek ongoing support group treatment for the accountability factor. The opportunity to attend a tobacco use and addiction support group once a week is all the support that some need to stay on track and engaged in the quit process.

It is important to note the difference between group therapy and Nic Anonymous, a 12-step facilitation (TSF) group. Alcoholics Anonymous (AA) was the first twelve-step self-help group that started in the 1930s. Since that time, TSF has become a worldwide fellowship of individuals with common problems that provide support, individually and in the meetings, to others that seek help. Many have reported benefits from attending Nic Anonymous but it is not beneficial for all individuals who are trying to quit, or maintain their abstinence from, tobacco.

HYPNOTHERAPY AND ACUPUNCTURE FOR QUITTING SMOKING: WHAT SHOULD WE TELL OUR PATIENTS?

Charl Els

The body of evidence to date does not support a difference in efficacy between either hypnotherapy or acupuncture versus control. Due to a range of methodological problems in the trials, it is difficult to draw definitive conclusions from the limited studies to date. Of note is that neither the Canadian Clinical Practice Guidelines for smoking cessation (CAN-ADAPTT) nor the USDHHS Clinical Practice Guideline (Treating Tobacco Use and Dependence) supports the use of these alternative methods of smoking cessation.

However, a recent meta-analysis of randomized controlled trials to determine the efficacy of alternative methods included a total of 14 trials conducted to assess the efficacy of three alternative smoking cessation interventions: 1. Acupuncture (6 trials; n=823), which consists of stimulating acupuncture points on the respondents' ear, 2. Hypnotherapy (4 trials, n=273), which consists of inducing an altered state of consciousness, and 3. Aversive smoking (4 trials, n=99), which consists of rapid smoking in a brief time period. The results of this analysis reported mean treatment effects for acupuncture (odds ratio [OR], 3.53; 95% confidence interval [CI], 1.03-12.07), hypnotherapy (OR, 4.55; 95% CI, 0.98-21.01), and aversive smoking (OR, 4.26; 95% CI, 1.26-14.38).

This single meta-analysis suggests that these alternative methods may help smokers quit. The positive effects may be explained by a Hawthorne effect, and not because of the actual intervention. However, more research is required to guide our decisions in this regard. In the absence of more robust evidence in support of these methods, especially in the presence of safe alternatives that are proven to work, patients are generally advised to access methods endorsed by the rigorously established clinical practice guideline sets.

REFERENCES

1   Tahiri M, et al. Alternative smoking cessation aids: A meta-analysis of randomized controlled trials. The American Journal of Medicine. 2012. Available from: http://www.medicine.mcgill.ca/epidemiology/Joseph/publications/Methodological/tahiri2012.pdf

2   CAN-ADAPTT The Canadian Action Network for the Advancement, Dissemination and Adoption of Practice-informed Tobacco Treatment. https://www.nicotinedependenceclinic.com/English/CANADAPTT/Pages/Home.aspx

3   Fiore MC, Jaén C, Baker T, Bailey W., Benowitz N. et.al. Clinical Practice Guideline: Treating Tobacco Use and Dependence, 2008 Update. U.S. Department of Health and Human Services. Available at: http://www.surgeongeneral.gov/tobacco

TOBACCO CESSATION QUITLINES

A tobacco cessation quitline provides counselling services, mainly via telephone, to tobacco users who want to quit.[22] Quitlines are available in every province, territory, and state in Canada and the US, and are staffed by individuals trained in smoking cessation techniques. The two most common types of available quitlines are reactive and proactive. Reactive quitlines respond to incoming calls whereas with proactive quitlines, the counsellor calls the patient and offers counselling in a systematic manner, similar to cessation clinics. Quitlines can also vary in size and complexity with a variety of approaches. Callers may speak directly with a quitline specialist, or they may hear a brief recorded daily message with the option of speaking with a specialist directly. In the case of a specialist answering, the caller would be screened first to collect demographic and smoking history information to determine the patient's needs. The trained specialist will then develop a quit plan, may recommend medications (e.g. nicotine replacement therapy), and possibly provide several proactive follow-up calls. Brief counselling would ensue followed by referrals to community resources, and mailing out self-help material. In-depth counselling with practical quitting information such as confidence building, motivational enhancement, social support, and coping skills may also be essential for some callers.

Quitlines offer an accessible way of delivering evidence-based treatment and can be cost effective in reaching a potentially large population of people who use tobacco.[23] They provide a centralized resource for simple access to evidence-based information and effective counselling services to assist tobacco users in stopping. It has been shown that quitlines can increase healthcare provider adherence to conduct routine brief tobacco interventions with tobacco users.[1,24-26] Quitlines are free, confidential, and could be tailored to meet the needs of the individual motivated to quit. Quitlines assist in overcoming challenges in seeking tobacco treatment, and with them anxiety around transportation, childcare, financial or geographical obstacles are nonexistent.

A systematic review of 48 randomized/quasi-randomized clinical trials demonstrated that proactive telephone counselling helped smokers to quit, particularly in trials where the smokers were motivated to quit. It also concluded that 3 or more calls increased the likelihood of quitting versus negligible interventions (i.e. self-help materials, brief advice, strictly pharmacotherapy). There were no significant differences in two studies comparing different counselling approaches during a single quitline contact. Cessation rates were also increased when the counselling was not initiated by calls to the quitlines.[27] In summary, quitlines appear to be an effective way to reach large numbers of people at potentially lower costs than in-person interventions, particularly with proactive quitline approaches if successfully engaging patients around contracting multiple phone sessions.

WEB-ASSISTED TOBACCO INTERVENTIONS

Web-assisted tobacco interventions (WATI) are technology-enabled behavioural change interventions.[28] WATI provide smoking cessation programs and support health professional training in tobacco control. These resources have been developed to focus on 1 or more of 4 key areas: cessation, prevention, social support, and professional development/training. They can be used as a stand-alone intervention, a complement to other resources, or as an integrated component within a larger intervention.[28]

WATI designed specifically for tobacco prevention and cessation can readily be found on the Internet. Given the Internet's widespread use worldwide and in Canada (approximately 80% of households),[29] even small changes attributed to a web-based intervention can translate into a large-population health effect. As of 2007, over 60% of Canadian and American quitlines offered some sort of web-based cessation support;[30] these websites offered services ranging from self-sufficient interventions, chat rooms, interactive counselling and emails with cessation counsellors, and interactive maps on cessation information and services. Many of the web-based programs also offered message boards, information, literature, and updates on tobacco cessation subjects and events. WATI are affordable, effective, and easily accessible tools that can be customized to the individual.

A systematic review failed to demonstrate adequate evidence when assessing the efficacy of web-based interventions in adolescents, adults, and college and university students.[31] A 2010 review found that that there was some evidence that tailored and interactive sites were more effective than those that were static; still this finding was not consistent across all trials that investigated this factor.[32] Results did suggest that some Internet-based interventions assist with smoking cessation particularly if the information was tailored to the users, and it could provide frequent automated contacts; however, these findings were inconsistent.[32] In another systematic review of 22 randomized controlled trials, the intervention group had a significant effect on smoking cessation.[33] Similar findings were observed in 9 trials using WATI and in 13 trials using a computer-based intervention. The meta-analysis indicated that there was sufficient clinical evidence to promote the use of WATI smoking cessation programs for adult smokers.

CONTINGENCY MANAGEMENT

A behavioural intervention that has recently gained momentum for its use in tobacco addiction treatment is contingency management (CM). Based on principles of operant conditioning, CM provides patients with tangible reinforcers if they achieve certain performance or target behaviours, such as smoking abstinence or reducing to quit.[34] CM interventions may be effective in encouraging recruitment in a smoking cessation program or reward cessation achieved at predefined stages.[35] Moreover, specific populations have been known to respond favourably to incentive-based programming, such as pregnant and post-partum women, adolescents, and individuals addicted on other illicit substances.[36-38] The success rates of CM are further enhanced when combined with other psychosocial or pharmacological interventions.[39-41]

In order to use CM as a behavioural intervention for smoking cessation, 4 conditions must be met. First a target behaviour must be selected at the beginning of treatment in consultation with a therapist or clinician. Examples of target behaviours could be smoking abstinence or reducing to quit. However, if a patient chooses to reduce to quit, their reduction must be specific and measurable. Secondly, the quit process needs to be closely monitored for measures of success (i.e. the reduction of biological markers of smoking).[42] Standard measures of success look at biochemically verified reports such as exhaled carbon monoxide levels of less than 10 ppm or urinary or salivary cotinine (a metabolite or byproduct of nicotine, thus a biomarker for exposure to tobacco). It is important to keep track of these changes in order to ensure that this intervention is appropriate for the patient.

Thirdly, the selected target behaviour must be supported with some kind of tangible reinforcement, one that must be subjectively experienced by the patient as being as or more reinforcing than smoking cigarettes.[43] Reinforcements used in CM can consist of financial incentives such as cash, or material incentives such as vouchers, prizes, or special privileges. When engaging the patient in a CM intervention, it is essential that the reinforcement not only be perceived as desirable to the patient but also relevant to their current situation. For example, if working with an adolescent male who was trying to quit smoking, a computer or gaming system might be perceived as more desirable and more relevant to their current lifestyle than a gift certificate to a furniture store. Finally, if a patient relapses during the quit process, the reinforcement must be withheld.[43]

Several factors limit the use of CM as a behavioural intervention in tobacco dependence treatment, including the costs associated with supporting financial and material incentives.[44] The amount of time and effort required of patients and practitioners to consistently monitor the reduction of biological markers of smoking can also minimize the use of contingency management.[45] If a smoking cessation program does not have the funding or labour resources necessary to operate incentive-based programming, CM is not a suitable intervention. Another limitation in the use of CM as a behavioural intervention for smoking cessation is the inability for patients to sustain their quit after the contingencies have ended.[35,46] According to a recent systematic review, researchers found that with the exception of one trial, incentive-based programming for smoking cessation did not show to enhance long-term cessation. Early success tended to disappear once the reinforcements were no longer available.[35]

A number of the studies under this review showed that incentives could increase participation in smoking cessation programs; however, these results need to be interpreted with caution. Increasing enrollment in cessation programming does not necessarily guarantee long-term quit rates. For instance, non-smokers may join incentive-based cessation programming to receive the benefits of a material or financial incentive even though they are abstinent. Furthermore, incentive-based programming tends to attract individuals who are motivated differently from those who sign up for more conventional cessation methods; this can also attribute to the lack of long-term effectiveness. Therefore, although CM may have a value mechanism for cessation induction, its long-term effectiveness in sustaining abstinence requires further review.[47]

CONCLUSION

There are many different counselling models and psychosocial support options that are effective in assisting individuals to achieve abstinence from tobacco. There are still many barriers around accessing these treatments in Canada. Challenges still remain around the ability to make psychosocial support and counselling interventions more widely available. At the same time, further research is needed to identify strategies for increasing adherence to current evidence-based treatment models. Healthcare practitioners need to be provided with brief and intensive tobacco cessation training opportunities in order develop competencies in this area and to ensure accountability and continuity of care. In addition, further research is needed to explore the optimal methods for integrating new technology such as internet-based treatments into comprehensive plans of care.[4]

Optimal tobacco use and addiction treatment consists of a menu of different treatment approaches offered across different healthcare settings and provided by a variety of different healthcare professionals. Ideally, individuals should be able to access a variety of evidence-based treatment modalities to address tobacco reduction and cessation whenever needed. At the same time, the healthcare system should be constantly reaching out by systematically screening and offering assistance to all individuals that use tobacco all of the time.

REFERENCES

1   Fiore MC, Jaén CR, Baker TB, Bailey, WC, Benowitz, NL, Curry, SJ, et al. Treating tobacco use and dependence: 2008 update. Clinical practice guideline. Rockville MD: U.S. Department of Health and Human Services. Public Health Service; 2008 May [cited 2012 Mar 16]. Available from: http://www.surgeongeneral.gov/tobacco/treating_tobacco_use08.pdf.

2   CAN-ADAPTT. Canadian smoking cessation clinical practice guideline. Toronto: Canadian Action Network for the Advancement, Dissemination and Adoption of Practice-informed Tobacco Treatment, Centre for Addiction and Mental Health; 2011 [cited 2012 Mar 16]. Available from: http://www.can-adaptt.net/English/Guideline/Introduction.aspx.

3   Perkins KA, Conklin CA, Levine MD. Cognitive-behavioral therapy for smoking cessation: a practical guidebook to the most effective treatments. New York: Routledge Taylor & Francis Group; 2008.

4   Fiore MC, Baker TB. Treating smokers in health care settings. N Engl J Med. 2011;365:1222-31.

5   West R, Shiffman S. Fast facts: smoking cessation. Oxford UK: Health Press Ltd; 2007 [cited 2012 Mar 16]. Available from: http://www.fastfacts.com/_files/samplefiles/FF_SmokingCessation_sample.pdf.

6   Saitz R. Unhealthy alcohol use. N Engl J Med. 2005;352(6):596-607.

7   Henry-Edwards S, Humeniuk R, Ali R, Monteiro M, Poznyak V. Brief Intervention for substance use: a manual for use in primary care (draft version 1.1 for field testing). Geneva: World Health Organization; 2003 [cited 2012 Mar 15]. Available from: http://www.who.int/substance_abuse/activities/en/Draft_Brief_Intervention_for_Substance_Use.pdf.

8   Yahne CE, Miller WR, Irvin-Vitela L, Scott Tonigan J. Magdalena Pilot Project: motivational outreach to substance abusing women street sex workers. J Subst Abuse Treat. 2002;23(1):49-53.

9   McEwen A, Hajek P, McRobbie H, West R. Manual of smoking cessation: a guide for counsellors and practitioners. Oxford UK: Blackwell Publishing Ltd; 2006.

10   Abrams DB, Niaura R, Brown RA, Emmons KM, Goldstein MG, Monti, PM. The tobacco dependence treatment handbook: a guide to best practices. New York: Guilford Press; 2003.

11   Herie MA, Watkin-Merek L. Structured Relapse Prevention (SRP): An outpatient counselling approach. 2nd ed. Toronto: Centre for Addiction and Mental Health; 2006.

12   DiClemente CC. Addiction and change: how addictions develop and addicted people recover. New York: Guilford Press; 2006.

13   Hettema J, Hendricks P. Motivational interviewing for smoking cessation: a meta-analytic review. J Consult Clin Psychol. 2010;78(6):868-84.

14   Baca C, Yahne C. Smoking cessation during substance abuse treatment: what you need to know. J Subst Abuse Treat. 2009;36:205-19.

15   Rollnick S, Butler C, Kinnersley P, Gregory J, Mash B. Practice: Motivational interviewing. BMJ. 2010;340:1900.

16   Miller R, Rollnick S. Motivational interviewing. 2nd ed. New York: Guilford Press; 2002.

17   Ingersoll KS, Wagner CC, Gharib S. Motivational groups for community substance abuse programs. Richmond VA: Mid-Atlantic Addiction Technology Transfer Center; 2002 [cited 2012 Mar 16]. Available from: http://people.uncw.edu/ogler/MI%20Groups%20for%20Com%20SA%20Prog.pdf.

18   Peterson A, Kealey K, Mann S, Marek P, Ludman E, Liu J, Bricker J. Group randomized trial of a proactive, personalized telephone counseling intervention for adolescent smoking cessation. JNCI. 2009;101(20):1378-92.

19   Rollnick S, Miller W, Butler C. Motivational interviewing in health care: helping patients change behaviour. New York: Guilford Press; 2008.

20   Stead LF, Lancaster T. Group behaviour therapy programmes for smoking cessation (review). Cochrane Database Syst Rev. 2006;1:1-114.

21   Khara M, Okoli CTC. Tobacco dependence treatment in an addiction services outpatient setting. Am J Addict. 2011;20(1):45-55.

22   World Health Organization. Developing and improving national toll-free tobacco quit line services: a World Health Organization manual. Geneva: WHO; 2011 Nov [cited 2012 Mar 23]. Available from: http://www.who.int/tobacco/publications/smoking_cessation/quit_lines_services/en/index.html

23   Cummins SE, Bailey L, Campbell S, Koon-Kirby C, Zhu S. Tobacco cessation quitlines in North America: a descriptive study. Tob Control. 2007 Dec;16(Suppl 1): i9-15.

24   McAfee TA. Quitlines a tool for research and dissemination of evidence-based cessation practices. Am J Prev Med. 2007 Dec;33(6 Suppl):S357-67.

25   Bentz, CJ., Bayley KB, Bonin KE, Fleming L, Hollis JF, Hunt JS, et al. Provider feedback to improve 5A's tobacco cessation in primary care: a cluster randomized clinical trial. Nicotine Tob Res. 2007 Mar;9(3):341-9.

26   An LC, Zhu SH, Nelson DB, Arikian NJ, Nugent S, Partin MR, Joseph AM. Benefits of telephone care over primary care for smoking cessation: a randomized trial. Archives of Internal Medicine 2006 Mar 13;166(5):536–42.

27   Stead LF, Perera R, Lancaster T. Telephone counselling for smoking cessation. Cochrane Database Syst Rev. 2006; Issue 3. Art. No.:CD002850.

28   Norman C. Using information technology to support smoking-related behaviour change: web-assisted tobacco interventions. Smoking Cessation Rounds 2007 [cited 2012 Mar 23]. Available from: www.smokingcessationrounds.ca/crus/smokingceseng_08_07.pdf.

29   Canadian Internet Use Survey. The daily: Wed, May 25, 2011 [cited 2012 Mar 23]. Available from: http://http://www.statcan.gc.ca/daily-quotidien/110525/dq110525b-eng.htm

30   Web-assisted tobacco interventions (WATI): the future of tobacco cessation? North American Quitline Consortium; 2007 [cited 2012 Mar 23]. Available from: www.naquitline.org/resource/resmgr/docs/factsheet-wati_2007.pdf

31   HE, Wilson LM, Apelberg BJ, Tang EA, Odelola O, Bass EB, et al. A systematic review of randomized controlled trials: web-based interventions for smoking cessation among adolescents, college students, and adults. Nicotine Tob Res 2011 Apr;13(4):227–38.

32   Civljak M, Sheikh A, Stead LF, Car J. Internet-based interventions for smoking cessation. Cochrane Database Syst Rev. 2010; Issue 9. Art. No.:CD007078.

33   Myung SK, McDonnell DD, Kazinets G, Seo HG, Moskowitz JM. Effects of web- and computer-based smoking cessation programs: meta-analysis of randomized controlled trials. Arch Intern Med 2009 May 25;169(10):929–37.

34   Cavallo DA, Cooney JL, Duhig AM, Smith AE, Liss TB, McFetridge AK, et al. Combining cognitive behavioral therapy with contingency management for smoking cessation in adolescent smokers: a preliminary comparison of two different CBT formats. Am J Addict 2007;16:468–74.

35   Cahill K, Perera R. Competitions and incentives for smoking cessation. Cochrane Database of Syst Rev 2011;4:1–51.

36   Dunn KE, Saulsgiver KA, Sigmon SC. Contingency management for behaviour change: applications to promote brief smoking cessation among opioid-maintained patients. ExpClinPsychopharmacol. 2011; 19(1): 20-30.

37   Gray D, Stearne A, Wilson M, Doyle M. Indigenous-specific alcohol and other drug interventions. Australian National Council on Drugs research paper no. 20. Canberra: Australian National Council on Drugs; 2010.

38   Higgins ST, Heil SH, Solomon LJ, et al. A pilot study on voucher-based incentives to promote abstinence from cigarette smoking during pregnancy and postpartum. Nicotine Tob Res 2004; 6:1015-20.

39   Cavallo DA, Cooney JL, Duhig AM, Smith AE, Liss TB, McFetridge AK, et al. Combining cognitive behavioral therapy with contingency management for smoking cessation in adolescent smokers: a preliminary comparison of two different CBT formats. Am J Addict 2007;16:468-74.

40   Lamb RJ, Morral AR, Kirby KC, Galbicka G, Javors MA, Iguchi M. Contingencies for change in complacent smokers. Exp Clin Psychopharmacol. 2007;15(3):245-55.

41   Krishnan-Sarin S, Duhig AM, McKee SA, et al. Contingency management for smoking cessation in adolescent smokers. Exp Clin Psychopharmacol. 2006;14:306-10.

42   Sigmon SC, Lamb RJ, Dallery J. Tobacco. In: Higgins ST, Silverman K, Heil SH, editors. Contingency management in substance abuse treatment. New York: Guilford Press; 2008. p. 99-119.

43   Ledgerwood DM. Contingency management for smoking cessation: where do we go from here? Curr Drug Abuse Rev. 2008;1: 340-9.

44   Sindelar J, Elbel B, Petry NM. What do we get for our money? cost-effectiveness of adding contingency management. Addiction. 2007;102:309-16.

45   Glenn IM, Dallery J. Effects of internet-based voucher reinforcement and a transdermal nicotine patch on cigarette smoking. J Appl Behav Anal. 2007;40:1-13.

46   Prendergast M, Podus D, Finney J, Greenwell L, Roll JM. Contingency management for treatment of substance use disorders: a meta-analysis. Addiction. 2006;101:1546-60.

47   Hughes JR, Keely JP, Niaura RS, Ossip-Klein DJ, Richmond RL, Swan GE. Measures of abstinence in clinical trials: issues and recommendations. Nicotine Tob Res. 2003;5(1):13-25.

9

Pharmacotherapies

CAN-ADAPTT Summary Statements for Pharmacotherapy

CAN-ADAPTT SUMMARY STATEMENTS FOR PHARMACOTHERAPY

1. Offer efficacious pharmacotherapy to every patient who smokes 10 or more cigarettes daily and is willing to make a quit attempt.
2. Healthcare providers should tailor smoking cessation pharmacotherapy to the patient's clinical needs and preferences.
3. Varenicline improves smoking cessation rates at 6 and 12 months when compared with placebo.
4. Bupropion improves smoking cessation rates at 6 months and may improve cessation rates at 12 months when compared with placebo.
5. Nicotine patch improves smoking cessation rates at 6 and 12 months when compared with placebo.
6. Nicotine gum may improve smoking cessation rates at 6 and 12 months when compared with placebo.
7. Nicotine lozenge may improve smoking cessation rates at 6 and 12 months when compared with placebo.
8. Nicotine nasal spray improves smoking cessation rates at 6 and 12 months when compared with placebo.
9. Nicotine oral inhaler may improve smoking cessation rates at 6 and 12 months when compared with placebo.
10. Nicotine sublingual tablet may improve smoking cessation rates at 6 and 12 months when compared with placebo.
11. There is insufficient evidence to make a recommendation regarding the use of Clonidine for smoking cessation.
12. There is insufficient evidence to make a recommendation regarding the use of Nortriptyline for smoking cessation.

Source: CAN-ADAPTT. Canadian smoking cessation clinical practice guideline. Toronto: Canadian Action Network for the Advancement, Dissemination and Adoption of Practice-informed Tobacco Treatment, Centre for Addiction and Mental Health; 2011. Available from: www.can-adaptt.net. Reprinted with permission.

9.1

Nicotine Replacement Therapies

JOHN HUGHES

NICOTINE REPLACEMENT THERAPIES (NRTS) AVAILABLE IN CANADA INCLUDE NICOTINE gum, inhaler, lozenge, oromucosal (mouth) spray, and patch. All are available over-the-counter (OTC). Overall, NRT increases long-term cessation by a factor of 1.6.[1] Quit rates do not differ across individual NRTs and there is no verified method to match patients to specific NRT products. Currently, NRTs are classified as "lifestyle" medications, and are not covered in most Canadian insurance plans.[2]

Most NRT is used for cessation. In 2007, among Canadians who tried to quit smoking in the last year, 45% had used a medication to quit[3] and most of this was OTC NRT. In Canada, NRT can also be used to reduce prior to quitting, or for relief of withdrawal during short periods of enforced abstinence. Recent Canadian studies suggest many individuals may be using NRT for non-cessation reasons including temporary abstinence from smoking or reducing the number of cigarettes smoked.[4]

FORMATS AVAILABLE

Nicotine gum (2 and 4 mg), nicotine inhaler (10 mg), nicotine lozenge (2 and 4 mg), oromucosal spray (1mg/spray), 16-hour nicotine patch (5, 10, and 15 mg), and 24-hour nicotine patch (7, 14, and 21mg) are available in Canada. Nicotine microtabs and nasal spray are not available and will not be discussed.

MECHANISM OF ACTION

Nicotine can induce addiction and dependence because it stimulates nicotinic receptors to release dopamine in the "reward centres" of the brain.[5] In addition, nicotine increases the release of norepinephrine, serotonin, endorphins, and ACTH which increase attention and performance, and decrease hunger, impulsivity, anger, and others. Nicotine increases peripheral vasoconstriction, tachycardia, and blood pressure. Tolerance to some of these effects occurs. Cessation of nicotine can cause a withdrawal syndrome, with anxiety, craving, depression, difficulty concentrating, hunger, insomnia, irritability, and restlessness.

Replacing nicotine via medications reduces abstinence-induced craving and withdrawal symptoms which makes it easier to cut down and to stop smoking. Nicotine via NRT also decreases post-cessation weight gain while NRT is being used. In addition, because NRTs maintain tolerance to nicotine, they can blunt the effects of the first cigarettes during a lapse, and thereby decrease the probability that a slip will progress to a return of regular smoking. Nicotine is not a major cause of the medical problems from smoking.[5]

PHARMACOKINETIC COMMENTS

Nicotine from gum, mouth spray, and lozenge are absorbed buccally.[6] Although the term nicotine "inhaler" suggests respiratory absorption, nicotine from the inhaler is absorbed buccally. Nicotine from patch is readily absorbed across the skin. Oral nicotine (e.g. via a pill) is not used because almost all of the nicotine undergoes first-pass metabolism in the liver.

The time to maximal effect for the mouth spray is about 10 minutes for nicotine gum, lozenge and inhaler is about 30 minutes and for nicotine patch is about 6 hours. The usual nicotine levels from using inhaler are less than that from gum or lozenge and are greatest for the nicotine patch. The usual levels from the mouth spray are not known. Usually blood levels from all NRTs stabilize after 2–3 days of use and are 50% or less than that from smoking. Acidic liquids (e.g. coffee, juices, soda) can interfere with buccal absorption of nicotine and should not be used for 30 minutes before or after using NRTs. The elimination of nicotine after cessation of gum, inhaler, lozenge or mouth spray is about 3–5 hours;[5] however, it is 12–24 hours after cessation of patch.

TABLE 1: Recent Findings about Nicotine Replacement Therapies

1. Use of over-the-counter NRT (i.e. in the absence of any talk therapy) appears effective.[10]
2. Combining nicotine patch plus gum, inhaler, or lozenge is so much more effective than monotherapy that many believe combined use is first line treatment. [1] Combined NRT appears as effective as prescription smoking cessation treatments.[11]
3. Smoking while using NRT does not appear to be dangerous.[12]
4. New flavors of nicotine gum and lozenge may increase treatment adherence.
5. Among smokers not currently planning to quit, the use of NRT to reduce cigarettes per day, increases the probability of a later quit attempt and abstinence.[13]
6. Among smokers currently trying to quit, the use of NRT as part of a gradual cessation quit attempt appears effective.[14]
7. Whether the use of NRT among continuing smokers reduces the harm from smoking is unclear.[13]
8. Continued use of NRT during an initial post-abstinence lapse increases the ability to reestablish abstinence.[8]
9. Use of NRT to relieve withdrawal during periods of temporary abstinence does not appear to undermine motivation to quit smoking.[15]
10. True addiction to NRT (i.e. inability to stop) is rare.[16]
11. Given that NRT produces a slower onset of nicotine and much lower levels of nicotine from cigarettes, use of it is "contraindication" can often be justified.[17]

INDICATIONS AND CLINICAL USE

Nicotine medications are indicated as an "aid to smoking cessation." In the last decade, several recent findings have better delineated the pros and cons of NRT (Table 1). The higher-dose forms of NRT are for the more dependent smokers, as indicated by smoking within 30 minutes of arising, or scores of 7 and above on the Fagerström Test for Nicotine Dependence (see Chapter 6). All NRTs can be used for abrupt cessation. With this use, NRT begins on the first day of abstinence (i.e. the quit day). Several studies suggest starting NRT prior to the quit day to accommodate adverse events, and having good blood levels on the quit date, increases quit rates; other studies have failed to replicate this finding.[7] Because NRT can prevent slips from becoming full relapses, it is important for smokers to continue NRT even during a few slips.[8] Although the recommended duration of NRTs is typically 10 weeks, some may benefit from longer-duration use;[1] however, NRT use beyond 6 months should occur under a physician's care. Except for patch, abrupt cessation of NRT can produce withdrawal symptoms and, thus, NRTs should be gradually weaned by using fewer times per day or using lower doses. It is logical that NRT products should also help smokeless tobacco users to quit; however, the evidence for this is mixed.[9]

NICOTINE GUM

Nicotine gum has nicotine bound to a polyacrylic matrix[18] that is released upon chewing. The gum should be used 10–12 times a day (i.e. once every 1–2 hours) and whenever a craving occurs or in anticipation of craving. The gum should be chewed slowly and intermittently (e.g. by "parking" the gum after a few chews) to avoid adverse effects. Smokers should not eat or drink acidic beverages while using the gum or any oral NRT (i.e. inhaler, lozenge, or mouth spray). The recommended duration of use of the gum is 6 weeks followed by tapering over another 6 weeks and then, if needed, 1–2 times/day for the next 12 weeks. The gum is the only NRT that can be used both for abrupt and gradual cessation.

The gradual or "reduce-to-quit" method for nicotine gum recommends individuals have a goal of decreasing smoking by 50% within 4 months of treatment before quitting. The decision to quit can be decided at any point in this process. Nicotine gum is also approved to be used not for smoking cessation but to decrease craving and withdrawal symptoms during enforced temporary abstinence periods.[19] Some have worried that such use would undermine motivation to quit smoking (because individuals would no longer have to suffer withdrawal or leave work or home to smoke); however, the only study on this found gum use for temporary abstinence increased, not decreased, later quitting.[15]

NICOTINE INHALER

The nicotine inhaler is a plastic cylinder with a mouthpiece and looks like a small cigarette.[18] The cylinder contains a cartridge impregnated with nicotine that volatilizes when warm air is passed over the cartridge. The nicotine inhaler has poor absorption when ambient air is < 10°C. Smokers should not eat or drink acidic beverages while using the inhaler. Smokers should puff on the inhaler multiple times over a 20–minute period. They should be able to detect the inhaler is no longer effective within 20 minutes and begin a new inhaler cartridge. Smokers may use 6–12 cartridges/day. The recommended duration is 6 weeks followed by tapering over another 6 weeks and, if needed, use of 1–2 pieces/day during the next 12 weeks.

NICOTINE LOZENGE

Nicotine lozenge is a small white lozenge that comes in two flavours.[18] The lozenge is not to be chewed but simply placed in the mouth and switched from side to side as needed. Patients should be encouraged to use 8–12 times a day (i.e. once every 1–2 hours) and when a craving occurs. The recommended duration of use is 6 weeks followed by tapering over another 6 weeks and then, if needed, 1–2 times a day for the next 12 weeks. Eating and drinking acidic beverages should be avoided while using the lozenge. The lozenge takes about 30 minutes to dissolve.

NICOTINE MOUTH SPRAY

The mouth spray is a nicotine aerosol that is used to relieve cravings to smoke. It has a faster onset than gum, inhaler, or lozenge. A similar mouth spray from a different manufacturer produces faster craving relief than nicotine gum. Upon quitting smoking, smokers are to use 1 or 2 sprays to replace each cigarette (if one smoked 15 cigs then one should use the mouth spray 15 times at 1–2 spray/time). This regime should occur for the first 6 weeks and then smokers should slowly decrease use over the next 6 weeks. The maximum use is 4 sprays/hour or 64/day.

NICOTINE PATCH

The nicotine patch is a thin rectangle of 10–30 cm^2 area impregnated with nicotine.[18] An adhesive in the patch regulates the delivery of nicotine to the skin. The patch sold in Canada is for 15, 10, or 5 mg/16 hrs, as well as a 24-hour-delivery format with strengths of 21 mg, 14 mg, or 7 mg. The patch is to be administered each morning and the 16-hour patch is worn only while awake. This method avoids the problem of insomnia seen with 24-hour patches but probably has less efficacy for morning cravings. On the other hand, little relapse occurs in the early-morning hours. The recommended duration for the 16-hour patch is 15 mg for 6 weeks, then 10 mg for 2 weeks, then 5 mg for 2 weeks. For the 24-hour patch it is 21mg for 6 weeks, then 14 mg for 2 weeks, then 7 mg for 2 weeks.

TABLE 2. Typical long-term quit rates

Medication	Psychosocial Treatment		
	None (OTC)	Brief Advice	Counselling
No Medication	4%	8%	15%
Single NRT	8%	15%	25%
Combined NRTs	?	?	30%
Rx Cessation Medications	?	?	30%

COMBINED NICOTINE PATCH AND NICOTINE GUM/INHALER/ LOZENGE/MOUTH SPRAY

Combining a nicotine patch (to produce steady nicotine levels) with a short-acting NRT (to abate sudden cravings) increases quit rates by a factor of 1.4 over single NRT treatment.[1] Currently, only combined patch and 2 mg gum is approved in Canada; however, there is good reason to believe similar results would occur with inhaler, lozenge, or mouth spray. Adverse events from combining patch and other NRTs are minor. Whether combining NRT with non-nicotine smoking cessation medications (e.g. bupropion or varenicline) increases efficacy is unclear.[20]

COMBINED NRT + PSYCHOSOCIAL TREATMENT VS OTC NRT

Psychosocial treatments for smoking cessation include quitlines, individual face-to-face counseling, group therapy, and internet sites (see Chapter 8).[18] Overall such programs increase quitting by a factor of 1.3–2.8.[21] The different formats to delivering psychosocial treatments appear equally effective. Although labelling states NRT is an "adjunct to a smoking cessation program," psychosocial treatments are not essential for OTC NRT to work.[10] However, overall quit rates are lower when NRT is used without a psychosocial treatment than with a psychosocial treatment (Table 2). Thus, smokers should be encouraged to use both NRT and a psychosocial treatment; however, < 10% of NRT users do so.[22]

CONTRAINDICATIONS

Product labelling states that NRT is contraindicated in smokers who are adolescents, pregnant or breastfeeding, have active temporomandibular joint disease (gum only), life-threatening arrhythmias, worsening or severe angina, or have recently had a cardiac infarct or cerebrovascular accident. However, because the nicotine in NRT is absorbed less rapidly and produces much lower levels than smoking, many experts believe there are no absolute contraindications for NRT in smokers because the benefits of NRT often outweigh the contraindication risks (see Adverse Effects below).[17,23]

Very few studies have examined NRT in adolescents and these produced mixed efficacy results, but did not find an unusual side-effect profile.[24] Given that nicotine dependence develops rapidly within the first few years, many experts see no reason NRT should not be effective in nicotine dependent, daily adolescent smokers.[17] Whether NRT is effective in non-daily smokers has not been tested.

Smoking is associated with low birth-weight and several perinatal complications.[25] Whether this is due to nicotine or carbon monoxide is unclear. The few studies of NRT use during pregnancy have not found significant adverse events.[26] Recent expert opinion papers have argued for use of NRT among pregnant smokers who cannot stop on their own.[17] Nicotine is secreted in breast milk; whether this causes problems is unstudied. Children of smokers are more likely to have sudden infant death syndrome, and animal studies suggest nicotine may be a causal agent by interfering with cell differentiation in respiratory centers; however, tests of nicotine per se as a cause of this syndrome in humans have not been reported.[25]

Cigarette smoking increases cardiovascular events, hypertension, and arrhythmias via several mechanisms, some of which could be due to nicotine.[27] However, there are several non-nicotine components in tobacco smoke (e.g. carbon monoxide, and oxidants) that could be causal instead. Multiple studies of NRT use among smokers with cardiovascular disease have not found increased risk in those with stable heart disease. Whether NRT is safe to use in the immediate post-cardiac infarct or post-cerebrovascular accident period, with life-threatening arrhythmia, or with severe or worsening angina, is unclear.[27]

WARNINGS AND PRECAUTIONS

Smokers who have high blood pressure, hyperthyroidism, insulin-dependent diabetes, kidney disease, liver disease, pheochromocytoma, or an ulcer are advised to see a physician before using NRT, because nicotine has the potential to worsen these disorders. Adequate studies demonstrating such worsening have not been published. Many experts believe the benefits of use of NRT in these conditions often outweighs their risk.[17] Nicotine from NRT could produce symptoms of nicotine intoxication. Nicotine can be fatal in children or pets; thus, patients should keep them out of the reach of children and pets.

Some package labels advise patients to not use NRT and smoke concurrently. An early anecdotal report concluded that smoking while using NRT could cause heart attacks. Many more rigorous studies since then have found concurrent use is safe.[12] For example, 15 studies have examined concurrent use of smoking and NRT in over 5,000 smokers and none have reported serious adverse events plausibly due to concurrent use.[12] Also, one study asked individuals to smoke their usual amount while wearing three nicotine patches delivering 63 mg of nicotine (cf 15 mg in usual patch) and found no serious adverse events.[28] Smokers with dental plates and cavities should be warned that, like any gum, nicotine gum could loosen such fixtures. Smokers with asthma or chronic obstructive pulmonary disease should be warned that the inhaler has the potential to cause bronchospasm. The nicotine patch labels lists allergies to glue or bandages, atopic or eczematous dermatitis, and using the patch while exercising, as warnings.

EFFICACY

The NRTs were superior to placebo or no treatment in 102 of the 111 trials involving in total over 40,000 smokers.[1,21,29] Overall, NRTs increase quit rates 1.6-fold and the different NRTs appear to have similar effectiveness. Higher doses of gum are more effective for more dependent smokers. The efficacy of OTC NRT does not appear to be inferior to that of prescription non-nicotine medications; however, few comparisons are available. Using NRT to reduce smoking increases the probability of a later quit attempt, but whether reduction in cigarettes per day decreases the risk of smoking is unclear.[13] Typical long-term quit rates are illustrated in Table 1.

NRT is effective across subgroups of smokers (e.g. those with lung disease, psychiatric patients, and African Americans).[1] Its efficacy compared with placebo is independent of the amount of concomitant psychosocial treatment, and setting (specialty clinics vs. primary care clinics).

ADVERSE REACTIONS

Less than 5% of NRT users have to stop NRT due to adverse events.[30] Serious adverse events are very rare. Long-term use of NRT has not been associated with adverse outcomes. The most common adverse events for nicotine gum and lozenge are nausea, heartburn, hiccups, dyspepsia, and throat irritation.[30] The most common adverse events for the patch are erythema and pruritus. The most common adverse events for inhaler are headache, dyspepsia, and nausea.

Nicotine does not appear to cause cancer.[31] Although some animal studies have suggested nicotine might promote cancer growth, their clinical relevance is unclear. Also, the relative role of nicotine, carbon monoxide, oxidants, and other chemicals in smoking-related cardiovascular disease is unclear.[27]

A minority of smokers use nicotine gum for longer than recommended and this is could be the case for nicotine lozenge as well. However, much of that use appears to be due to seeking the therapeutic effect of nicotine, not because they are unable to stop NRT use.[16] Estimates are that < 5% gum users become addicted to nicotine gum. Rates are probably even lower with nicotine patch and inhaler. These low incidences are probably because nicotine is absorbed slower and to smaller levels with NRT than with cigarettes. Use of NRTs in never-smokers is very rare.

Smoking increases the metabolism of several medications (the most common are psychiatric and cardiac medications) and, thus, cessation of smoking can increase levels of these medications and cause adverse events.[32] This pharmacokinetic interaction is not due to nicotine and, thus, NRT should not influence it. Nicotine may increase insulin resistance and thereby decrease the efficacy of insulin.

DOSAGE AND ADMINISTRATION

Most NRTs have been tested in individuals smoking ≥ 10 cigarettes per day but may be effective for any daily smokers.[33] Higher doses are for those who are more addicted, i.e. smoke sooner after rising or have higher dependence scores. Lower-dose patches are used for those weighing <100 pounds.

OVERDOSAGE

As the doses of nicotine in NRT are low and because high doses of nicotine cause nausea and vomiting, unintentional overdose from NRT is very rare.[34] Signs of nicotine toxicity are abdominal pain, dizziness, headache, nausea, palpitations, sweating, and weakness. More severe signs include delirium, hypotension, circulatory collapse, respiratory failure, and death. Treatment includes activated charcoal to eliminate any swallowed nicotine, and supportive care.

THE FUTURE OF NRT

Several nicotine products are being developed or tested for smoking cessation. Many believe the rapid absorption of nicotine via pulmonary absorption is key to the reinforcing effects of nicotine. Thus, several companies are developing a true nicotine pulmonary inhaler. Several "electronic cigarettes" that vapourize nicotine have been marketed. How much they deliver pulmonary nicotine is unclear and, thus far, only one trial of efficacy has been published.[35] Whether these are more effective than traditional NRTs is unclear. A formulation of nicotine water is available but has not been scientifically tested. A nicotine buccal pouch and buccal strip are currently being developed.

SUMMARY

Nicotine replacement therapies continue to be widely used and have retained their status as safe and effective first-line treatments.

PATIENT HANDOUT: NICOTINE GUM

Ron Pohar

What are the benefits of this medication?   Nicotine gum can help individuals to reduce or quit smoking by gradually weaning off nicotine. Nicotine gum helps to reduce the symptoms of nicotine withdrawal (irritability, frustration, anxiety, restlessness, difficulty concentrating) and to control cravings for nicotine. Those who use nicotine gum when attempting to quit are about twice as likely to be successful as those who do not.

How should this medication be used?   When you are ready to stop smoking, set a target quit date. On that day, nicotine gum can be started. In general, most people will start with 10–20 pieces per day (1–2 pieces every 1–2 hours) and then slowly reduce the number of pieces chewed each day. The nicotine gum is available over the counter. Consultation with a healthcare provider can help to determine the appropriate strength of nicotine gum (2 mg or 4 mg based on the number of cigarettes smoked per day and the time to first cigarette) and schedule for reducing the number of pieces of gum chewed each day. For those individuals not yet prepared to quit smoking altogether, a "reduce-to-quit" approach can be used whereby the number of cigarettes smoked daily is gradually reduced. Nicotine gum is not like ordinary chewing gum and must be chewed a specific way in order for it to be maximally effective and to reduce the chance of having side effects. Use the "bite-and-park" technique: the gum should be bitten (chewed) once or twice and then "parked" between the cheek and gum for about 1 minute. The gum is then repeatedly chewed then parked for about 30 minutes, after which time all of the nicotine will have been released. Eating or drinking 30 minutes before use or during use or the consumption of caffeinated or acidic beverages while chewing nicotine gum should be avoided.

What are the common side effects with this medication?   The most common side effects of nicotine gum include feeling light-headed, nauseous, and having hiccups. Often these side effects are related to incorrect chewing technique and will subside if the chewing technique is corrected.

What symptoms would indicate that I should stop taking this medication?   If you experience chest pain, irregular heartbeat, leg pain, fainting, or severe stomach upset, consider stopping use of the gum and contacting your healthcare provider.

What can happen if I smoke while taking this medication?   Smoking while using nicotine gum is part of the reduce-to-quit strategy and may help those who have previously been unable to quit do so.

Can I use other forms of nicotine replacement therapy while using nicotine gum? Yes, nicotine gum can be used in combination with nicotine patches on an as-needed basis when cravings occur and may provide faster relief of cravings than the patch, which can take up to 2–4 hours.

What can happen if I consume caffeine while taking this medication? It is generally advised to reduce caffeine (e.g. in tea, coffee, colas, energy drinks, etc.) intake when quitting smoking because the tar in cigarette smoke helps the liver to process caffeine more quickly. When you stop smoking, the liver's ability to process caffeine returns to its normal level and the effect of caffeine will feel stronger and may produce symptoms similar to nicotine withdrawal (for example, irritability and anxiety).

How will nicotine gum affect other medications? Nicotine gum does not directly affect blood levels of other medications. However, quitting smoking does affect the blood levels of some medications. The potential need for dose adjustments of other medications should be discussed with a healthcare provider.

PATIENT HANDOUT: NICOTINE PATCH

Ron Pohar

How would I benefit from using this medication? Nicotine patches slowly deliver nicotine through the skin and into the blood. Nicotine patches can help individuals reduce or quit smoking by gradual weaning off nicotine. Nicotine patches help to reduce the symptoms of nicotine withdrawal and control cravings for nicotine. Those who use nicotine patches when attempting to quit smoking are roughly twice as likely to be successful as those who do not.

How should I use this medication? A target quit date is set and then the nicotine patch is started on that day. Some people may benefit using the patch before the quit date. The nicotine patch is available over the counter. There are different strengths and brands of nicotine patches available. Nicotine patches are generally applied in the morning to a clean, dry, hairless application site on the upper arm, hip, back, or shoulder. Some brands of nicotine patches are left on for 24 hours, then removed and replaced with a new patch. Other brands are designed to deliver nicotine over a 16-hour period and are removed at bedtime to allow for a nicotine-free period. Consultation with a healthcare provider can help to determine the appropriate starting strength of nicotine patch and schedule for reducing the strength of patch.

What are the common side effects with this medication? The most common side effects of nicotine patches include itching or burning at the site of application. This usually goes away in about an hour following application but can persist if an individual is allergic to the patch components. Applying the patch to a new site and avoiding using the same site within 1 week can reduce the risk of skin irritation. Sometimes switching to a different brand of patch may reduce skin irritation in those with persistent skin reactions. For those who experience difficulty sleeping while using nicotine patches, removing the patch 1–2 hours prior to bedtime may help.

What symptoms would indicate that I should stop taking this medication? If you experience chest pain, irregular heartbeat, leg pain, fainting, or severe stomach upset, consider stopping the patch and contacting your healthcare provider.

Can I use other forms of nicotine replacement therapy while using nicotine patches? Yes, nicotine patches can be used with other forms of nicotine replacement therapy for those individuals who do not have adequate craving control when using nicotine patches. Nicotine gum, for example, can be used with the patch on an as needed basis when cravings occur and may provide faster relief of cravings than the patch, which can take up to 2–4 hours.

What can happen if I consume caffeine while taking this medication? It is generally advised to reduce caffeine (e.g. in tea, coffee, colas, energy drinks, etc.) intake when quitting smoking because the tar in cigarette smoke helps the liver to process caffeine more quickly. When you stop smoking, the liver's ability to process caffeine returns to its normal level, and the effect of caffeine will feel stronger and may produce symptoms similar to nicotine withdrawal (for example, irritability and anxiety). Reducing caffeine consumption prior to quitting can help to avoid unpleasant effects of excessive caffeine.

How will nicotine patch affect other medications? Nicotine replacement therapy does not directly affect blood levels of other medications. However, quitting smoking does affect the blood levels of some medications. The potential need for dose adjustments of other medications should be discussed with a healthcare provider.

PATIENT HANDOUT: NICOTINE INHALER

Ron Pohar

How would I benefit from using this medication? The nicotine inhaler can help individuals to reduce or quit smoking by gradually weaning off nicotine. The nicotine inhaler helps to reduce the symptoms of nicotine withdrawal (irritability, frustration, anxiety, restlessness, difficulty concentrating) and to control cravings for nicotine. The nicotine inhaler is also helpful because it can serve as a substitute for the hand-to-mouth ritual that is part of cigarette smoking. Those who use nicotine inhalers when attempting to quit are about twice as likely to be successful as those who do not.

How should I use medication? Set a target quit date for stopping smoking. On that day, use of the nicotine inhaler can be started. The nicotine inhaler is available over the counter. The nicotine inhaler requires assembly of a mouthpiece and cartridge. After assembling the inhaler and cartridge, the mouthpiece is placed in the mouth and the user inhales deeply into the back of the throat or puffs in short breaths. This allows the nicotine to be absorbed through the lining of the mouth and throat and into the bloodstream. Nicotine from the inhaler is absorbed into the body more slowly than nicotine from a cigarette, which is absorbed from the lungs. Because of this, it takes about 3–4 times longer to notice an effect with the nicotine inhaler than with a cigarette. Each cartridge is designed to provide 80 inhalations over a 20-minute period but the entire cartridge does not have to be used at one time. For example, if you use the inhaler for 5 minutes at a time, the cartridge can last for 4 uses. Generally, 6–12 cartridges are used each day for 3 months, and then the number of cartridges is gradually reduced over a 6–12 week period. The inhaler should be kept between 15°C to 30°C, so avoid storing them in a car during extreme temperatures.

What are the common side effects with this medication? The most common side effects of the nicotine inhaler include a mild irritation in the mouth and/or throat and cough. Stomach upset can also occur. With continued use of the nicotine inhaler, these side effects tend to subside.

What symptoms would indicate that I should stop taking this medication? If you experience chest pain, irregular heartbeat, leg pain, fainting or severe stomach upset, consider stopping the use of the inhaler and contacting your healthcare provider.

Can I drink beverages with caffeine while taking this medication? It is generally advised to reduce caffeine (e.g. in tea, coffee, colas, energy drinks, etc.) intake when quitting smoking because the tar in cigarette smoke helps the liver to process caffeine more quickly. When you stop smoking, the liver's ability to process caffeine returns to its normal level, and the effect of caffeine will feel stronger and may produce symptoms similar to nicotine withdrawal (for example, irritability and anxiety). Reducing caffeine consumption prior to quitting can help to avoid unpleasant effects of excessive caffeine. Also, coffee, tea, citrus juice, soft drinks, and alcohol are best avoided 30 minutes before and after using the nicotine inhaler because these may prevent the medication from working properly.

How will the nicotine inhaler affect other medications? Generally, the nicotine inhaler does not directly affect blood levels of other medications. However, quitting smoking does affect the blood levels of some medications. The potential need for dose adjustments of other medications should be discussed with a healthcare provider.

PATIENT HANDOUT: NICOTINE LOZENGE

Ron Pohar

How would I benefit from using this medication? Nicotine lozenges can help individuals to reduce or quit smoking by gradually weaning off nicotine. Nicotine lozenges help to reduce the symptoms of nicotine withdrawal (irritability, frustration, anxiety, restlessness, difficulty concentrating) and to quickly control cravings for nicotine. Those who use nicotine lozenges when attempting to quit are about twice as likely to be successful as those who do not.

How should I use this medication? Set a target quit date for stopping smoking and start using nicotine lozenges that day. Nicotine lozenges are available over the counter. Nicotine lozenges are placed in the mouth and left to dissolve, delivering nicotine through the lining of the mouth while the lozenge dissolves. The lozenge is occasionally moved from one side of the mouth to the other until it dissolves completely, which takes about 20 to 30 minutes. Lozenge tablets should not be chewed or swallowed as this will reduce absorption of nicotine. Avoid eating or drinking 15 minutes before and during use of nicotine lozenges. Nicotine lozenges are available in two strengths (2 mg and 4 mg). Consultation with a healthcare provider can help you determine which strength is appropriate based upon the number of cigarettes smoked each day and how soon after awakening the first cigarette is smoked. Generally, 1 to 2 lozenges are used every 1 to 2 hours to a maximum of 15 lozenges per day. Smoking cessation is most successful when at least 8 lozenges are used daily. Nicotine lozenges are continued for up to 6 months, during which time the dose is reduced. During the tapering period, it might be helpful to substitute sugarless candy for the lozenges.

What are the common side effects with this medication? A hot or tingling sensation usually occurs as the lozenge dissolves. Mouth or throat irritation can occur, as can nausea, heartburn, headaches, and hiccups. Side effects are more common when lozenges are taken one after the other and tend to subside with continued use of the nicotine lozenge.

What symptoms would indicate that I should stop taking this medication? If you experience chest pain, irregular heartbeat, leg pain, fainting, or severe stomach upset, consider stopping use of the lozenge and contacting your healthcare provider.

Can I drink beverages with caffeine while taking this medication? It is generally advised to reduce caffeine (e.g. in tea, coffee, colas, energy drinks, etc.) intake when quitting smoking because the tar in cigarette smoke helps the liver to process caffeine more quickly. When you stop smoking, the liver's ability to process caffeine returns to its normal level, and the effect of caffeine will feel stronger and may produce symptoms similar to nicotine withdrawal (for example, irritability and anxiety). Reducing caffeine consumption prior to quitting can help to avoid unpleasant effects of excessive caffeine.

How will nicotine lozenges affect other medications? Nicotine lozenges do not directly affect blood levels of other medications. However, quitting smoking does affect the blood levels of some medications. The potential need for dose adjustments of other medications should be discussed with a healthcare provider.

PATIENT HANDOUT: NICOTINE MOUTH SPRAY

Ron Pohar

How would I benefit from using this medication? Nicotine mouth spray can help individuals to reduce or quit smoking by gradually weaning off nicotine. The spray helps to reduce the symptoms of nicotine withdrawal (irritability, frustration, anxiety, restlessness, difficulty concentrating) and to control cravings for nicotine. Those who use nicotine mouth spray when attempting to quit are about twice as likely to be successful as those who do not.

How should I use this medication? Set a target quit date for stopping smoking. On that day, the nicotine mouth spray can be started. The nicotine mouth spray is available over the counter. During the first 6 weeks, use 1 or 2 sprays when you would usually smoke and when craving cigarettes. Generally 1–2 sprays are used every 30–60 minutes. The maximum dose of nicotine mouth spray is 2 sprays at 1 time, 4 sprays in 1 hour, and 64 sprays in 24 hours. During weeks 7–9, reduce the number of sprays that you use each day, with the goal of reaching half the amount originally used by the end of week 9. By week 12, you should be using about 2–4 sprays each day. Nicotine mouth spray is generally used for 3–6 months.

Nicotine mouth spray must be unlocked prior to use according to the package insert. Before using nicotine mouth spray for the first time, the pump must be loaded (primed) by spraying it into the air a few times until a fine spray comes out. To administer the spray, hold it as close to your open mouth as possible and press the top of the device to activate one spray. Avoid inhaling during spraying and avoid contact with the lips. Do not swallow for a few seconds following administration. A second spray can be used if needed. It is then recommended to close the spray pump (according to directions found in the package insert) to avoid accidental administration. The pump must be primed again prior to administration if it has not been used for more than 2 days.

What are the common side effects with this medication? The most common side effects of nicotine mouth spray include hiccups, headache, nausea, tingling, or burning in the mouth, dry mouth, increased production of saliva, and stomach upset.

What symptoms would indicate that I should stop taking this medication? If you experience chest pain, irregular heartbeat, leg pain, fainting, or severe stomach upset, consider stopping the use of the nicotine mouth spray and contacting your healthcare provider.

Can I drink beverages with caffeine while taking this medication? It is generally advised to reduce caffeine (e.g. in tea, coffee, colas, energy drinks, etc.) intake when quitting smoking because the tar in cigarette smoke helps the liver to process caffeine more quickly. When you stop smoking, the liver's ability to process caffeine returns to its normal level and the effect of caffeine will feel stronger and may produce symptoms similar to nicotine withdrawal (for example, irritability and anxiety). Reducing caffeine consumption prior to quitting can help to avoid unpleasant effects of excessive caffeine. Also, coffee, tea, citrus juice, soft drinks, and alcohol are best avoided 15 minutes before and after using nicotine mouth spray because they may prevent the medication from working properly.

How will nicotine mouth spray affect other medications? Generally, nicotine mouth spray does not directly affect blood levels of other medications. However, quitting smoking does affect the blood levels of some medications. The potential need for dose adjustments of other medications should be discussed with a healthcare provider. Nicotine mouth spray contains a small amount of alcohol (ethanol). Sixty-four doses per day of the mouth spray would contain about the same amount of alcohol as one teaspoonful of wine containing 12% ethanol.

9.2

Sustained-Release Bupropion (Bupropion SR)

PETER SELBY AND ANDRIY SAMOKHVALOV

BUPROPION 2-(T-BUTYLAMINO)-3'-CHLOROPROPIOPHENONE IS AN AMINOKETONE synthesized in 1968 as a new antidepressant agent.[37,38] Its chemical structure and mechanism of action are similar to phenylethylamines (e.g. amphetamine)[39] and its three-dimensional structure resembles other drugs with psychostimulant properties.[40]

Originally marketed as an antidepressant, bupropion initially showed minimal clinical effectiveness in the treatment of depression and had modest to no efficacy in other psychiatric conditions. Incidence of seizures resulted in its withdrawal from the market. The discovery that patients given this medication stopped smoking spontaneously led to the development of bupropion as a smoking cessation medication.[41] Currently bupropion is available under the trade names Wellbutrin™ and Zyban™ for the treatment of depression and smoking cessation respectively. In addition to immediate release formulation (taken 3 times a day), sustained release (SR, twice-a-day dosing) and extended release (XL, once daily administration) forms are available. For smoking cessation, however, there is no XL-formulation available, and bupropion is supplied in a sustained-release form for twice a day dosing for this indication.

MECHANISM OF ACTION

Bupropion does not mediate smoking cessation by treating symptoms of clinical depression,[42,43] though it reduces the negative affective state associated with quitting smoking in the first few weeks.[44-46] This was found to be a mediating mechanism for achieving abstinence in 20% of the cases in a randomized controlled trial while effects of bupropion were independent of change in positive affect and withdrawal symptoms.[47] Other studies have shown that bupropion may reduce symptoms of nicotine withdrawal[42,48] and may also lead to a reduction in craving when compared with placebo persisting up to one year.[48] It is hypothesized that bupropion primarily attenuates nicotine withdrawal symptoms by mimicking the effects of nicotine on dopaminergic and noradrenergic receptors when smokers quit. Its ability to antagonize nicotinic receptors prevents relapse by attenuating the rewarding properties of nicotine.[49]

PHARMACOKINETICS

When taken orally, bupropion is absorbed completely and peak plasma concentration is reached within 1–3 hours with a biphasic decline. About 84% of the compound is protein-bound,[50] and the half-life ($t\frac{1}{2}$) of the initial (alpha) phase is approximately 1.5 hours and that of the second (beta) phase approximately 14 hours.[15] Bupropion is metabolized in the liver almost exclusively by CYP P450 2B6 into 3 active metabolites: hydroxybupropion, threohydrobupropion, and erythrohydrobupropion.[51-55] Hydroxybupropion is the most potent of the metabolites with a half-life of 20–25 hours. Finally, bupropion is excreted mainly through the urine.

Though the $t\frac{1}{2}$ is 15% longer in females, there is no need for dosage adjustments (minor differences in peak concentrations are not clinically significant). In a small study in the elderly, there was evidence of accumulation of metabolites with repeated dosing,[56] so dose reductions may be required to prevent toxicity. Although bupropion is not used in persons with active alcohol withdrawal, there are no significant effects of alcohol levels on bupropion or vice versa.[57] Alcoholic liver disease also does not significantly alter the kinetics of the drug.[58]

INDICATIONS AND CLINICAL USE

For smoking cessation, bupropion is prescribed in sustained-release (SR) form. To ensure tolerability, and to test for adverse reactions, the initial dose of bupropion is 150 mg once a day. This is increased to 150 mg twice a day within 3 days if no clinically significant side effects are observed. Although some evidence suggests efficacy in persons not ready to quit smoking, clinical prerequisites for bupropion are motivation (readiness) to quit and it is used in persons smoking 10 or more cigarettes per day. Normally a quit date is set for 7–14 days after starting the medication. However, delayed responses are seen up to 4 weeks after starting the medication.

CONTRAINDICATIONS

Absolute contraindications are the following:

1. Hypersensitivity: the risk of anaphylactic-type reactions is 1–3 in 1000 and usually appears within 7–14 days of starting bupropion.
2. Concurrent use of an MAOI due to high risk of hypertensive crisis.
3. Presence of a seizure disorder.
4. Concomitant use of another formulation of bupropion (e.g. combining Zyban™ with Wellbutrin™).

In the general population, the risk of seizure with immediate release formations is estimated to be 1 in 1000 with doses of 300 mg of bupropion per day where no single dose exceeds 150 mg. The estimated risk of seizure increases 10-fold with doses between 450 and 600 mg per day.[59] If post-marketing surveillance studies are included, the risk of seizures is 1 in 3000 and in half the cases, the patients had pre-existing seizure disorders or distinct risk factors for seizures.[60]

Relative contraindications include high risk for seizures due to underlying conditions or concomitant use of medications. Bupropion is not recommended for patients with head trauma, eating disorders, acute withdrawal from other sedative-hypnotics including alcohol, or other drugs that reduce the seizure threshold. It is advisable in these situations to weigh the risks versus benefits of all modes of smoking cessation before prescribing bupropion.

ADVERSE REACTIONS

Bupropion is relatively free of side effects. The most common recorded are insomnia (30–45%), headache (29.3%), dose-dependent incidence of dry mouth (5–15%), dizziness (7.3%), nausea (7.3%), anxiety (6.9%), constipation (6.7%), irritability (6.2%), concentration disturbance (5.2%), depression (4.2%), and dream abnormality (2.9%).[61,62] In clinical trials, only 10% of patients discontinued medication due to adverse effects.[63]

There are clinical trial and postmarketing reports with SSRIs and other newer antidepressants, including bupropion, in both pediatrics and adults, of severe agitation-type adverse events coupled with self-harm or harm to others. The agitation-type events include: akathisia, agitation, disinhibition, emotional lability, hostility, aggression, depersonalization. In some cases, the events occurred within several weeks of starting treatment. Rigorous clinical monitoring for suicidal ideation or other indicators of potential for suicidal behaviour is advised in patients of all ages. This includes monitoring for agitation-type emotional and behavioural changes.

OVERDOSE

Bupropion has low abuse potential. Overdose-related deaths are very uncommon and most individuals recover with supportive care following an overdose.

DRUG INTERACTIONS

There are a few drugs that interact with bupropion due to its primary metabolism by CYP450 2B6. The hydroxylation of bupropion is inhibited in vitro by medication used in HIV/AIDS treatment, e.g. nelfinavir, ritonavir, and efavirenz.[64] Medications such as carbamazepine, phenytoin, and phenobarbital may induce bupropion's metabolism. In vitro, bupropion inhibits CYP450 2D6, the isoenzyme responsible for metabolism of certain CNS and cardiovascular drugs. Lowering of the dose of these drugs may be warranted when prescribing bupropion.

USE DURING PREGNANCY AND LACTATION

In animal studies no teratogenicity has been found even at high doses of bupropion. There are, however, no well-controlled trials in pregnant smokers. Bupropion accumulates in breast milk but in some mother–infant pairs no bupropion or its metabolites were detected in the serum of the infants.[65,66]

EFFECTS ON WEIGHT

In short-term smoking cessation studies, weight gain has been minimal but not maintained once medication was stopped.[42,43] There appears to be an inverse dose response relationship with weight gain.[43] Patients on combined bupropion and nicotine patch therapy have the least weight gain.[42] The use of bupropion appears to postpone the usual weight gain associated with smoking cessation.

EFFICACY

There have been at least 7 randomized placebo controlled trials of bupropion for smoking cessation in over 8,000 patients. In a recent review, it was concluded that there was approximately twice the likelihood to achieve abstinence when receiving bupropion vs. placebo in the short term (i.e. 4–9 weeks post quit) with a moderate decline in efficacy to 75% in the long term (abstinence at 52 weeks).[67] In a recent meta-analysis comparing first-line smoking cessation therapies, bupropion was superior to placebo but half as efficacious as varenicline in 4-week continuous abstinence. There was no difference at 12 months.[68]

In a dose-finding study (N=615), the rate of continuous abstinence at the end of 7 weeks of treatment was significantly better for those who received 300 mg of bupropion (44.2%) than those who received 150 mg (38.6%) and in the placebo group (19%). The continuous abstinence at 1 year showed no statistical difference between groups receiving bupropion (300 mg; 23.1%, 100 mg; 22.9%) but were greater than placebo (12.4%).[43] It can be concluded that bupropion is superior to placebo, and that the 300 mg dose has initial but not sustainable benefit when compared with the 150-mg dose.

RE-TREATMENT

A study examined 450 smokers who had previously used bupropion 300 mg per day for at least 2 weeks but had not quit or had only stopped smoking for a short period of time. They were found to be more likely to respond to bupropion versus placebo (OR=13.2, 95% CI, 3.9–44.2 for those who had not responded at all and OR 8.6, 95%CI 2.8-25.8 for those who had stopped for less than 28 days). Those who had stayed in treatment for more than 7 weeks in their prior experience with bupropion were also more likely to stop smoking regardless of treatment assignment during this study.[69]

RELAPSE PREVENTION

In a double-blind study, 429 subjects who achieved abstinence using bupropion 300 mg/day for 7 weeks were randomized to continue receiving bupropion or placebo for 45 weeks. The continuous abstinence rate was higher in the bupropion group than in the placebo group at study week 24 (17 weeks after randomization) (52.3% vs. 42.3%; P = 0.03) but did not differ between groups afterwards. The authors conclude that in persons who initially respond to bupropion, additional therapy for 12 months delayed smoking relapse. This effect appears to last up to 6 months after stopping the medication.[70]

DELAYED RESPONSE

A post hoc analysis was conducted to examine whether subjects had a delayed response to bupropion.[42,71] Among the 467 patients who continued to smoke in the first 3 weeks, an additional 58 quit by the end of week 9. These findings allow clinicians to encourage patients to continue with their medication if they have not stopped smoking completely in the first 3 weeks of treatment.

COMBINATION THERAPY

In a multi-centre study, 893 bupropion-naïve smokers were randomized to bupropion (n=244), nicotine patch (n=244), bupropion and a nicotine patch (n=245), or placebo (n=160 subjects). Abstinence rates at week 52 were 5.6% in the placebo group, 9.8% in the patch group, 18.4% in the bupropion group, and 22.5% in the combined group. The lowest rate of discontinuation was in the combination group and the highest in the placebo group. The study demonstrated that bupropion alone or in combination with nicotine replacement was better than nicotine replacement alone or placebo.[72]

SMOKELESS TOBACCO USERS

In a meta-analysis of all treatments for smokeless tobacco use, bupropion increased point prevalence of tobacco abstinence at 12 weeks [OR=2.1; 95% CI: 1.0-4.2].[73]

EFFECTIVENESS IN THE REAL WORLD

Gold et al. (2002) conducted a naturalistic study in a Veterans Affairs primary care clinic to evaluate the effectiveness of bupropion and NRT or both in the real world.[74] Consecutive consenting patients (n=189) self-selected one of three treatments: nicotine patch (n=27), bupropion (n=101), and bupropion plus nicotine patch (n=61). Six-month self-reported abstinence rates were 14.8%, 27.7%, and 34.4%, respectively. Odds ratios for 6-month abstinence, with the nicotine patch as reference, showed no statistical difference between groups but there was a trend similar to that found under controlled conditions. Due to several limitations in design and attrition, these data should be interpreted with caution.

WOMEN

Post hoc analysis of the Jorenby et al. (1999) study[42] showed that bupropion is more effective in women than men at the end of 52 weeks but not at the end of treatment (OR=4.6 vs 1.7).[75] Moreover, women in the bupropion group had similar rates of negative affect at the end of treatment as men. In the placebo group, the women complained of higher rates of negative affect than men. In a post hoc analysis of the Hays et al. (2001) relapse prevention study,[70] bupropion appeared to mitigate the effect of gender on smoking cessation.[76]

UNMOTIVATED SMOKERS

There is preliminary evidence for efficacy of bupropion in smokers unwilling, ambivalent, or not ready to quit. In a trial of bupropion vs. placebo for 7 weeks, in 214 smokers not ready to quit smoking, a third of the subjects were able to reduce their smoking by half and were then willing to make a quit attempt; 14% were abstinent at the end of treatment versus 8% in the placebo group (p=0.003).[77,78] The complete findings have not been published yet. A recent Canadian study showed that though bupropion has no effect on the number of cigarettes smoked in those unmotivated to quit, it lowers plasma cotinine levels, suggesting subconscious changes in the amount of nicotine being inhaled per puff.[79]

CONCLUSION

Bupropion is considered a safe and effective first-line option for smoking cessation. It has added qualities as an antidepressant, and may have particular application in persons with a history of depression wanting to quit smoking.

PATIENT HANDOUT: SUSTAINED-RELEASE (SR) BUPROPION

Ron Pohar

How would I benefit from using this medication? When used with supportive counselling, individuals who take bupropion are about twice as likely to quit smoking as those who do not. Bupropion helps to reduce symptoms of nicotine withdrawal and craving of cigarettes but does not contain nicotine and is not related to nicotine.

How should I take this medication? A date to stop smoking is set prior to starting treatment with bupropion. This date should be roughly during the second week of treatment because bupropion takes about 1 week to start working. Bupropion is only available by prescription. For the first 3 days of treatment, 150 mg of bupropion is taken in the morning. The dose is then increased to 150 mg twice daily with 1 tablet taken in the morning and the other in early evening at least 8 hours after the first tablet. Treatment with bupropion is generally continued for 12 weeks but may be taken longer if needed.

What are the common side effects with this medication? The most common side effects of bupropion include dry mouth and insomnia (difficulty sleeping). These side effects are most common in the first weeks of treatment and may go away with continued use. Sucking on sugarless candy or chewing sugarless gum can help with dry mouth. Taking the second dose of bupropion in the early evening (e.g. 6:00 pm) may help with insomnia. Less common side effects include hallucinations and behavioural changes such as increased impulsiveness, agitation, anxiety, aggression or hostility, and feeling suicidal or thinking of harming yourself or others. If you experience these feelings or any others that are concerning to you, consider stopping bupropion and contacting a healthcare provider. Similar mood and behaviour changes can, in fact, occur due to nicotine withdrawal and when quitting smoking without taking bupropion.

What is the risk of seizures when taking this medication? There is a risk of seizure (approximately 0.1%) when taking bupropion. Certain medical conditions (e.g. a seizure disorder, eating disorder, history of liver problems, or head injury) and medications can increase the risk of a seizure. Taking more than the recommended dose of bupropion also increases the risk of seizures. Do not take more than 150 mg twice daily of bupropion and if a tablet is missed, just take bupropion at the next scheduled dosing time. Do not double the dose of bupropion, as this may theoretically increase the seizure risk.

What symptoms would indicate that I should stop taking this medication? Changes in behaviour may suggest that bupropion should be discontinued. A healthcare provider should be contacted if behavioural changes occur.

What can happen if I smoke while taking this medication? Prior to the target quit date, you will continue to smoke while taking bupropion; however, smoking after the target quit date may reduce the chances of successfully quitting.

Can I use nicotine replacement therapy while taking this medication? Yes, bupropion can be used in combination with nicotine patches and other forms of nicotine replacement therapy (such as gum).

What can happen if I drink alcohol while taking this medication? Drinking alcohol while taking bupropion is not recommended as it may increase the chances of having a seizure or allergic reaction. As well, bupropion may make you more sensitive to the effects of alcohol.

Can I drink beverages with caffeine while taking this medication? It is generally advised to reduce caffeine intake when quitting smoking because the tar in cigarette smoke helps the liver to process caffeine more quickly. When you stop smoking, the liver's ability to process caffeine returns to its normal level, and the effect of caffeine will feel stronger and may produce symptoms similar to nicotine withdrawal (for example, irritability and anxiety). Reducing caffeine consumption prior to quitting can help to avoid unpleasant effects of excessive caffeine.

How will bupropion affect other medications? Bupropion can interact with a number of medications and quitting smoking can also affect the blood levels of some medications. The potential need for dose adjustments of other medications should be discussed with a healthcare provider.

9.3

Varenicline

JOTHAM COE

THE MOLECULAR AND PHARMACOLOGICAL JOURNEY TO VARENICLINE BEGAN IN THE early 90s. A science had emerged in the 1970s and 1980s that a spectrum exists between the extremes of receptor agonism and antagonism. Partial agonists reside between the extremes and were targeted as medicinal aids to smoking cessation.[80] The tools to measure partial agonist effects were developing concurrently. Stable human cell lines expressing nicotinic receptor subtypes were not yet commonplace, existing only in specialized laboratories. Even more challenging was the development of in vivo pharmacological measures that reliably gauged agonism and antagonism in animals. Methods were assembled and developed to aid the evaluation of the chemical pharmacopeia. Over 100,000 pharmaceutical compounds and natural products from plants and animals were initially evaluated, revealing few with robust signals as partial agonists. In the end, 5 natural products (anabasine, lobeline, nicotine, anabaseine, cytisine) offered medicinal chemistry starting points to pursue and optimize. Other pharmacological tools such as nicotinic antagonists (mecamylamine and hexamethonium) were used to support the initial research. From significant triage, cytisine emerged as the most promising chemical prototype, with a relatively stable architecture and reasonably promising in vitro partial agonist activity.[80]

More work revealed that although potent at the receptor, cytisine displayed weak in vivo potency and poor brain penetration insufficient to effectively block the effects of smoked nicotine on receptors in mice and humans.[81] The synthesis and pharmacological evaluation of hundreds of analogs ultimately led to the discovery of varenicline, a compound with excellent in vivo potency, duration, selectivity, and safety to progress into development.[82] By 1999, varenicline had entered human clinical trials for safety and PK (pharmacokinetic) evaluation then progressed through clinical trials to establish efficacy.

INDICATIONS

Varenicline tartrate is available for oral treatment as an aid to smoking cessation.

MECHANISM OF ACTION

Varenicline is an α4β2 nicotinic acetylcholine receptor (nAChR) partial agonist that binds potently and selectively to this subtype with a greater affinity than nicotine; it stimulates α4β2 receptor mediated activity, but to a lesser degree than nicotine, and can also block nicotine, a full agonist at α4β2 nAChRs, from binding to that receptor. Stimulation of this receptor leads to release of dopamine in the mesolimbic system, which is thought to be a component of the "reward" that reinforces smoking and relieves craving and withdrawal symptoms. The dual mechanism of partial agonist receptor stimulation to address craving and withdrawal symptoms while antagonizing nicotine binding to block reward upon smoking is a hallmark of the partial agonist profile.[82]

PHARMACOKINETICS

Varenicline is rapidly absorbed across the gastric mucosa, reaching a peak plasma concentration (C-max) in about 4 hours. With daily dosing, plasma concentrations reach a steady state after 4 days. Varenicline has a half-life of 17-24 hours; it is minimally metabolized and is excreted virtually unchanged by the kidneys.[83,84] After the recommended dose of 1.0 mg BID, steady state plasma levels are 6–10 ng/mL.[84]

CLINICAL STUDIES / EFFICACY

Comparison with bupropion   Two identically-designed randomized, double-blind, placebo-controlled trials established varenicline's efficacy by comparing 1.0 mg twice daily with bupropion SR 150 mg twice daily and with placebo. The primary outcome was biochemically confirmed measures of exhaled carbon monoxide (10 ppm) and self-reported continuous abstinence rate (CAR) for the last 4 weeks of treatment, weeks 9–12. At 12 weeks, the 4-week CAR in both studies was 18% with placebo, 30% with bupropion SR and 44% with varenicline. The smoking cessation rates for varenicline were significantly higher compared with both placebo and bupropion. Nine months after treatment had stopped, continuous smoking cessation rates in the 2 studies were 8% and 10% with placebo, 15% and 16% with buproprion SR, and 22% and 23% with varenicline.[85-87]

Comparison with NRT   Varenicline has also been compared with transdermal nicotine patch (NRT) in an open-label, randomized, multi-centre clinical trial for smoking cessation in a study comparing a 12-week standard regimen of varenicline (N = 376) with a 10-week standard regimen of transdermal nicotine replacement therapy (NRT N = 370). The continuous abstinence rate CAR for the last 4 weeks of treatment was significantly greater for varenicline (55.9%) than NRT (43.2%; odds ratio (OR) 1.70, 95% CI 1.26 to 2.28, p=0.001). After completion of treatment, subjects were followed for an additional 40 weeks up to week 52 to assess how many remained abstinent. The week 52 CAR (NRT, weeks 8–52; varenicline, weeks 9–52) was 26.1% for varenicline and 20.3% for NRT (OR 1.40, 95% CI 0.99 to 1.99, p=0.056). During treatment, varenicline significantly reduced craving, withdrawal symptoms and smoking satisfaction compared with NRT (p=0.001).[88]

Maintenance therapy A randomized controlled trial evaluated whether an additional 12 weeks of treatment with varenicline was beneficial for those who had stopped smoking during the first 12 weeks of treatment. A total of 1,928 subjects initially received open-label varenicline 1.0 mg twice daily. At 12 weeks, those who responded and had not smoked for at least 7 days (63%) were randomized to continue varenicline or switch to placebo. Continuous smoking cessation rates were significantly better with varenicline than with placebo at the end of the second 12 weeks of treatment (71% vs. 50%) and remained better from weeks 13–52 (44% vs. 37%).[89]

Studies have demonstrated that flexible quit dates exhibited similar efficacy and safety compared with the fixed day-8 quit date.[90]

Smokers from different regions of the world The efficacy and safety of varenicline as an aid to smoking cessation has been evaluated in smokers from Asia, Latin America, and the Middle East without comorbidities. Efficacy in Europeans and non-Europeans is the same.[91-94]

Smokers with cardiovascular disease In a randomized clinical trial of varenicline and placebo in 700 patients with cardiovascular disease who smoked, patients received varenicline 1.0 mg twice daily or placebo for 12 weeks, followed by a 40-week non-treatment period. All patients also received smoking cessation counselling throughout the study. Varenicline was efficacious in this study; there was a significantly higher 4-week continuous quit rate in patients who received the drug compared with placebo (47.0% vs. 13.9%; OR, 6.11; 95% [CI], 4.18 to 8.93). In addition, patients who received varenicline had a significantly higher continuous abstinence rate from week 9 through week 52 (19% vs. 7%).[95]

Smokers with chronic obstructive pulmonary disease (COPD) Varenicline was more efficacious than placebo for smoking cessation in patients with mild to moderate COPD and demonstrated a safety profile consistent with that observed in previous trials. CAR for weeks 9–12 was significantly higher for patients in the varenicline group (42.3%) than for those in the placebo group (8.8%) (OR, 8.40; 95% CI, 4.99-14.14; P<.0001). CAR in the patients treated with varenicline remained significantly higher than in those treated with placebo through weeks 9–52 (18.6% vs 5.6%) (OR, 4.04; 95% CI, 2.13-7.67; P<.0001).[96]

CONTRAINDICATIONS

The only contraindication listed in the package insert is history of serious hypersensitivity or skin reactions to varenicline.[97]

ADVERSE EFFECTS

The most frequent adverse effect of varenicline in clinical trials was dose-dependent nausea, which was generally mild to moderate in intensity and became less severe with continued use of the drug. The nausea is typically transient, lasting 30–60 minutes. It caused approximately 3% of patients to discontinue treatment prematurely. Other adverse events include: insomnia (18%), abnormal dreams (13%), constipation (8%), vomiting (5%), and flatulence (6%).[98] In a separate, 1-year safety study, 40% of patients treated with varenicline 1.0 mg twice daily reported nausea compared with 8% of placebo-treated patients.[99]

Abrupt discontinuation of varenicline was associated with an increase in irritability and sleep disturbances in up to 3% of patients. This suggests that, in some patients, varenicline may produce mild physical dependence which is not associated with addiction.[99]

Varenicline is classified by the FDA as category C (risk cannot be ruled out) for use during pregnancy. There are no adequate and well-controlled studies of varenicline use in pregnant women. Varenicline should be used during pregnancy only if the potential benefit justifies the potential risk to the fetus. For nursing mothers, it is not known whether varenicline is excreted in human milk. In animal studies varenicline was excreted in milk of lactating animals. Because many drugs are excreted in human milk and because of the potential for serious adverse reactions in nursing infants from varenicline, a decision should be made whether to discontinue nursing or to discontinue the drug, taking into account the importance of the drug to the mother.

Precautions and warnings The varenicline package insert has a boxed warning regarding post-marketing reports of neuropsychiatric events in patients taking varenicline:

Serious neuropsychiatric events, including, but not limited to depression, suicidal ideation, suicide attempt and completed suicide have been reported in patients taking varenicline. Some reported cases may have been complicated by the symptoms of nicotine withdrawal in patients who stopped smoking. Depressed mood may be a symptom of nicotine withdrawal. Depression, rarely including suicidal ideation, has been reported in smokers undergoing a smoking cessation attempt without medication. However, some of these symptoms have occurred in patients taking varenicline who continued to smoke.

In patients treated with varenicline, there have been post-marketing reports of neuropsychiatric symptoms such as depressed mood, agitation, aggression, hostility, changes in behaviour, suicide related events and worsening of pre-existing psychiatric disorders. However, no causal relationship has been established.

Williams et al. (2011) examined the post-marketing experience with varenicline, including case reports, clinical trials and secondary analyses of large clinical datasets and concluded that "despite case reports of serious neuropsychiatric symptoms in patients taking varenicline, including changes in behavior and mood, causality has not been established. Recent analyses of large datasets from clinical trials have not demonstrated that varenicline is associated with more depression or suicidality than other treatments for smoking cessation."[99] A large placebo- and active-controlled safety study of smokers with and without psychiatric disorders is underway to further evaluate varenicline for neuropsychiatric events in a controlled clinical setting.[100]

In a placebo-controlled study of varenicline in subjects with stable cardiovascular disease, with approximately 350 patients per treatment arm, certain cardiovascular events were reported more frequently in patients treated with varenicline than in patients treated with placebo. These events included angina pectoris (13 patients in the varenicline arm vs. 7 in the placebo arm), and the serious cardiovascular events of nonfatal myocardial infarction (4 vs. 1) and nonfatal stroke (2 vs. 0).[95] The package insert instructs physicians to "inform patients with cardiovascular disease of the symptoms of a heart attack and stroke, and instruct them to get emergency medical help right away if they experience any of these symptoms."[101]

Weight gain   Fear of weight gain prevents many tobacco-dependent patients from trying to stop smoking, and weight gain after stopping is a major cause of relapse. Unlike bupropion SR[102,103] and most nicotine medications,[104] varenicline does not reduce the weight gain commonly seen after stopping smoking. Among the patients who stopped smoking after 12 weeks' treatment, weight gain averaged about 7 lbs with placebo, 6 lbs with varenicline, and 4 lbs with bupropion SR.[85–87]

DRUG INTERACTIONS

Varenicline is excreted primarily unchanged in the urine and has negligible effects on the cytochrome P450 system. Since metabolism of varenicline represents less than 10% of its clearance, drugs known to affect the cytochrome P450 system are unlikely to alter the pharmacokinetics of varenicline. Varenicline is mediated by the human organic cation transporter OCT2. Although co-administration with inhibitors of OCT2, such as the H2-antagonist cimetidine, can decrease renal clearance of varenicline and increase its serum concentrations by 29%, this increase is not clinically meaningful and does not necessitate any dose adjustments. Co-administration of varenicline with transdermal nicotine did not affect nicotine pharmacokinetics. However, nausea, headache, vomiting, dizziness, dyspepsia, and fatigue occurred more frequently with the combination than with transdermal nicotine alone. The combination caused 8 of 22 patients (36%) to discontinue treatment prematurely, compared with 1 of 17 (6%) who discontinued transdermal nicotine plus placebo.[88] While there are no drug interactions with varenicline, smoking cessation, with or without treatment with varenicline, may alter the pharmacokinetics or pharmacodynamics of some drugs, such as theophylline, warfarin, and insulin. Dosage adjustment for these drugs may be necessary.[83,84,98]

DOSAGE

Smoking cessation therapies are more likely to succeed for patients who are motivated to stop smoking and who are provided additional advice and support. Patients should be provided with appropriate educational materials and counselling to support the quit attempt. Varenicline should be taken after eating and with a full glass of water.

As an aid to smoking cessation, the recommended initial dosage of varenicline is 0.5 mg once daily for 3 days followed by 0.5 mg twice daily for days 4–7. The dose is then increased to 1.0 mg twice daily for the remainder of the 12 weeks of treatment. Patients are advised to set a target quit date and start the drug one week before that date. Alternatively, the patient can begin varenicline titrating the dose as just discussed, and then quit smoking between days 8 and

35 of treatment. The dosage of varenicline should be reduced in patients with severe renal impairment. Patients who cannot tolerate adverse effects of varenicline may have the dose lowered temporarily or permanently. Patients should be treated with varenicline for 12 weeks. For patients who have successfully stopped smoking at the end of 12 weeks, an additional course of 12 weeks treatment with varenicline is recommended to further increase the likelihood of long-term abstinence. The package insert does not limit the total duration of use. Patients who do not succeed in stopping smoking during 12 weeks of initial therapy, or who relapse after treatment, should be encouraged to make another attempt once factors contributing to the failed attempt have been identified and addressed. In Canada, a daily dosage of either 1.0 mg per day (i.e. 0.5 mg twice a day) or 2.0 mg per day (1.0 mg twice a day) is approved, with each dosage strength having a titration dosing as already discussed. The choice of dosing regimen should be based on physician judgment and patient preference.[98,101]

OVERDOSAGE

In case of overdose, standard supportive measures should be instituted as required. Varenicline has been shown to be dialyzed in patients with end-stage renal disease; however, there is no experience in dialysis following overdose. One case report of overdose showed that after spontaneously vomiting and treatment with oral activated charcoal follow by an additional round of vomit, the patient resolved over 4 hours and was discharged.[105,106]

COMBINATION THERAPY

Varenicline has not been approved for use in combination with other treatments as an aid to smoking cessation. Such combinations are being investigated.[107,108]

CONCLUSION

Varenicline has been demonstrated to be an effective aid to smoking cessation with a positive benefit-risk profile.

PATIENT HANDOUT: VARENICLINE

Ron Pohar

How would I benefit from using this medication?   When used with supportive counselling, individuals who take varenicline are 2–3 times more likely to quit smoking than those who do not. Varenicline helps to reduce symptoms of nicotine withdrawal and craving of cigarettes by affecting receptors in the brain that are involved with nicotine addiction. Varenicline does not contain nicotine.

How should I take this medication?   A date to stop smoking is set prior to starting treatment with varenicline and should ideally be between 8 and 14 days after you start taking varenicline. Varenicline is only available by prescription. Treatment with varenicline is started with 0.5 mg daily on days 1–3, then increased to 0.5 mg twice daily for days 4–7 (one tablet with breakfast and one tablet with supper). After the first week of treatment, the dose of varenicline may remain at 0.5 mg twice daily or may increase to 1.0 mg twice daily (i.e. a total daily dose of 2 mg) depending on side effects and how well varenicline is working. Varenicline is continued for 12 weeks and possibly longer for those who have stopped smoking or substantially reduced their cigarette consumption during the first 12 weeks of treatment. Varenicline can also be used effectively at a total dose of 1.0 mg per day (i.e. 0.5 mg twice a day).

What are the common side effects with this medication?   The most common side effects of varenicline include those that affect the stomach (e.g. nausea and vomiting). As well, some individuals experience difficulty sleeping and vivid or unusual dreams. These side effects generally occur in the first weeks of treatment and may go away with continued use. Some individuals (those with and without previous issues with their mental health) have experienced changes in behaviour or mood while taking varenicline. However, similar mood and behaviour changes can occur due to nicotine withdrawal and when quitting smoking without taking varenicline.

What symptoms would indicate that I should stop taking this medication?   Changes in behaviour may suggest that treatment with varenicline be re-evaluated. Examples of behavioural changes that require further follow-up may include increased agitation, restlessness, anxiety, or aggression; development of hallucinations; inability to control impulses; and feeling hostile, symptoms of mania, feeling depressed, confused, paranoid, or suicidal. If you experience these feelings or any others that are concerning, consider stopping the use of varenicline and contacting a healthcare provider.

What can happen if I smoke while taking this medication?   Prior to the target quit date, you may continue to smoke while taking varenicline but may notice that varenicline may change the taste of cigarettes. Smoking after the target quit date, however, reduces the chances of successfully quitting.

What can happen if I drink alcohol while taking this medication?   Drinking alcohol may increase the chances of experiencing changes in behaviour when taking varenicline.

What can happen if I consume caffeine while taking this medication?   It is generally advised to reduce caffeine intake when quitting smoking because the tar in cigarette smoke helps the liver to process caffeine more quickly. When you stop smoking, the liver's ability to process caffeine returns to its normal level, and the effect of caffeine will feel stronger and may produce symptoms similar to nicotine withdrawal (for example, irritability and anxiety). Reducing caffeine consumption prior to quitting can help to avoid unpleasant effects of excessive caffeine.

How will varenicline affect my other medications?   No important drug interactions with varenicline have been identified to date but quitting smoking can affect the blood levels of some medications. The effect of quitting smoking on your other medications should be discussed with a healthcare provider.

9.4

Cardiovascular Complications of Pharmacotherapy for Smoking Cessation

SERENA TONSTAD

CIGARETTE SMOKING CONTRIBUTES TO ACUTE CARDIOVASCULAR EVENTS AND UNDER-lying atherosclerosis through promotion of thrombosis, endothelial dysfunction, inflammation, and coronary vasoconstriction. Aids to smoking cessation may potentially reduce cardiovascular disease (CVD) risk more than other pharma-cological preventive interventions.[109] Approved pharmacotherapies for smoking cessation include nicotine replacement therapy (NRT), bupropion and vareni-cline. All pharmacotherapies interact with nicotinic receptors, which are integral to the sympathetic nervous system, and have been examined in regard to their cardiovascular effects.

NICOTINE REPLACEMENT THERAPY

Nicotine replacement therapy stimulates nicotinic receptors leading to release of dopamine and other neurotransmitters in the brain and reduction in nico-tine withdrawal symptoms. The cardiovascular pharmacology of nicotine has been studied extensively.[110,111] Nicotine stimulates the sympathetic nervous sys-tem through peripheral chemoreceptors, direct effects on the brain stem and effects on more caudal portions of the spinal cord.[110] This leads to release of neurotransmitters that may contribute to hemodynamic and metabolic changes. The hemodynamic effects include an increase in heart rate and blood pressure and increased myocardial contractility. For example, nicotine acutely raises heart rate by 10 to 15 beats/minute and blood pressure by 5 to 10 mm Hg for about

30 minutes. Metabolic effects of nicotine include endothelial cell dysfunction, a more atherogenic lipid profile, and insulin resistance, though other components of cigarette smoke than nicotine play a primary causal role in these harms.[110,112]

While nicotine in cigarette smoke is delivered rapidly to central and peripheral nicotinic receptors, therapeutic nicotine results in low blood concentrations, and exhibits a flat dose-response relation and rapid development of tolerance.[110-114] Smoking a single cigarette for 5 minutes results in peak nicotine venous plasma levels within 5–8 minutes while use of a nicotine patch takes several hours to attain peak levels, which are much lower than peaks achieved with smoking. Nicotine patch produces less sympathetic activation than cigarette smoking. In an experimental study, nicotine patch was shown to be associated with a decrease rather than increase in the total exercise-induced myocardial perfusion defect size in smokers trying to quit.[115] An angiographic study of normal and diseased coronary artery segments found no enhancement of sympathetic stimulation of coronary vasoconstriction in subjects taking nicotine gum.[116]

Initial case reports of acute cardiac events in smokers using NRT have not been confirmed in observational, clinical and meta-analytic studies. The observational Lung Health Study followed up 5,887 smokers with chronic obstructive lung disease, of which about two-thirds were provided with nicotine gum.[117] No increase in hospital admissions for cardiovascular events was shown with nicotine gum treatment during 5 years of follow-up. In a population-based case control study among 68 hospitals, there was no association between myocardial infarction and use of nicotine patches.[118] Randomized controlled clinical trials of patients with cardiovascular disease have been conducted.[112] In a study using the transdermal nicotine patch in 156 patients with established CHD, NRT did not adversely impair cardiac symptoms or electrocardiogram findings.[119] A 10-week trial of transdermal nicotine in 584 outpatient military veteran smokers with CVD found a non-statistically significant decrease in cardiac events in NTR-treated subjects after 14 weeks of follow-up.[120] Other trials similarly found no increased cardiac risks with NRT.[112] A systematic review including trials with 9,253 mostly low CVD risk participants found no excess adverse CVD events with nicotine patch.[121] Event rates were similar in the nicotine (0.3–3%) and placebo groups (1–2%), with no indication of an increase or reduction in events in the NRT groups. In a case series of 33,247 individuals prescribed NRT, of whom 861 had had a myocardial infarction and 506 a stroke, there was a progressive increase in incidence of first myocardial infarction in the 56 days leading up to the first NRT prescription, but the incidence fell thereafter, and was not increased in the 56 days after NRT was started.[122]

There is no direct evidence regarding how soon after an acute cardiac event NRT may be safely administered, but if the alternative is continued smoking, NRT is most likely safer. An observational study of smokers admitted to hospital with acute coronary syndromes found no difference in short- or long-term mortality in patients receiving transdermal NRT or no patches.[123] On the other hand, some clinicians have suggested that NRT be formally contraindicated in patients with unstable coronary syndrome, pending prospective studies.[124] Label warnings and clinical guidelines[125] state that NRT should be discontinued during acute cardiovascular events and NRT is not recommended in smokers with a history of myocardial infarction within the past 2 weeks, uncontrolled hypertension, hypertension that emerges during treatment, severe arrhythmias, or serious or worsening angina. Despite this, smokers admitted to acute coronary care units are widely prescribed NRT to ameliorate symptoms of nicotine withdrawal as nicotine withdrawal may worsen cardiac status.[123] McRobbie and Hajek recommended use of short-acting ad libitum NRT-like gum in such situations to allow rapid discontinuation if needed.[126]

A retrospective, case-control study raised questions about the safety of administering NRT to smokers admitted to the intensive care unit.[127] A total of 90 NRT-treated patients were compared with 90 controls that were similar to the NRT-treated patients in terms of age, gender, ethnicity, and severity of illness. The hospital mortality rate was 20% in the NRT-treated cases versus 7% in the controls (p=0.0085) and the 28-day intensive care unit-free days were lower in NRT-treated cases compared to controls. A major limitation of the study was lack of matching for the degree and duration of smoking. Furthermore, the NRT group consisted of a tiny fraction of patients admitted during the study period indicating a strong element of selection bias.

In conclusion, most of the evidence suggesting cardiovascular safety of NRT comes from studies of smokers without cardiovascular disease diagnoses with some evidence available for outpatient smokers with established coronary heart disease (CHD). Nicotine Replacement Therapy should not be withheld from smokers with stabilized acute coronary symptoms who are routinely monitored in regard to cardiovascular vital signs. Use of NRT in a hemodynamically unstable patient, patients with serious arrhythmias, and those with worsening coronary symptoms requires the judgment and experience of the attending physician.

BUPROPION

Bupropion reduces nicotine withdrawal symptoms, mimics nicotinic effects on dopamine and noradrenaline, and may antagonize brain nicotinic receptors blocking the reinforcing effects of nicotine.[128] Adrenergic stimulation raises concerns about increased myocardial work and potential increase in blood pressure, effects that are more evident at high doses.

Clinical evidence has been obtained from uncontrolled post-marketing reports of hypertension, cardiovascular events, and deaths in smokers taking the drug for cessation and observational studies. A prescription-event monitoring study in England found no unexpected increase in cardiovascular events in patients taking the drug for smoking cessation.[130] A retrospective review of bupropion-only exposures reported to the Toxic Exposure Surveillance System in the US found that cardiac toxicity other than tachycardia was rare.[131] Uncontrolled studies of bupropion in depressed patients with CVD have shown increases in blood pressure, but no effects on heart rate, rhythm, or contractility.[129] The combination of nicotine patch and bupropion has been associated with a non-significant trend toward a greater incidence of new or worsening hypertension compared to placebo (6.1% vs. 3.1%).[132]

Three randomized controlled clinical trials of bupropion have been performed in smokers with CVD. In a trial of 629 outpatients with stable CVD, bupropion promoted smoking cessation rates after one year to 22% versus 9% with placebo.[133] There were 24 cardiovascular adverse events in the bupropion group versus 14 with placebo. These events were most commonly angina, hypertension, and palpitations. Two of the anginal events were classified as serious, but were also considered to be worsening of a preexisting condition. There were no adverse effects of bupropion on blood pressure or heart rate in the study. Two studies examined bupropion in patients with acute CHD.[129,134] Both studies appear underpowered in regard to efficacy when compared with the study in patients with stable CVD. In one study, 248 smokers admitted for acute CVD were followed for 1 year after 12 weeks of treatment with bupropion or placebo.[129] Cessation rates were more favourable with bupropion after 3 months, but not after 1 year. There were no cardiovascular deaths with bupropion versus 1 with placebo. The incidence of cardiovascular events was 13% with bupropion versus 14% with placebo during the period of ≤30 days of stopping drug, and 25% versus 17% in the respective groups after 12 months of follow-up (incidence rate ratio 1.56; 95% CI, 0.90–2.72). In 151 smokers with acute coronary syndrome abstinence rates were similar with 8 weeks of treatment with bupropion or placebo after short-term and 1-year follow-up.[134] There were 2 myocardial infarctions in the bupropion group versus 1 in the placebo group, 2 cases of acute coronary syndrome in the bupropion group versus 5 cases in the placebo group, and no deaths in either group. In both of these studies in patients with acute CHD, blood pressure was not increased by bupropion compared with placebo.

In conclusion, other than case reports of increases in blood pressure, bupropion seems to be safe in the CVD population. Efficacy in the population with acute CHD has not been established.

VARENICLINE

Varenicline is a partial agonist of the nicotinic a4β2 acetylcholine receptor, which is the major subtype of nicotinic acetylcholine receptors associated with nicotine addiction. Varenicline has a dual mechanism of action with agonist effects that ameliorate craving and antagonist effects that reduce reward associated with smoking. In addition, varenicline appears to be a full agonist of the a7 nicotinic acetylcholine receptor.[135]

Results of a multi-centre, double-blind, placebo-controlled study of 714 smokers with stable CVD showed high efficacy for varenicline and have been interpreted to support the safety of varenicline in smokers with stable CVD.[136] In this study, varenicline was over 2.5 times more effective than placebo in promoting continuous abstinence after 1 year (19.2% vs. 7.2%). Though the study was not powered to examine event rates, analysis of adjudicated events was done for the entire year of follow-up, including 9 months after use of varenicline or placebo. This revealed that varenicline and placebo treated groups did not differ significantly in regard to CVD mortality (0.3 vs. 0.6%; difference -0.3%; 95% confidence interval [CI] -1.3 to 0.7), cardiovascular events (7.1 vs. 5.7%; difference 1.4%; 95% CI -2.3 to 5.0), or all-cause mortality (0.6 vs. 1.4%; difference -0.8%: 95% CI -2.3 to 0.6). The study further showed that varenicline had no adverse effects on heart rate or blood pressure.

More than 18 months after publication of the study, the US Federal Drug Administration reviewed these results and suggested a potential increased risk of certain cardiovascular events in smokers with stable CVD. The following information was added to the labelling of the drug: "Patients with CVD should be instructed to notify their healthcare providers of new or worsening cardiovascular symptoms and to seek immediate medical attention if they experience signs and symptoms of myocardial infarction."[137] In Canada, the latest drug label revised July 4, 2011 states that "there have been reports of myocardial infarction (MI) and cerebrovascular accident (CVA) including ischemic and hemorrhagic events in patients taking varenicline. In the majority of the reported cases, patients had preexisting cardiovascular disease and/or other risk factors. Although smoking is a risk factor for MI and CVA, a contributory role of varenicline cannot be ruled out, based on temporal relationship between medication use and events." The updated product monograph issued December 14, 2011 reiterated these statements.

The CVD population study publication did not separate CV events into treatment-emergent ones (on-treatment or 30 days after treatment) or events that occurred more than 30 days after the cessation of varenicline or placebo.[136] This information was subsequent to the FDA report added to the varenicline US package insert as follows: "Treatment-emergent cardiovascular events reported with a frequency ≥ 1% in either treatment group in this study were angina pectoris (3.7% and 2.0% for varenicline and placebo, respectively), chest pain (2.5% vs. 2.3%), peripheral edema (2.0% vs. 1.1%), hypertension (1.4% vs. 2.6%), and palpitations (0.6 % vs. 1.1%). The following treatment-emergent adjudicated serious cardiovascular events occurred with a frequency >1% in either treatment group: nonfatal MI (1.1% vs. 0.3% for varenicline and placebo, respectively), and hospitalization for angina pectoris (0.6% vs. 1.1%). During non-treatment follow-up to 52 weeks, the adjudicated events were needed for coronary revascularization (2.0% vs. 0.6%), hospitalization for angina pectoris (1.7% vs.1.1%), and new diagnosis of peripheral vascular disease (PVD) or admission for a PVD procedure (1.1% vs. 0.6%). Some of the patients requiring coronary revascularization underwent the procedure as part of management of nonfatal MI and hospitalization for angina." This added information shows that a significant number of cardiovascular events occurred after 30 days of discontinuation of study medication.

Currently with this label change, a meta-analysis of 14 clinical trials that included 8,216 smokers with or without CVD looked at the primary outcome of any ischemic or arrhythmic adverse cardiovascular event including myocardial infarction, unstable angina, coronary revascularization, coronary artery disease, arrhythmias, transient ischemic attacks, stroke, sudden death, cardiovascular-related death, or congestive heart failure.[138] This study found these events occurred in 52 (1.06%) of 4,908 smokers treated with varenicline and in 27 (0.82%) of 3,308 smokers given placebo resulting in an odds ratio of 1.72 with a 95% CI of 1.09–2.71. The secondary outcome of the meta-analysis was death, which occurred in 0.143% of varenicline-treated subjects versus 0.212% of placebo-treated subjects (7 in each group). The numbers of deaths were considered too small for separate analysis. The authors acknowledged that the event rates were very low, resulting in imprecise estimates, differences in ascertainment due to symptoms of withdrawal that may mimic cardiac symptoms (which would be more common in the varenicline group due to their higher cessation rates) could not be considered, and that the events were not pre-specified. As an example of events that were included in the primary outcome of the meta-analysis that are not typically used to evaluate cardiovascular safety a respondent from the manufacturer, Pfizer, pointed to atrial arrhythmias, of which 7 were observed in the varenicline group versus 1 in the placebo group.[139] It is not known how excluding such events would affect the statistical significance of the results, but that is likely. Other respondents noted further potential weaknesses including a different method to calculate the odds ratio (which did not find statistically significant increased risk with varenicline).[140] Other problems that the meta-analysis did not address were that the rate of patients lost to follow-up was higher in the placebo than the varenicline groups in most of the studies, and that the timing of events (whether occurring within 30 days of stopping the drug, or in the subsequent follow-up period) was not considered. Currently a new meta-analysis is being conducted by the manufacturer in conjunction with the US Food and Drug Administration to address some of these methodological issues. A meta-analysis recently conducted independent of the manufacturer sheds further light on these uncertainties.[141] This meta-analysis studied the same endpoints as did the previous meta-analysis[138] but did not include events reported after 30 days of study medication discontinuation. Also a larger number of studies were included (22 trials versus 14 trials in the Singh et al meta-analysis). This meta-analysis found no relationship between use of varenicline and treatment emergent CVD events. The summary estimate for the risk difference was 0.27% (p=0.15), a difference that was not clinically or statistically significant. Furthermore the authors also estimate risk using different methods, and none of the methods revealed risk associated with varenicline use.

Other information on usage of varenicline in patients with cardiovascular disease is a poster presentation by Willers.[142] This study reported that in 204 patients, mostly with heart and lung disease, treatment with varenicline resulted in an abstinence rate of 38% at 12 months with generally mild side effects.

Activation of nicotinic acetylcholine receptors could in theory be associated with sympathetic activation. It has been postulated that activation of the a7 receptor in the brainstem may modulate of parasympathetic output from the brainstem to the heart.[138] Any clinically significant hemodynamic or pro-arrhythmic effects of such modulation are not known. Nicotinic acetylcholine receptor subtypes that potentially could contribute to cardiovascular effects include ganglionic α3b4 and a7 nicotinic acetylcholine receptors, and/or central a7 and a4β2 nicotinic acetylcholine receptors.[143] A recent abstract indicated that therapeutic varenicline concentrations are insufficient to activate α3b4 nicotinic acetylcholine receptors or a7 nicotinic acetylcholine receptors, do not desensitize the α3b4 nicotinic acetylcholine receptor, and can only desensitize a small fraction of a7 nicotinic acetylcholine receptors at the high end of the therapeutic concentration range.[143] Additionally, though therapeutic concentrations of varenicline, as nicotine from NRT use, cause substantial desensitization and minimal activation of central a4β2 nicotinic acetylcholine receptors (the mechanism thought to underlie clinical efficacy for smoking cessation) these concentrations are unlikely to have CV effects, since CV effects of a4β2 nicotinic acetylcholine receptors were only shown in pharmacological studies after extremely high nicotine concentrations.[143]

The study in the population with stable cardiovascular disease showed that varenicline had no adverse effects on heart rate or systolic blood pressure, though there was a slight increase in diastolic blood pressure (1.6 mmHg, 95% confidence interval, 0.04-3.1) in the group treated with varenicline.[136] This was not analyzed in regard to any concomitant change in body weight. Varenicline treatment has not been reported to be associated with increased blood pressure or heart rate in other 12-week placebo-controlled studies.[144,145] Likewise, in a study of long-term treatment for 1 year, there were no differences in blood pressure or pulse between the varenicline and placebo groups.[146] Four cases of tachycardia in varenicline-treated subjects were reported in this study, but only 1 was considered serious and was not considered treatment-related by the investigator. In a study performed in 36 HIV-infected smokers, systolic blood pressure was unchanged but diastolic blood pressure increased by a mean of 6 mmHg after 12 weeks of treatment with varenicline.[147] Diastolic but not systolic pressure remained increased by 4 mm Hg after the end of the 12-week treatment with varenicline. There was no control group, and the effects of change in weight were not taken into account. Stopping smoking is associated with lower heart rate, but not consistently with decreased blood pressure – in fact lower blood pressure may be observed in smokers. Because varenicline treated subjects are more likely to quit, smoking status may confound study of hemodynamic changes of cessation. Hypertension may be associated with varenicline in individual patients.[148]

Studies of single doses of varenicline in smokers found no indication of autonomic cardiovascular dysfunction indicated by heart rate variability.[149] In a case series of cardiovascular events collected during postmarketing surveillance of varenicline in New Zealand reports of hypotension that were thought to be possibly related to varenicline were identified.[150]

In conclusion data does not support the notion that varenicline treatment leads to CVD. The number of events is small, the incidence of events is very low, and differences between varenicline and placebo were not clinically or statistically significant in recent meta-analysis.

CONCLUSION

All medications used to aid smoking cessation, a primary way to reduce cardiovascular risk, have been questioned in regard to cardiovascular safety. Medications for smoking cessation are usually used for a period of up to 12 weeks, and there is no convincing evidence that CVD is increased during their use or within 30 days following discontinuation of the drug. Both bupropion and varenicline effectively increase cessation rates in smokers with CVD; and CVD event rates are expected to be lower following cessation. However, certain events have been observed numerically more often during the period of follow-up. This is possibly due to the relatively small numbers of subjects that have been studied.

9.5

Neuropsychiatric Considerations

CHARL ELS

SEVERAL NEUROPSYCHIATRIC ADVERSE EVENTS HAVE BEEN REPORTED IN PERSONS taking either bupropion or varenicline. In 2010 Health Canada compelled the makers of varenicline to carry a boxed warning label. A year prior, in the US, similar boxed warnings were introduced for *both* varenicline and bupropion. These warnings are usually reserved for drugs that have been linked the most serious safety issues or adverse events.[151]

Neuropsychiatric events under discussion in the context of smoking cessation include: abnormal dreams, mood changes, hostility, sleep disturbances/disorders, suicidal ideation, suicide, psychotic reactions, and self-harm events. The possible relation between the use of medication and the neuropsychiatric effects has become a focus of interest.

The fact that smokers are at a 2-3 times higher risk of suicide confounds the issue.[152] Abstinence from smoking may profoundly impact on mental status, irrespective of which drug is used to achieve abstinence. Three salient mechanisms postulated to potentially be involved in mental status changes may include nicotine withdrawal (see chapter 10), the withdrawal of the B-carbolines, and the issue of caffeine intoxication when individuals quit smoking. Tobacco plants contain biologically active compounds (β-Carbolines, i.e. harman and nor-harman), which act like weak monoamine oxidase inhibitors (and which act in an antidepressant fashion). Quitting smoking is hence the equivalent of discontinuing a naturally occurring antidepressant. The scheme demonstrates the inhibition of monoamine oxidase enzyme and compares smokers with non-smokers.

Smokers consume greater quantities of coffee (containing caffeine) compared to non-smokers. Caffeine is a substrate for cytochrome P450 1A2, which is induced by tar in tobacco smoke (and not by nicotine, nicotine replacement therapy, bupropion, or varenicline). Quitting smoking may lead to a decreased activity level of this enzyme, which leads to increased caffeine levels in smokers who quit while consuming caffeine as they did before quitting smoking.

The only neuropsychiatric side-effects that are currently considered causally linked to the use of all smoking cessation medications include abnormal dreams and sleep disturbances. Current evidence does not support a direct causal link between the use of smoking cessation medications and other neuropsychiatric adverse effects like depression and suicide.[153]

Despite this absence of evidence for a causal link between medication and depression and suicide, health providers are challenged with incorporating sufficient levels of vigilance to neuropsychiatric adverse events into their routine cessation treatment. Given the high degree of comorbidity between depression and smoking, prudence suggests screening for mood issues in patients who consume tobacco products regardless of their readiness to quit or whether prescribing cessation medications.[151]

IMAGE 1. Whole-body images of MAO distribution in a nonsmoker versus in a smoker.

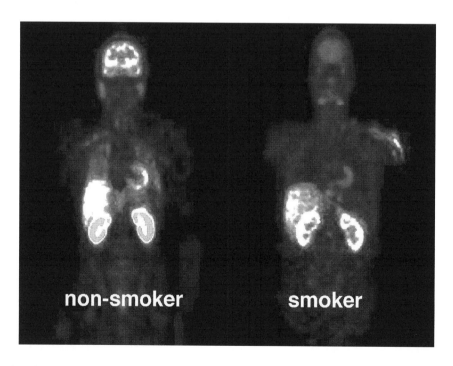

Smokers have been shown to have reduced levels of brain MAO leading to speculation that MAO inhibition by tobacco smoke may underlie some of the behavioral and epidemiological features of smoking.[154] Reproduced with permission of Dr. J. Fowler; Brookhaven National Laboratory.

REFERENCES

1   Stead L, Perera R, Bullen C, Mant D, Lancaster T. Nicotine replacement therapy for smoking cessation. Cochrane Database Syst rev; 2008.

2   McIvor A. Tobacco control and nicotine addiction in Canada: current trends, management and challenges. Canadian Respiratory Journal. 2009;16;21-6.

3   Borland R, Li L, Driezen P, Wilson N, Hammond D, Thompson M, Fong G, Mons U, Willemsen M, McNeill A, Thrasher J, Cummings K. Cessation assistance reported by smokers in 15 countries participating in the International Tobacco Control (ITC) policy evaluation surveys. Addiction. 2012 (forthcoming).

4   Hammond D, Reid J, Driezen P, Cummings K, Borland R, Fong G, McNeill A. Smokers' use of nicotine replacement therapy for reasons other than stopping smoking: findings from the ITC Four Country Survey. Addiction. 2008;103:1696-703.

5   Benowitz N. Nicotine Addiction. N Engl J Med. 2010;362:2295-303.

6   Benowitz N. Clinical pharmacology of nicotine: implications for understanding, preventing, and treating tobacco addiction. Clin Pharmacol Ther. 2008;83:531-41.

7   Bullen C, Howe C, Lin R, Grigg M, Laugesen M, McRobbie H, Clover M, Walker N, Wallace-Bell M, Whittaker R, Rodgers A. Pre-cessation nicotine replacement therapy: pragmatic randomized trial. Addiction. 2010;105:1474-83.

8   Shiffman S, Scharf D, Shadel W, Gwaltney C, Dang Q, Paton S, Clark D. Analyzing milestones in smoking cessation: illustration in a nicotine patch trial in adult smokers. J Consult Clin Psychol. 2006;74:276-85.

9   Ebbert J, Montori V, Erwin P, Stead L. Interventions for smokeless tobacco use cessation. Cochrane Database Syst rev; 2011.

10   Hughes JR, Shiffman S, Callas P, Zhang J. A meta-analysis of the efficacy of over-the-counter nicotine replacement. Tob Control. 2003;12:21-7.

11   Doggrell S. Which is the best primary medication for long-term smoking cessation - nicotine replacement therapy, bupropion or varenicline? Expert Opin Pharmacother. 2007;8:2903-15.

12   Fagerström K-O, Hughes JR. Nicotine concentrations with concurrent use of cigarettes and nicotine replacement: a review. Nicotine Tob Res. 2002;8:S73-79.

13   Hughes JR, Carpenter MJ. Does smoking reduction increase future cessation and decrease disease risk? A qualitative review. Nicotine Tob Res. 2006;8:739-49.

14   Moore D, Aveyard P, Connock M, Wang D, Fry-Smith A, Barton P. Effectiveness and safety of nicotine replacement therapy assisted reduction to stop smoking: systematic review and meta-analysis. BMJ. 2009;338:b1024.

15   Beard E, McNeill A, Aveyard P, Fidler J, Michie S, West R. Association between use of nicotine replacement therapy for harm reduction and smoking cessation: a prospective study of English smokers. Tob Control. 2011 doi:10.1136/tobaccocontrol-2011-050007. Abstract.

16   Hughes J. Significance of off-label use of NRT. Addiction. 2008;103:1704-5.

17   Kozlowski L, Giovino G, Edwards B, DiFranza J, Foulds J, Hurt R, Niaura R, Sachs D, Selby P, Dollar K, Bowen D, Cummings K, Counts M, Fox B, Sweanor D, Ahern F. Advice on using over-the-counter nicotine replacement therapy-patch, gum, or lozenge-to quit smoking. Addict Behav. 2007;32:2140-50.

18   Hatsukami DK, Stead LF, Gupta P. Tobacco addiction. Lancet. 2008;371:2027-38.

19   Foulds J. Use of nicotine replacement therapy to treat nicotine withdrawal syndrome and aid temporary abstinence. Int J Clin Pract. 2010;64:292-4.

20   Hughes J, Stead L, Lancaster T. Antidepressants for smoking cessation. Cochrane Database Syst rev; 2009.

21   Fiore M, Jaen C, Baker T, Bailey W, Benowitz N, Curry S, Dorfman S, Froelicher E, Goldstein M, Healton C, Henderson P, Heyman R, Koh H, Kottke T, Lando H, Mecklenburg R, Mermelstein R, Mullen P, Orleans C, Robinson L, Stitzer M, Tommasello A, Villejo L, Wewers M. Treating tobacco use and dependence: clinical practice guideline. Washington DC: US Public Health and Human Services; 2008.

22   Shiffman S, Brockwell SE, Pillitteri JL, Gitchell JG. Use of smoking-cessation treatments in the United States. Am J Prev Med. 2008;34:102-11.

23   Zapawa LM, Hughes J, Benowitz N, Rigotti N, Shiffman S. Cautions and warnings on the US OTC label for nicotine replacement: what's a doctor to do? Addict Behav. 2011;36:327-32.

24   Grimshaw GM, Stanton A. Tobacco cessation interventions for young people. Cochrane Database Syst rev; 2006.

25   Rogers J. Tobacco and pregnancy. Reprod Toxicol. 2009;28:152-60.

26   Coleman T, Chamberlain C, Cooper S, Leonardi-Bee J. Efficacy and safety of nicotine replacement therapy for smoking cessation in pregnancy: systematic review and meta-analysis. Addiction. 2010;106:52-61.

27   Ford CL, Zlabek JA. Nicotine replacement therapy and cardiovascular disease. Mayo Clin Proc. 2005:80:652-6.

28   Zevin S, Jacob III P, Benowitz N. Dose-related cardiovascular and endocrine effects of transdermal nicotine. Clin Pharmacol Ther. 1998;64:87-95.

29   Hughes J. How confident should we be that smoking cessation treatments work? Addiction. 2009;104:1637-40.

30   Mills E, Wu P, Lockhart I, Wilson K, Ebbert J. Adverse events associated with nicotine replacement therapy (NRT) for smoking cessation. A systematic review and meta-analysis of one hundred and twenty studies involving 177,390 individuals. Tobacco Induced Diseases. 2010;8:1-15.

31   Shields P. Long-term nicotine replacement therapy: cancer risk in context. Cancer Prevention Research. 2011;4:1719-23.

32   Kroon L. Drug interactions with smoking. Am J Health Syst Pharm. 2007;64:1917-21.

33   Cinciripini PM, Wetter DW, McClure JB. Scheduled reduced smoking: effects on smoking abstinence and potential mechanisms of action. Addict Behav. 1997;22:759-67.

34   Solarino B, Rosenbaum F, RieBelmann B, Buschmann C, Tsokos M. Death due to ingestion of nicotine-containing solution: case report and review of the literature. Forensic Sci Int.
2010;195:e19-22.

35   Polosa R, Caponnetto P, Morjaria J, Papale G, Campagna D, Russo C. Effect of an electronic nicotine delivery device (e-cigarette) on smoking reduction and cessation: a prospective
6-month pilot study. BMC Public Health. 2011;11:1-12.

36   McRobbie H, Thornley S, Bullen C, Lin R-B, Senior H, Laugesen M, Whittaker R, Hajek P. A
randomized trial of the effects of two novel nicotine replacement therapies on tobacco withdrawal
symptoms and user satisfaction. Addiction. 2010;105:1290-8.

37   Baltzly R, Mehta NB. N-sec- and N-t-alkyl derivatives of methoxamine and related compounds. J Med Chem. 1968;11(4):833-44.

38   Soroko FE, Mehta NB, et al. Bupropion hydrochloride ((+/-) alpha-t-butylamino-3-chloropro-
piophenone HCl): a novel antidepressant agent. J Pharm Pharmacol. 1977;29(12):767-70.

39   Dufresne RL, Weber SS, et al. Bupropion hydrochloride. Drug Intell Clin Pharm.
1984;18(12):957-64.

40   Froimowitz M, George C. Conformational analysis and a crystal structure of bupropion, an antidepressant with dopamine reuptake blocking activity. J Chem Inf Comput Sci.
1998;38(3):506-10.

41   Ferry LH, Robbins AS, et al. Enhancement of smoking cessation using the antidepressant
bupropion hydrochloride [abstract 2670]. Circulation. 1992;86(4 Suppl 1):I-671.

42   Jorenby DE, Leischow SJ, et al. A controlled trial of sustained-release bupropion, a nicotine
patch, or both for smoking cessation. N Engl J Med. 1999;340(9):685-91.

43   Hurt RD, Sachs DPL, et al. A comparison of sustained-release bupropion and placebo for
smoking cessation. N Engl J Med. 1997;337(17):1195-1202.

44   Balfour DJ. The pharmacology underlying pharmacotherapy for tobacco dependence: a
focus on bupropion. Int J Clin Pract. 2001;55(1):53-7.

45   Lerman C, Roth D, et al. Mediating mechanisms for the impact of bupropion in smoking
cessation treatment. Drug Alcohol Depend. 2002;67(2):219-23.

46   Strong DR, Kahler CW, et al. Impact of bupropion and cognitive-behavioral treatment for
depression on positive affect, negative affect, and urges to smoke during cessation treatment.
Nicotine Tob Res. 2009;11(10):1142-53.

47   Shiffman S, Johnston JA, et al. The effect of bupropion on nicotine craving and withdrawal.
Psychopharmacol. 2000;148(1):33-40.

48   Durcan MJ, Deener G, et al. The effect of bupropion sustained-release on cigarette craving
after smoking cessation. Clin Ther. 2002;24(4):540-51.

49   Warner C, Shoaib M. How does bupropion work as a smoking cessation aid? Addict Biol.
2005;10(3):219-31.

50   Findlay JW, Van Wyck Fleet J, et al. Pharmacokinetics of bupropion, a novel antidepressant
agent, following oral administration to healthy subjects. Eur J Clin Pharmacol. 1981;21(2):127-35.

51   Lai AA, Schroeder DH. Clinical pharmacokinetics of bupropion: a review. J Clin Psychiatry. 1983;44(5 Pt 2):82-4.

52   Ferris RM, Cooper BR. Mechanisms of antidepressant activity of bupropion. J Clin Psychiatry. 1993;11:2-14.

53   Hsyu PH, Singh A, et al. Pharmacokinetics of bupropion and its metabolites in cigarette smokers versus non-smokers. J Clin Pharmacol. 1997;37(8):737-43.

54   Hesse LM, Venkatakrishnan K, et al. CYP2B6 mediates the in vitro hydroxylation of bupropion: potential drug interactions with other antidepressants. Drug Metab Dispos. 2000;28(10):1176-83.

55   Faucette SR, Hawke RL, et al. Evaluation of the contribution of cytochrome P450 3A4 to human liver microsomal bupropion hydroxylation. Drug Metab Dispos. 2001;29(8):1123-9.

56   Sweet RA, Pollock BG, et al. Pharmacokinetics of single- and multiple-dose bupropion in elderly patients with depression. J Clin Pharmacol. 1995;35(9):876-84.

57   Posner J, Bye A, et al. Alcohol and bupropion pharmacokinetics in healthy male volunteers. Eur J Clin Pharmacol. 1984;26(5):627-30.

58   DeVane CL, Laizure SC, et al. Disposition of bupropion in healthy volunteers and subjects with alcoholic liver disease. J Clin Psychopharmacol. 1990;10(5):328-32.

59   Dunner DL, Zisook S, et al. A prospective safety surveillance study for bupropion sustained-release in the treatment of depression. J Clin Psychiatry. 1998;59(7):366-73.

60   West R. Bupropion SR for smoking cessation. Expert Opin Pharmacother. 2003;4(4):533-40.

61   Hays JT, Ebbert JO. Bupropion for the treatment of tobacco dependence: guidelines for balancing risks and benefits. CNS Drugs. 2003;17(2):71-83.

62   Johnston JA, Fiedler-Kelly J, et al. Relationship between drug exposure and the efficacy and safety of bupropion sustained release for smoking cessation. Nicotine Tob Res. 2001;3(2):131-40.

63   Hughes JR, Stead LF, et al. Antidepressants for smoking cessation. Cochrane Database Syst rev;2003;2:CD000031.

64   Hesse LM, von Moltke LL, et al. Ritonavir, efavirenz, and nelfinavir inhibit CYP2B6 activity in vitro: potential drug interactions with bupropion. Drug Metab Dispos. 2001;29(2):100-102.

65   Briggs GG, Samson JH, et al. Excretion of bupropion in breast milk. Ann Pharmacother. 1993;27(4):431-3.

66   Baab SW, Peindl KS et al. Serum bupropion levels in 2 breastfeeding mother-infant pairs. J Clin Psychiatry. 2002;63(10):910-1.

67   Fagerström K. Clinical treatment of tobacco dependence: the endurance of pharmacologic efficacy. J Clin Psychiatry Monograph. 2003;18(1):35-40.

68   Eisenberg MJ, Filion KB, et al. Pharmacotherapies for smoking cessation: a meta-analysis of randomized control trials. CMAJ. 2008;179(2):135-44.

69   Gonzales DH, Nides MA, et al. Bupropion SR as an aid to smoking cessation in smokers treated previously with bupropion: a randomized placebo-controlled study. Clin Pharmacol Ther. 2001;69(6):438-44.

70   Hays JT, Hurt RD, et al. Sustained-release bupropion for pharmacologic relapse prevention after smoking cessation: a randomized controlled trial. Ann Intern Med. 2001;135(6):423-33.

71   Jamerson BD, Nides M, et al. Late-term smoking cessation despite initial failure: an evaluation of bupropion sustained release, nicotine patch, combination therapy, and placebo. Clin Ther. 2001;23(5):744-52.

72   Jorenby D. Clinical efficacy of bupropion in the management of smoking cessation. Drugs. 2002;62(Suppl 2):25-35.

73   Ebbert JO, Rowland LC, et al. Treatments for spit tobacco use: a quantitative systematic review. Addiction. 2003;98(5):569-83.

74   Gold PB, Rubey RN, et al. Naturalistic, self-assignment comparative trial of bupropion SR, a nicotine patch, or both for smoking cessation treatment in primary care. Am J Addict. 2002;11(4):315-31.

75   Smith SS, Jorenby DE, et al. Targeting smokers at increased risk for relapse: treating women and those with a history of depression. Nicotine Tob Res. 2003;5(1):99-109.

76   Gonzales D, Bjornson W, et al. Effects of gender on relapse prevention in smokers treated with bupropion SR. Am J Prev Med. 2002;22(4):234-9.

77   Hatsukami D, Rennard S, et al. A multicentre study examining the effects of Zyban (bupropion SR) vs placebo as an aid to smoking reduction leading to cessation among smokers unwilling or unable to quit smoking [abstract]. Eighth Annual Conference of the Society for Research on Nicotine and Tobacco, Savannah GA;2002.

78   Tonstad S. Use of sustained-release bupropion in specific patient populations for smoking cessation. Drugs. 2002;62 Suppl 2:37-43.

79   Hussain S, Zawertailo L, et al. The impact of chronic bupropion on plasma cotinine and on the subjective effects of ad lib smoking: a randomized controlled trial in unmotivated smokers. Addict Behav. 2010;35(2):164-7.

80   Coe JW, Rollema H, O'Neill BT. Case history: Chantix™/Champix™ (Varenicline Tartrate), a nicotinic acetylcholine receptor partial agonist as a smoking cessation aid. Annu Reports Med Chem. 2009;44:71-101.

81   Rollema H, Shrikhande A, Ward KM, Tingley FD III, Coe JW, O'Neill BT, et al. Pre-clinical properties of the alpha4beta2 nicotinic acetylcholine receptor partial agonists varenicline, cytisine and dianicline translate to clinical efficacy for nicotine dependence. Br J Pharmacol. 2010 May;160(2):334-45.

82   Rollema H, Chambers LK, Coe JW, Glowa J, Hurst RS, Lebel LA, et al. Pharmacological profile of the alpha4beta2 nicotinic acetylcholine receptor partial agonist varenicline, an effective smoking cessation aid. Neuropharmacol. 2007 Mar;52(3):985-94.

83   Obach RS, Reed-Hagen AE, Krueger SS, Obach BJ, O'Connell TN, Zandi KS, Miller S, Coe JW. Metabolism and disposition of varenicline , a selective α4β2 acetylcholine receptor partial agonist, in vivo and in vitro. Drug Metab Dispos. 2006;34(1):121-30.

84   Faessel HM, Obach RS, Rollema H, Ravva P, Williams KE, Burstein AH. A review of the clinical pharmacokinetics and pharmacodynamics of varenicline for smoking cessation. Clin Pharmacokinet .2010;49(12):799-816.

85   Gonzales D, Rennard SI, Nides M, Oncken C, Azoulay S, Billing CB, Watsky EJ, Gong J, Williams KE, Reeves KR. Varenicline, an alpha4beta2 nicotinic acetylcholine receptor partial agonist, vs. sustained-release bupropion and placebo for smoking cessation: a randomized controlled trial. JAMA. 2006;296(1):47-55.

86   Jorenby DE, Hays JT, Rigotti NA, Azoulay S, Watsky EJ, Williams KE, Billing CB, Gong J, Reeves KR. Efficacy of varenicline, an alpha4beta2 nicotinic acetylcholine receptor partial agonist, vs placebo or sustained-release bupropion for smoking cessation: a randomized controlled trial. JAMA. 2006;296(1):56-63.

87   Nides M, Glover ED, Reus VI, Christen AG, Make BJ, Billing CB Jr, Williams KE. Varenicline versus bupropion SR or placebo for smoking cessation: a pooled analysis. Am J Health Behavior. 2008;32(6):664-75.

88   Aubin HJ, Bobak A, Britton JR, Oncken C, Billing CB Jr, Gong J, et al. Varenicline versus transdermal nicotine patch for open-label trial smoking cessation: results from a randomized open-label trial. Thorax. 2008;63(8):717-24.

89   Tonstad, S, Tønnesen, P, Hajek, P, Williams, KE, Billing, CB, Reeves, KR Effect of Maintenance Therapy with varenicline on Smoking Cessation, A Randomized Controlled Trial Journal of the American Medical Association, (2006) July 5;296(1):64–71.

90   Rennard S, Hughes J, Cinciripini PM, Kralikova E, Raupach T, Arteaga C, St Aubin LB, Russ C; Flexible Quit Date Study Group. A randomized placebo-controlled trial of varenicline for smoking cessation allowing flexible quit dates. Nicotine Tob Res. 2012 Mar;14(3):343-50.

91   Nakamura M, Oshima A, Fujimoto Y, Maruyama N, Ishibashi T, Reeves KR. Efficacy and tolerability of varenicline, an alpha4beta2 nicotinic acetylcholine receptor partial agonist, in a 12-week, randomized, placebo-controlled, dose-response study with 40-week follow-up for smoking cessation in Japanese smokers. Clinical Therapeutics 2007 Jun;29(6):1040-56.

92   Tsai ST, Cho HJ, Cheng HS, Kim CH, Hsueh KC, Billing CB Jr, Williams KE. A randomized, placebo-controlled trial of varenicline, a selective alpha4beta2 nicotinic acetylcholine receptor partial agonist, as a new therapy for smoking cessation in Asian smokers. Clin Ther. 2007 Jun;29(6):1027-39.

93   Wang C, Xiao D, Chan KP, Pothirat C, Garza D, Davies S. Varenicline for smoking cessation: a placebo-controlled, randomized study. Respirology. 2009 Apr;14(3):384-92.

94   Bolliger, Chris T, Jaqueline S Issa, Rodolfo Posadas-Valay, Tarek Safwat, Paula Abreu, Eurico A Correia, Peter W Park, and Pravin Chopra. Effects of Varenicline in Adult Smokers: A Multinational, 24-week, Randomized, Double-blind, Placebo-controlled Study. Clin Ther. 2011 Apr;33(4):465-77.

95   Rigotti NA, Pipe AL, Benowitz NL, Arteaga C, Garza D, Tonstad S. Efficacy and safety of varenicline for smoking cessation in patients with cardiovascular disease: a randomized trial. Circulation. 2010 Jan;121(2):221-9.

96   Tashkin DP, Rennard S, Hays JT, Ma W, Lawrence D, Lee TC. Effects of varenicline on smoking cessation in patients with mild to moderate COPD: a randomized controlled trial. Chest. 2011 Mar;139(3):591-9.

97   US label insert.

98   Williams KE, Reeves KR, Billing CB Jr, Pennington AM, Gong J. A double-blind study evaluating the long-term safety of varenicline for smoking cessation. Curr Med Res Opin. 2007 Apr;23(4):793-801.

99   Williams JM, Steinberg MB, Steinberg ML, Gandhi KK, Ulpe R, Foulds J. Varenicline for tobacco dependence: panacea or plight? Expert Opin Pharmacother. 2011 Aug;12(11):1799-812.

100   Clinical trials.gov no. NCT01456936. Available from: http://clinicaltrials.gov/ct2/show/NCT01456936.

101   Canadian package insert.

102   Jorenby DE, Leischow SJ, Nides MA, Rennard SI, Johnston JA, Hughes AR, Smith SS, Muramoto ML, Daughton DM, Doan K, Fiore MC, Baker TB. A controlled trial of sustained-release bupropion, a nicotine patch, or both for smoking cessation. N Engl J Med. 1997;337(17):685-91.

103   Hurt RD, Sachs DP, Glover ED, Offord KP, Johnston JA, Dale LC, Khayralla MA, Schroeder DR, Glover PN, Sullivan CR, Croghan IT, Sullivan PM. A comparison of sustained-release bupropion and placebo for smoking cessation. N Engl J Med. 1997;337(17):1195-202.

104   Dale LC, Schroeder DR, Wolter TD, Croghan IT, Hurt RD, Offord KP. Weight change after smoking cessation using variable doses of transdermal nicotine replacement. J Gen Intern Med. 1998;13(1):9-15.

105   Hedlund AJ, Broderick M, Shah N, Cantrell L. Varenicline overdose in a teenager. Clin Toxicol 2009;47(4):371.

106   Rollema Hans; Faessel Helene M; Williams Kathryn E. Varenicline overdose in a teenager- a clinical pharmacology perspective. Clinical Toxicology. 2009;47(6):605.

107   Ebbert JO, Croghan IT, Sood A, Schroeder DR, Hays JT, Hurt RD. Varenicline and bupropion sustained-release combination therapy for smoking cessation. Nicotine Tob Res. 2009;11(3):234-9.

108   Ebbert JO, Burke MV, Hays JT, Hurt RD. Combination treatment with varenicline and nicotine replacement therapy. Nicotine Tob Res. 2009;11(5):572-6.

109   Aveyard P, Moore D, Connock M, Wang D, Fry-Smith A, Barton P. Authors respond to criticism that treatment is ineffective. BMJ. 2009;338:1227.

110   Benowitz NL, Gourlay SG. Cardiovascular toxicity of nicotine: implications for nicotine replacement therapy. J Am Coll Cardiol. 1997;29:1422-31.

111   Benowitz NL. Cardiovascular toxicity of nicotine: pharmacokinetic and pharmcodynamic considerations. In NL Benowitz (Ed), Nicotine safety and toxicity (pp 19-27), New York: Oxford University Press; 1998.

112   Joseph AM, Fu SS. Safety issue in pharmacotherapy for smoking in patients with cardio-vascular disease. Prog Cardiovasc Dis. 2003;45:429-41.

113   Hukkanen J, Jacob P III, Benowitz NL. Metabolism and disposition kinetics of nicotine. Pharmacol Rev. 2005;57;79-115.

114   Zevin S, Jacob P, Benowitz NL. Dose-related cardiovascular and endocrine effects of trans-dermal nicotine. Clin Pharmacol Ther. 1998;64:87-95.

115   Mahmarian JJ, Moye LA, Nasser GA et al. Nicotine patch therapy in smoking cessation reduces the extent of exercise-induced myocardial ischemia. J Am Coll Cardiol. 1997;30:125-30.

116   Nitenberg A, Antony I. Effects of nicotine gum on coronary vasomotor responses during sympathetic stimulation in patients with coronary artery stenosis. J Cardiovasc Pharmacol. 1999;34:694-9.

117   Murray RP, Bailey WC, Daniels K et al. Safety of nicotine polacrilex gum used by 3,094 participants in the Lung Health Study. Chest. 1996;109:438-45.

118   Kimmel SE, Berlin JA, Miles C et al. Risk of acute myocardial infarction and use of nicotine patches in a general population. J Am Coll Cardiol. 2001;37:1297-1302.

119   Working Group for the study of transdermal nicotine in patients with coronary artery dis-ease. Nicotine replacement therapy for patients with coronary artery disease. Arch Intern Med. 1994;154:989-95.

120   Joseph AM, Norman SM, Ferry LH, Prochazka AV, Westman EC, Steele BG et al. The safety of transdermal nicotine as an aid to smoking cessation in patients with cardiac disease. N Engl J Med. 1996;335:1792-8.

121   Greenland S, Satterfield MH, Lanes SF. A meta-analysis to assess the incidence of adverse effects associated with the transdermal nicotine patch. Drug Safety. 1998;8;297-308.

122   Hubbard R, Lewis S, Smith C, et al. Use of nicotine replacement therapy and the risk of acute myocardial infarction, stroke, and death. Tob Control. 2005; 14:416-21.

123   Meine TJ, Patel MR, Washam JB et al. Safety and effectiveness of transdermal nicotine patch in smokers admitted with acute coronary syndromes. Am J Cardiol. 2005;95:976-8.

124   Mathew TP, Herity NA. Acute myocardial infarction soon after nicotine replacement therapy. Q J Med. 2001;94:503-6.

125   Fiore M, Baker T, Jaen C et al. Treating tobacco use and dependence: 2008 update. Clini-cal Practice Guideline. Rockville, MD: US Department of Health & Human Services, Public Health Service; 2008.

126   McRobbie H, Hajek P. Nicotine replacement therapy in patients with cardiovascular disease: guidelines for health professionals. Addiction. 2001;96;1547-51.

127   Lee AH, Afessa B. The association of nicotine replacement therapy with mortality in a medi-cal intensive care unit. Crit Care Med. 2007;35:1517-21.

128   Warner C, Shoaib M. How does bupropion work as a smoking cessation aid? Addict Biol. 2005;10:219-31.

129   Rigotti NA, Thorndike AN, Regan S et al. Bupropion for smokers hospitalized with acute cardiovascular disease. Am J Med. 2006;119:1080-7.

130   Boshier A, Wilton LV, Shakir SAW. Evaluation of the safety of bupropion (Zyban) for smoking cessation from experience gained in general practice use in England in 2000. Eur J Clin Pharmacol. 2003;59:767-73.

131   Belson MG, Kelley TR. Bupropion exposures: clinical manifestations and medical outcome. J Emerg Med. 2002;23:223-30.

132   Jorenby DE, Leischow SJ, Nides MA et al. A controlled trial of sustained-release bupropion, a nicotine patch, or both for smoking cessation. N Engl J Med. 1999;340:685-91.

133   Tonstad S, Farsang C, Klaene G et al. Bupropion SR for smoking cessation in smokers with cardiovascular disease: a multicentre, randomised study. Eur Heart J. 2003;24:946-55.

134   Planer D, Lev I, Elitzur Y, Sharon N, Ouzan E, Pugatsch T, Chasid M, Rom M, Lotan C. Bupropion for smoking cessation in patients with acute coronary syndrome. Arch Intern Med. 2011;171:1055-60.

135   Mihalak KB, Carroll FI, Leutje CW. Varenicline is a partial agonist at alpha 4 beta 2 and a full agonist at alpha 7 neuronal nicotinic receptors. Mol Pharmacol. 2006;70:801-5.

136   Rigotti NA, Pipe AL, Benowitz NL et al. Efficacy and safety of varenicline for smoking cessation in patients with stable cardiovascular disease: a randomized trial. Circulation. 2010;121:221-9.

137   FDA Drug Safety Communication: Chantix (varenicline) may increase the risk of certain cardiovascular adverse events in patients with cardiovascular disease. Rockville MD: US Food and Drug Administration; 2011. Available from: www.fda.gov/Drugs/DrugSafety/ucm259161.htm

138   Singh S, Loke YK, Spangler JG, Furberg CD. Risk of serious adverse cardiovascular events associated with varenicline: a systematic review and meta-analysis. CMAJ. 2011;183:1359-66.

139   Samuels L. Varenicline: cardiovascular safety. CMA.J 2011;183:1407-8.

140   Varenicline: quantifying the risk. CMAJ. 2011;183:1404-5.

141   Prochaska JJ, Hilton JF. Risk of cardiovascular serious adverse events associated with varenicline use for tobacco cessation: systematic review and meta-analysis. BMJ. 2012 May 4;344:e2856. doi: 10.1136/bmj.e2856.

142   Willers S. Smoking cessation treatment using varenicline in a patient population with mostly heart and lung disease. Society for Research on Nicotine and Tobacco 16-19 February 2011 Westin Harbour Castle, Toronto, Canada.

143   Rollema H, Lee TC, Bertrand D. Interactions of nicotine and varenicline with nAChR subtypes: implications for the cardiovascular system., SRNT Annual Mtg, Poster #106, March 16, 2012, Houston TX (http://srnt.org/conferences/2012/pdf/2012_Abstracts_H.pdf, p. 155).

144   Nides M, Oncken C, Gonzales D et al. Smoking cessation with varenicline, a selective a4β2 nicotinic receptor partial agonist. Arch Intern Med. 2006;166:1561-8.

145   Tonstad S, Tønnesen P, Hajek P, Williams KE, Billing CB, Reeves KR; Varenicline phase 3 study group. Effect of maintenance therapy with varenicline on smoking cessation. A randomized controlled trial. JAMA. 2006;296:64-71.

146 Williams KE, Reeves KR, Billing CB, Pennington AM, Gong J. A double-blind study evaluating the long-term safety of varenicline for smoking cessation. Curr Med Res Opin. 2007;23;793-801.

147 Cui Q, Robinson L, Elston D et al. Safety and tolerability of varenicline tartrate (Champix/Chantix) for smoking cessation in HIV-infected subjects: a pilot open-label study. AIDS Patient Care STDs. 2012;26:12-9.

148 Physician's desk reference. 64th ed. Montvale NJ: Thomson; 2010: 2715.

149 Ari H, Celiloğlu N, Ari S, Coşar S, Doanay K, Bozat T. The effect of varenicline on heart rate variability in healthy smokers and non-smokers. Autonomic Neuroscience. 2011;164:82-6.

150 Harrison-Woolrych M, Maggo S, Tan M, Savage R, Ashton J. Cardiovascular events in patients taking varenicline: a case series from intensive postmarketing surveillance in New Zealand. Drug Saf. 2012;35:33-43.

151 Els C, Kunyk D, Sidhu H. Smoking cessation and neuropsychiatric adverse events: Are physicians between a rock and a hard place? Canadian Family Physician. 2011;67: 647-649.

152 Hemmingsson T, Kriebel D. Smoking at age 18–20 and suicide during 26 years of follow-up—how can the association be explained? Int J Epidemiol. 2003;32:1000–4.

153 Tonstad S and Els C. Varenicline: Smoking Cessation in patients with medical and psychiatric comorbidity. Clinical Medical Insights: Therapeutics 2010;2:681-695.

154 Fowler JS, Volkow ND, Wang GD, et al. (1996) Brain monoamine oxidase A inhibition in cigarette smokers. PNAS 1996;93;14065-14069.

10

Detoxification: Treatment of the 'Other' Tobacco Use Disorder

CHARL ELS, DIANE KUNYK, YORAM BARAK, EILEEN THOMAS AND DEBRA SCHARF

WITH THE GROWING BODY OF EVIDENCE CONFIRMING THE HARMFUL EFFECTS OF SEC-
ondhand smoke, healthcare facilities are increasingly becoming smokefree for the
purposes of protecting patients, employees, visitors, volunteers, and contractors. It is
critical to note that the purposes of smokefree policies are about the provision of clean
air for occupational health and safety reasons, and these are not enacted for the purposes of forcing individuals to quit smoking. When unable to smoke without restric-
tion, however, individuals are faced with a decision. Some will simply abstain from
smoking to comply with the policy and others may smoke outside (with some policies
requiring this be off hospital property). There are some patients who may be unable
to make the choice to go out of doors to smoke, for example, as a result of imminent
risk of harm to self or others because of a psychiatric illness, immobility due to state
of consciousness or surgery, or risk of spread of communicable diseases. In these situations, involuntary abstinence without adequate support may lead to nicotine withdrawal in tobacco-addicted patients. A pragmatic approach is needed to balance the
needs of patients' right to self-determination (i.e. who choose not to quit smoking
during hospitalization) with protection from exposure to secondhand smoke.

BACKGROUND

An expanding number of healthcare and other organizational facilities are enacting smokefree environments, also referred to as tobacco-free policies.[1] These

measures are motivated primarily by the fundamental right of all persons to receive care or work in a healthy (i.e. free of exposure to secondhand smoke) environment and to be provided an opportunity to achieve their highest attainable standard of health. The motivation to ban smoking from indoor spaces is motivated by occupational health and safety reasons. As designated smoking rooms, including those with the most advanced ventilation technology available, do not protect from exposure to secondhand smoke,[2] the development of 100% indoor smoke-free environments are essential to protect individuals, visitors, staff members, families, volunteers, and others against the negative health consequences of secondhand smoke in facilities.

Smokefree healthcare institutions provide patients an opportunity to reduce or quit smoking in a supportive environment (Chapter 10). With the introduction of smokefree indoor environments, there has also been a subsequent and increased visibility of individuals consuming tobacco in outdoor spaces. When in smokefree spaces, those who are unable or unwilling to abstain from tobacco use are placed in situations whereby they may feel compelled to either break the policy or to go out of doors to smoke. In these situations, the provision of options for smoking cessation alone is not sufficient as many confined persons in smokefree environments may not be willing or ready to stop their tobacco use. As a result, these individuals are forced to abstain from tobacco involuntarily and, if addicted to tobacco, some may suffer with symptoms of tobacco (nicotine) withdrawal.

There is an alternative solution to this conundrum. It is proposed that the minimum standard of care for health not only include the provision of support and opportunities for smoking cessation but that it also provide the necessary detoxification (withdrawal) interventions for ensuring safe and comfortable transition to smoke-free environments. In these situations, this intervention would include the prevention and management of nicotine withdrawal in patients. A supportive experience of not smoking may also increase readiness to make a quit attempt.

CASE STUDY: THE SPECIAL CASE OF PSYCHIATRIC FACILITIES

For decades the use of tobacco products has been tolerated, and even facilitated, in many psychiatric settings. Some facilities have offered access to discounted tobacco products by accommodating programming to include 'smoke breaks,' and by the provision of designated smoking rooms, spaces, or total facilities. Hospital staff members in some settings have been known to purchase and store products for patients, some may have supported inpatients to purchase contraband cigarettes reportedly to reduce its costs, and some healthcare agencies (and their partnering academic institutions) have been known to partner with tobacco industries. The tobacco industry's efforts to recruit smokers in marginalized populations—the homeless and mentally ill— has been well-documented including forming alliances with organizations that provide services to these populations. In Canada, up to fairly recently, there were mental health consumer societies / associations receiving funding from the tobacco industry. Violations of the Canada Tobacco Act and the Canada Customs Act have been reported in Canadian psychiatric facilities, and there have been anecdotes of psychiatric facilities balancing their budgets from the sale of tobacco products to offer programming for their severe and persistently mentally ill patients.

Smoking rates are disproportionately high in persons with mental illness, and up to 70–90% of persons with severe mental illness smoke (Chapter 11). At the time of publication in 2012, there exist almost 20,000 psychiatric hospital facilities globally. Psychiatric facilities have traditionally been the bastion of smoking, and smoking has been ingrained within the culture of psychiatry and well documented within the settings of mental health facilities. Instead of offering cessation support to hospitalized mentally ill persons, smoking has been widely neglected and in many cases actively facilitated.[3,4]

The establishment of psychiatric facilities dates back centuries. The peak of the tobacco epidemic, however, only occurred in the middle of the 20th century made possible in part by the invention of the cigarette-rolling machine in the late 19th century. Johnston (1952) described in the *Lancet*:

"The increase in prevalence of smoking resulted in the progressive elimination of one non-smokers' sanctuary after another—drawing rooms, bedroom, workroom, place of entertainment, conveyance, and finally of late years, hospital ward and sanatorium, even when and where patients seriously ill from respiratory diseases are under treatment".[5]

He goes on to describe that the right to breathe clean air is as basic as the right to drink clean water. To this day, in many psychiatric facilities, the exposure to secondhand smoke continues in settings where indoor smoking is still allowed. The movement towards going smoke-free in hospital facilities hence represents a return to an earlier status.

Lawn and Pols (2005) reviewed the findings from 26 international studies reporting on the effectiveness of smoking bans in inpatient psychiatric settings.[3] Their findings suggest that staff generally expected more problems than what actually occurred. This finding is supported by the experiences of the authors. Echoing the earlier findings of el-Guebaly et. al. (2002) (22 examples of smoking bans),[6] there were no increases in aggression, use of seclusion, discharge against medical advice or increased use of as-needed (prn) medication following the ban. Consistent with what is expected, many patients continued to smoke post-admission, supporting the notion that smoke-free facilities' policies are not effective or intended as long-term cessation interventions. Smoking cessation strategies should be an inherent component of policies that ban smoking. Voci and co-workers (2010) suggest that a smoke-free policy can be implemented in a large psychiatric hospital with a high degree of support from staff and no substantial negative impact on patient behavior.[7] They further suggest that the proportion of staff who supported the policy increased from pre-implementation (82.6%) to post-implementation (89.1%), and a high level of support was maintained 2 years after policy enactment (90.1%). Among hospitals that changed to a smoke-free policy, the proportion that reported adverse events decreased by 75% or more in three areas: smoking or tobacco use as a precursor to incidents that led to seclusion or restraint, smoking-related health conditions, and coercion or threats among patients and staff.[8]

NICOTINE WITHDRAWAL SYNDROME

The *DSM-IV-TR* describes the syndrome of Nicotine Withdrawal (anticipated to change to Tobacco Withdrawal in the proposed *DSM 5* changes) that occurs when the brain of a person who has adapted to the use of nicotine is deprived of ongoing exposure to nicotine. The symptoms may result when the substance of nicotine (i.e. through smoking) is reduced or discontinued, thereby leading to the recognized diagnosis of the substance-related disorder of Nicotine Withdrawal.[9]

Symptoms of nicotine withdrawal vary but may include cravings, irritability, restlessness, difficulty concentrating, depression, frustration, anxiety, insomnia, fatigue, and increased appetite. Most symptoms reach maximum intensity at 24–48 hours and are relieved within a few weeks but some individuals may be unable to concentrate and have strong cravings to smoke for weeks or months after quitting smoking. As these symptoms are not specific to nicotine withdrawal when these are not identified, their expression may complicate patient diagnoses and the treatment of other medical diseases (e.g. a comatose patient in intensive care treatment). Following a review, Hughes (2002) concluded that anger, anxiety, depression, difficulty concentrating, impatience, insomnia, and restlessness were valid withdrawal symptoms that peak within the first week and usually last 2–4 weeks.[10,11] Also noted are constipation, cough, dizziness, increased dreaming, and mouth ulcers, described as possible abstinence effects (Table 1). The presence of drowsiness, fatigue, and several physical symptoms were not considered abstinence effects.

TABLE 1. Symptoms of nicotine withdrawal and length of time these are experienced

Symptom	Duration:	Prevalence:
Increase appetite	Up to 10 weeks	70%
Urges to smoke (cravings)	Up to 2 weeks	70%
Depression	Up to 4 weeks	60%
Restlessness	Up to 4 weeks	60%
Poor concentration	Up to 2 weeks	60%
Irritability or aggression	Up to 4 weeks	50%
Mouth ulcers	Up to 4 weeks	40%
Sleep disturbance	Up to 1 week	25%
Constipation	Up to 4 weeks	17%
Light-headedness	Up to 48 hours	10%

Sources: Adapted from: Jarvis MJ. Why people smoke. BMJ 2004;328:277-279 and Hughes JR. Effects of abstinence from tobacco: valid symptoms and time course. Nicotine Tobacco Research. 2007:9(3): 315-27.

FORCING PATIENTS TO QUIT SMOKING?

As it is not the case that every patient admitted to a smoke-free facility is ready or interested in making a quit attempt, only offering cessation services puts some tobacco-addicted inpatients in an impossible position. Furthermore this conundrum places healthcare professionals in a very difficult position. There is often an erroneous perception or expectation that the induced requirement of smokefree policies is to help patients to quit smoking. This approach ignores the existence of the bona fide *DSM* diagnosis of Nicotine Withdrawal: one managed quite differently from smoking cessation. The development of elaborate (and often expensive) smoking cessation programs without offering detoxification (or withdrawal management) is at best misguided and at worst potentially negligent. This paradigm also understandably often evokes resistance from:

- Administrators struggling to free capacity and resourcing to provide these from an already stretched and stressed system,
- Healthcare professionals under pressure to compress the management of tobacco use and addiction into short hospital stays, and
- Patients interpreting policy messaging as requiring involuntary quitting. Resistance to this messaging may exacerbate resistance to necessary hospitalization for treatments.

Healthcare professionals recognize that their patients ought not to be forced to quit smoking and, thereby, they and their patients are left in an untenable situation. However, the philosophy of addiction treatment in general can be translated to this situation, and hence opens up alternative approaches applicable to tobacco addiction under these circumstances. Detoxification (as applied in other drugs of abuse) provides an alternative for patients and healthcare providers in this situation where they're not ready to quit.

NICOTINE DETOXIFICATION

Nicotine withdrawal is recognized as a bona fide medical condition. Hospital settings are well experienced with managing the withdrawal from other substances (i.e. alcohol or benzodiazepines). Typically detoxification is not considered rehabilitation (addiction) treatment and by itself does not contribute to long-term abstinence from tobacco. Rather, detoxification is considered a precursor to engagement in addiction treatment with the patient receiving referral upon discharge. Similarly tobacco addiction can be managed by implementing a detoxification model as a precursor to later addiction treatment for the purposes of achieving long-term abstinence from tobacco. This would be similar to what would be offered for an individual who is at risk of alcohol detoxification who would also be offered opportunities to quit drinking once he or she has been medically stabilized through an alcohol detoxification regime. The management of nicotine detoxification should be offered irrespective of the patient's level of interest or engagement in smoking cessation. Consistent with their right to self-determination, patients should also have the right to refuse detoxification management. Should this involuntary and untreated abstinence contribute to an increased risk of disorganized behaviour, this may be dealt with in exactly the same fashion as disorganized behaviour resulting from other causes.

Educating key opinion leaders within the healthcare environment and community is essential to help distinguish between withdrawal management and tobacco use and addiction treatment (i.e. smoking cessation). The authors posit that this distinction allows for lowering of resistance against such policies for both patients and staff members, and prevents inconsistencies with prescribing. Engagement and adherence to policies are essential to safe and successful introduction and maintenance of smokefree indoor spaces that in turn protect against harmful exposure to secondhand smoke.

DETOXIFICATION MANAGEMENT

Effective detoxification requires screening for patients' tobacco use upon admission, repeated opportunities to receive nicotine replacement therapies (including a range and combination of products). The standard for withdrawal management is to offer nicotine replacement therapy (NRT), at sufficient doses, and without the expectation and pressure for making a commitment to quit smoking. Combinations of slow-acting and rapid-acting nicotine preparations are considered a standard of care for management of withdrawal, as well as the possibility to carefully exceed doses of NRT displayed in monographs if needed in selected cases.

Effective detoxification further requires repeated daily opportunities to receive NRT (including a range and combination of products), and provision of a supportive environment including omission of cues to smoke. In order to quickly intervene, systematic measures are required to ensure rapid treatment delivery. Standing orders of NRT when a physician is not immediately available, ward stock for quick access, and supplies of a broad spectrum of these products on hospital formulary to meet the needs of patients are necessary. Having NRT available with full coverage (i.e. no out-of-pocket cost to the patient) is critical for successful implementation of smoke-free policies in institutional facilities.

Although addressing tobacco use has been found to be a constant part of daily practice, the delivery of effective treatment is not considered to be routine. In a qualitative study of smoke-free policies in Canadian hospitals, it was concluded that the focus was instead on managing the behaviour of the patients.[12]

Nicotine detoxification should be viewed as a part of a larger comprehensive tobacco-control strategy. The provision of adequate pharmacotherapy for the treatment of withdrawal and cravings can enhance the likelihood of attempts to quit. As most individuals who smoke would like to quit, successful management during enforced withdrawal may increase their receptivity to opportunities for stopping their tobacco use. It is proposed that withdrawal management should dovetail with adequately matched longitudinal cessation interventions, preferably offered no later than discharge from the institutional facility and that may include bridging regimes.[13] The Safety-Sensitive Algorithm (Chapter 1) offers the integration of detoxification management as a separate step in the tobacco reduction and cessation process. One Online example of orders for treating nicotine detoxification in hospitalized patients is the Centre for Addiction and Mental Health's Physician's Order sheet for nicotine treatment freely available at:

https://www.nicotinedependenceclinic.com/English/teach/resources/SitePages/Tobacco%20Cessation%20and%20Behaviour%20Change.aspx

THE CHALLENGE WITH OUTDOOR SMOKING

While the tactics to ban indoor smoking in hospitals has been effective, outdoor smoking may at time result in a new set of complications. There is limited information available that offers an understanding of how this affects the daily nicotine intake of patients who have opportunities to leave the units. Many patients smoking opportunities fluctuate, thereby affecting their day-to-day cigarette consumption. When unable to smoke for long periods, acute nicotine withdrawal may be induced. If considered an active smoker, the patient may not be offered nicotine replacement medication or may not make recognize their need for assistance. Intense cravings can provoke patients to violate indoor smoking policies such as smoking in the washrooms.

Some hospitals offer smoking breaks, and may even escort patients out to smoke. It is argued that this enables tobacco addiction. It also sends a message of health professionals condoning cigarette smoking. In many psychiatric settings where smoking is allowed on hospital property, smoke breaks for patients are used as an incentive not unlike in the past when cigarettes were offered as a reward for desirable behavior.

Other factors to consider when smoking on property is allowed are the environmental cues. The stimulus of observing other patients going outside to smoke, or watching smokers out the window, or having smoking paraphilia in sight can make it difficult for those not allowed to smoke to manage their cravings and desire to smoke. If the smokefree policy does not address all aspects of a supportive non-smoking environment, further discussion is recommended.

LEGAL IMPLICATIONS

Legal and legislative debates reveal the cultural and organizational challenges that have to be dealt with to make healthcare services health-promoting.[14] Smoking has not yet been determined as a human right and that, consistent with providing a safe occupational health setting, a healthcare facility has the right to govern their indoor environment and declare it as smoke-free. Smoke-free policies in facilities have been legally challenged in a number of jurisdictions, and the decisions upheld. In the landmark case of *Vaughan et al. v. Mental Health Centre Penetanguishene*, the Court rejected an injunction application to block implementation of a smoking ban at Oak Ridge (a maximum-security psychiatric facility housing patients who have been violent and are regarded as a risk to others and to themselves), which is a part of the Mental Health Centre Penetanguishene (MHCP). Justice Lang stated:

> *"Smoking, on the evidence before the court, compromises the health and well being of the facility's staff and the other patients. The dangers inherent in smoking, and even more so in exposure to second-hand smoke, are not alleviated, on the evidence, by smoking rooms and smoking outdoors. The MHCP's evidence is not contradicted that the smoking rooms do not successfully curtail the leakage of smoke into the common areas".[15]*

In Canada, since 2004, Bill C-45 is federal legislation that amends the Canadian Criminal Code. The bill established new legal duties for workplace health and safety, imposing serious penalties for violations that result in injuries or death. The new Section 217.1 in the Criminal Code reads:

> Everyone who undertakes, or has the authority, to direct how another person does work or performs a task is under a legal duty to take reasonable steps to prevent bodily harm to that person, or any other person, arising from that work or task.[16]

It also establishes rules for attributing criminal liability to organizations, including corporations, for the acts of their representatives, and creates a legal duty for all persons directing work to take 'reasonable steps' to ensure the safety of workers and the public. The safety hazards related to exposure to secondhand smoke are well-established but claims of secondhand smoke-related damages to the health of staff have not been tested under C-45.

10 KEY MESSAGES REGARDING SMOKEFREE HEALTHCARE FACILITIES

1. Secondhand smoke is toxic, and designated smoking rooms do not protect against secondhand smoke exposure.
2. Patients, staff, physicians, visitors, and volunteers have the right to breathe clean air, and it is the hospital's duty and legal obligation to ensure such.
3. Hospitals have the legal right to introduce smoke-free policies on their premises.
4. Exceptions to the policy (including partial policy measures or making exceptions for 'special' sub-populations) complicate successful implementation.
5. Supported and treated abstinence from tobacco does not compromise health or safety and does not increase risk of patients leaving against medical advice.
6. Withdrawal management is not the equivalent to smoking cessation and represents a distinctly different process of managing a different disorder.
7. Nicotine agonist treatment (NRT, in sufficient doses) represents the gold standard of treating nicotine withdrawal during involuntary abstinence.
8. Tobacco addiction is a chronic, relapsing yet treatable medical condition. Cessation should not be offered as the only option upon hospital admission, and in some cases its treatment may be deferred, while still offering withdrawal management for those unable or unwilling or uninterested in quitting smoking.
9. Health professionals are expected to adhere to hospital-mandated policies and have a duty to treat both tobacco addiction and nicotine withdrawal. It should be emphasized that there is a need to achieve staff cooperation and increased motivation to adhere to such policies, through psychoeducation of all staff members.
10. Hospital administrators have a legal duty to provide a clean air environment.

SUMMARY

Progressively more hospitals are declaring/reclaiming smokefree status. Going smokefree is feasible and requires the optimal management of two different and distinct *DSM*-recognized psychiatric conditions: tobacco withdrawal and tobacco addiction. Yet Sellman (2005) suggests it is disappointing that it may take litigation to for psychiatry to wake up to the reality of nicotine dependence as a mental disorder[17] Failure to address detoxification can negatively impact on successful policy implementation, induce suffering for patients addicted to tobacco, and deprive patients of opportunities to attempt to quit smoking in a supportive environment.

REFERENCES

1   Parle D, Parker S, Steeves D. Making Canadian healthcare facilities 100% smoke-free: a national trend emerges. Healthcare Quarterly. 2005;8:53-7.

2   Repace J, Kawachi I, Glantz S. Fact sheet on secondhand smoke. 2nd European Conference on Tobacco or Health, 1st Ibero-American Conference on Tobacco or Health; 1999. Available from: http://www.repace.com/SHSFactsheet.pdf.

3   Lawn S, Pols R. Smoking bans in psychiatric settings? A review of the research. Aust N Z J Psychiatry. 2005;39:866-85.

4   Lawn S. Cigarette smoking in psychiatric inpatient settings: occupational health, safety, welfare, and legal concerns. Aust N Z J Psychiatry. 2005;39:886-91.

5   Johnston L. Cure of tobacco-smoking. Lancet. 1952:480-2.

6   El-Guebaly N, Cathcart J, Currie S, et al. Public health and therapeutic aspects of smoking bans in mental health and addiction settings. Psychiatr Serv. 2002;53:1617-22.

7   Voci S, Bondy S, Zawertailo L, Walker L, George TP, & Selby P. Impact of a smoke-free policy in a large psychiatric hospital on staff attitudes and patient behavior. Gen Hosp Psychiatry. 2010 Nov-Dec;32(6):623-30. Epub 2010 Oct 14.

8   Hollen V, Ortiz G, Schacht L, Mojarrad MG, Lane GM Jr, & Parks JJ. Effects of adopting a smoke-free policy in state psychiatric hospitals. Psychiatr Serv. 2010;61:899-904.

9   American Psychiatric Association. Diagnostic and statistical manual of mental disorders, 4th edition, text revision. Arlington VA: American Psychiatric Association; 2000.

10   Hughes JR. Effects of abstinence from tobacco: valid symptoms and time course. Nicotine Tob Res. 2007;9(3):315-27.

11   Hughes JR, Higgings ST, Bickel WK. Nicotine withdrawal versus other drug withdrawal syndromes: similarities and dissimilarities. Addiction. 1994;89:1461-70.

12   Schultz A, Finegan B, Nykiforuk C, Kvern M. A qualitative investigation of smoke-free policies on hospital property. CMAJ. 2011;183(18):E1335-43.

13   Kunyk D, Els C, Predy G, Haase M. Development and introduction of a comprehensive tobacco control policy in a Canadian Regional Health Authority. Preventing Chronic Disease: Public Health Research, Practice, and Policy. 2007;4(20):3-8.

14   Jochelson K. Smoke-free legislation and mental health units: the challenges ahead. Br J Psychiatry. 2006;189(6):479-80.

15   Vaughan et al. v. Mental Health Centre Penetanguishene (Ontario Superior Court of Justice, May 8, 2003, court file 252/03), para. 15-16.

16   Criminal Code of Canada, sect. 217.1. Available from: http://yourlaws.ca/criminal-code-canada/2171-duty-persons-directing-work.

17   Sellman D. Clinical neglect of nicotine dependence. Aust N Z J Psychiatry. 2005;39:847-8.

18   Jarvis MJ. Why people smoke. BMJ 2004;328:277-279.

11

Hospital-Initiated Smoking Cessation: The Ottawa Model for Smoking Cessation

ROBERT REID, KERRI-ANNE MULLEN AND ANDREW PIPE

IT IS ESTIMATED THAT 600,000 PATIENTS ADMITTED ANNUALLY TO CANADIAN HOSPITALS currently smoke tobacco.[1] Hospital care for smoking-related illnesses adds considerably to the healthcare burden in Canada; patients who smoke average more than twice as many hospital days compared with those who have never smoked.[2] Tobacco smoking plays a causative role in the development of several of the leading causes of hospitalization including cardiovascular and respiratory diseases as well as many forms of cancer.[3]

Stopping tobacco use helps hospitalized patients improve their recovery and overall health. For example, by quitting smoking, cardiac patients can reduce the likelihood of dying or suffering another heart attack,[4] lung, head, and neck cancer patients can reduce their risk of a second cancer,[5] patients with chronic obstructive lung/pulmonary disease (COLD/COPD) can slow the decline in lung function associated with their illness and improve their odds of survival,[6] and surgical patients can experience fewer post-surgical complications and improved bone and wound healing.[7-9]

Sixty-five to 82% of patients identified as smoking during index hospitalizations in Ontario continue to smoke in the following year.[10,11] This trend can be mitigated. Effective interventions exist to help hospitalized patients stop smoking. Intensive counselling interventions that begin during the hospital stay, and continue with supportive contacts for at least one month after discharge, increase smoking cessation rates after discharge when compared with control conditions

(Odds Ratio (OR) = 1.65, 95% confidence interval (CI) 1.44 to 1.90; 17 trials).[14] Data suggest that nicotine replacement therapy (NRT) and bupropion may be effective in the hospital setting not only to help reduce symptoms of nicotine withdrawal during hospitalization but also to increase the likelihood of longer-term abstinence.[15] These interventions appear to be effective regardless of the patient's reason for admission (i.e. smoking-related illness or not).[15] There is also emerging evidence to suggest that intensive hospital-initiated interventions can reduce healthcare utilization.[4,8]

In this chapter, clinical practice guidelines for hospital-initiated interventions and their operationalization in the Ottawa Model for Smoking Cessation (OMSC) are described.[11] Experiences implementing the OMSC in Canadian hospitals, including challenges and barriers to program implementation and sustainability, are also reported.

CLINICAL PRACTICE GUIDELINES AND BEST PRACTICES FOR HOSPITAL-INITIATED INTERVENTIONS

Clinical practice guidelines for hospital-initiated interventions have been developed by several organizations.[15-18] The Registered Nurses Association of Ontario recommends that "organizations and regional health authorities should consider smoking cessation as integral to nursing practice, and thereby integrate a variety of professional development opportunities to support nurses in effectively developing skills in smoking cessation intervention and counselling. All corporate hospital orientation programs should include training to use brief smoking cessation interventions as well as information on pharmacotherapy to support hospitalized persons who smoke."[17 (p.31)]

The New Zealand Ministry of Health smoking cessation guidelines include the following recommendations relevant to hospitalized smokers: 1) provide brief advice to stop smoking to all hospitalized people who smoke; 2) arrange multi-session intensive support, medication, and follow up for at least one month for all hospitalized patients who smoke; and 3) briefly advise people awaiting surgery who smoke to stop smoking and arrange support (such as NRT) prior to surgery.[16]

The US Department of Health and Human Services conducted a series of systematic reviews and meta-analyses of existing studies in forming their guidelines regarding hospitalized patients who smoke. They recommend the following actions: 1) ask every patient on admission if he or she uses tobacco and document their tobacco use status; 2) for current tobacco users, list tobacco use status on the admission problem list and as a discharge diagnosis; 3) use counselling and medications to help all tobacco users maintain abstinence and to treat withdrawal symptoms; 4) provide advice and assistance on how to quit during hospitalization and remain abstinent after discharge; and 5) arrange for follow-up regarding smoking status. Supportive contact should be provided for at least one month after discharge.[15]

More recently, Canadian guidelines for smoking cessation interventions in the hospital setting have been developed by the Canadian Action Network for the Advancement, Dissemination and Adoption of Practice-informed Tobacco Treatment (CAN-ADAPTT).[18] These guidelines build on the US guidelines but place additional emphasis on raising awareness regarding hospital smoke-free policies and initiating treatment for tobacco dependence (addiction) prior to hospitalization in patients being admitted to hospital on an elective basis (e.g. for planned surgical procedures).

CAN-ADAPTT SUMMARY STATEMENTS FOR HOSPITAL-BASED POPULATIONS

1. All patients should be made aware of hospital smoke-free policies.
2. All elective patients who smoke should be directed to resources to assist them to quit smoking prior to hospital admission or surgery, where possible.
3. All hospitals should have systems in place to:
   a. Identify all smokers;
   b. Manage nicotine withdrawal during hospitalization,
   c. Promote attempts toward long-term cessation and,
   d. Provide patients with follow-up support post hospitalization.
4. Pharmacotherapy should be considered:
   a. To assist patients to manage nicotine withdrawal in hospital;
   b. For use in-hospital and post-hospitalization to promote long term cessation

Source: CAN-ADAPTT. Canadian smoking cessation clinical practice guideline. Toronto: Canadian Action Network for the Advancement, Dissemination and Adoption of Practice-informed Tobacco Treatment, Centre for Addiction and Mental Health; 2011. Available from: www.can-adaptt.net. Reprinted with permission.

Despite the positive effects of smoking cessation on health and health outcomes among hospitalized patients who smoke and the presence of clinical practice guidelines relevant to hospital-initiated cessation programs, most hospitals in Canada do not provide tobacco dependence assistance. The OMSC provides one example of an organizational change for smoking cessation process that is customized to the hospital setting.

THE OTTAWA MODEL FOR SMOKING CESSATION

The Ottawa Model for Smoking Cessation (OMSC) is a systematic process for identifying smoking status, initiating treatment for tobacco dependence, and linking smoker-patients to post-discharge follow-up. It was first developed to assist cardiac patients at the University of Ottawa Heart Institute.[10] Adapted versions are available for primary care and outpatient specialty clinic (e.g. stroke prevention, cancer treatment, diabetes, HIV, COPD) settings.[11] This process is intended to create an environment where healthcare professionals and other staff can easily and routinely meet hospitalized patients' needs related to the management of acute nicotine withdrawal and/or long-term smoking cessation. Trained outreach facilitators assist hospitals to implement 10 "best practices" for tobacco dependence treatment (Table 1); best practices are introduced using principles of organizational change and implementation science. Between 2006 and 2012, more than 50,000 patient-smokers admitted to Canadian hospitals participated in OMSC-based interventions. Outreach facilitators use several organizational change strategies to optimize tobacco-dependence treatment practices (Table 2). These strategies are delivered in two phases: 1) a start-up phase involving preparation for program delivery; and 2) an operational phase during which program operations commence and refinements occur.

TABLE 1. Best practices for hospital-initiated smoking cessation interventions

Number	Best practice
1	Tobacco use queried and documented for all admissions and visits.
2	Training (i.e. workshops, in-services, and new staff orientation) for tobacco dependence treatment regularly offered to staff.
3	Program responsibilities designated to staff (i.e. program coordination, counselling, education, consultation).
4	Tobacco dependence treatment included on clinic forms, treatment pathways, care maps, Kardexes, etc.
5	Self-help materials readily available to patients, family members, and staff.
6	Referral to community resources readily available.
7	Pharmacotherapy (NRT, buproprion, varenicline) available with prescription or through hospital formulary.
8	Processes to follow-up tobacco users for at least one month after initial consultation.
9	Processes to evaluate degree to which healthcare providers are identifying, documenting, and treating patients who use tobacco.
10	Processes to provide feedback to healthcare providers about performance and program effectiveness.

Source: University of Ottawa Heart Institute. Ottawa Model for Smoking Cessation in-patient workplan. Ottawa: Author; 2010.

TABLE 2: OMSC program activities and intervention strategies

Activities and intervention strategies	Description
Meet with key hospital officials	• Meet with administrative, medical, and nursing leadership • Record hospital characteristics • Sign partnership agreement
Baseline audit and feedback	• Review current policies and practices related to tobacco-dependence treatment for hospitalized patients who smoke • Survey patient smoking prevalence • Present to leadership baseline policies and practices in relation to best practices and smoking prevalence data
Consensus building	• Set goals to improve practice gaps • Review ways for integrating care for hospitalized patients who smoke into routine practice
Accountability	• Designate care provider most responsible for delivering tobacco-dependence treatment
Practice tools	• Standardized smoker consult form • Standard orders for smoking cessation medications • Patient education materials • Interactive voice-response-mediated follow-up system
Reminder systems	• Standardized smoking status questions on intake histories • Tobacco-dependence treatment on care maps, clinical pathways, and Kardex systems
Educational outreach visits	• Regular meetings between program facilitators and implementers to solve the problem and assist with practice-change activities
Training	• Train physicians, frontline staff, clerks
Ongoing audit and feedback	• Present quarterly program results to unit managers and hospital leadership • Present results to frontline staff

Source: Reid RD, Mullen KA, Slovinec D'Angelo ME, Aitken DA, Papadakis S, Haley PM, et al. Smoking cessation for hospitalized smokers: an evaluation of the "Ottawa Model." Nicotine Tob Res. 2010;12(1):11–18.

Phase 1: Start-up Implementation commences with a meeting with key hospital officials to secure high-level commitment to the program. A hospital smoking cessation task force is developed consisting of medical, nursing, pharmacy, respiratory therapy, and other 'champions,' as well as a designated internal program coordinator. Facilitators then work with the hospital task force to review current tobacco-dependence treatment policies and practices. Information on policy/practice gaps and smoking prevalence (gathered during pre-implementation data collection) are presented to hospital leaders. Facilitators and hospital champions establish goals to reduce practice gaps and ensure an optimal environment for tobacco-dependence treatment. The internal program coordinator and other task force members attend an intensive two-day training program in which they learn about tobacco dependence treatment and how to operationalize the process within their hospital. Facilitators work with internal coordinators to introduce clinical practice tools, including a standardized smoking cessation consult form, standard orders for smoking cessation medications, patient education materials, and an automated telephone follow-up system and database.[19] Point-of-care reminders are introduced including standard smoking status questions on admission and patient history forms (i.e. "Have you used any form of tobacco in the past six months?" "Have you used any form of tobacco in the past seven days?"), and interventions for smoker-patients are added to patient care maps and other clinical management systems. Frontline physicians and nurses are trained during a one-hour session addressing principles of tobacco dependence treatment and smoking cessation medications; they are given instructions regarding the smoking cessation consult form and standard orders for cessation medications. For hospitals using paper charting, clerks are trained to enter patient information into the automated follow-up system and database. In preparing hospitals to begin using the OMSC intervention (typically, the preparation phase lasts six months), facilitators hold regular meetings (approximately every two to three weeks) with staff-level implementers to assist with practice change activities. Smoking cessation program delivery then commences.

Phase 2: Operational Phase At hospital admission, smoking status is documented on patient history forms or in the electronic medical record. If the patient is identified as currently smoking tobacco, the consult form is triggered using clinical management systems. At the bedside, patients are advised to quit smoking in a clear and supportive manner by their attending physician and nurse (e.g. "Given your current health condition, the most important thing you can do is to quit smoking. Someone is going to come by and talk to you while you're here about how we might be able to help you"). The cessation intervention is completed by a designated healthcare professional; in some hospitals it is the patient's attending nurse and in others it is dedicated tobacco cessation specialists or respiratory therapists who provide the intervention. The bedside intervention is delivered in accordance with the standardized smoking cessation consult form which contains questions and prompts concerning smoking history, previous quit attempts, confidence in quitting, readiness to quit smoking, nicotine withdrawal symptoms, and contact information for follow-up. The designated healthcare professional discusses medication options with the patient and, as appropriate, completes the standard order for cessation medication to be signed by an attending physician. Patients are informed about the automated telephone follow-up system in hospital and can choose whether to receive follow-up calls post-discharge. A clerk enters information from the smoking cessation consult form into the program database. For hospitals with electronic medical records, data can be automatically and securely linked to the system database. Data are sent to a secure server hosted by a third-party service provider. For patients agreeing to telephone follow-up, the automated calls are generated from this system.

The automated telephone follow-up system places follow-up calls to patients 3, 14, 30, 60, 90, 120, 150, and 180 days post-discharge. It delivers a set of prerecorded questions to establish patient identity, smoking status, current use of smoking cessation therapies, and, for relapsed smokers, interest in making another quit attempt. Trained counsellors that monitor the telephone system contact patients that appear to be experiencing difficulty. Data collected by the automated telephone system supports performance monitoring and feedback for quality assurance purposes, as well as program evaluation.

The OMSC has been examined for effectiveness. In an evaluation conducted at nine hospitals in Ontario, there was an 11.1% improvement in six-month continuous abstinence rates following implementation of the OMSC (18.3% pre-OMSC versus 29.4% post-OMSC; OR = 1.71, 95% CI = 1.11– 2.64; Z = 2.43; I 2 = 0%; p = .02).[11]

CHALLENGES AND SYSTEMIC BARRIERS TO IMPLEMENTATION AND SUSTAINABILITY

Hospital-initiated tobacco cessation interventions like the OMSC can be effective in helping patients to quit smoking but long-term sustainability of such programs is needed in order to see significant population-level impacts on health and healthcare utilization. In previous studies of tobacco cessation interventions, constraints on financial and staff resources, lack of system supports for the recommended cessation activities, and the need for continued staff support and performance feedback have been identified as major barriers to program implementation and sustainability.[20]

The sustainability of the OMSC intervention was recently assessed in a qualitative study by evaluators from the University of Waterloo.[21] High- and low-performing hospitals that had implemented the program were compared. Key factors associated with program sustainability in high-performing hospitals included: the perception of tobacco use as an important patient issue and tobacco-dependence treatment a fit with organizational priorities; leadership by medical, nursing, and administrative 'champions' (i.e. individuals who promote the program to hospital staff); initiating the program in conjunction with the hospital's smoke-free property initiative; framing of tobacco-dependence treatment as an organizational standard of care and holding staff accountable for delivering this standard; allocation of hospital staff time to support the program (e.g. educate staff, ensure that patients are counselled, communicate program results); dedicated funding; evidence that the intervention was having a positive impact on patient comfort during hospitalization (less irritation, restlessness) and on long-term abstinence; and using frontline healthcare professionals to deliver the intervention rather than tobacco dependence specialists. Hospital leaders identified the facilitation provided by OMSC staff as instrumental in helping them address issues of implementation and sustainability. Important barriers to sustainability included: concerns from hospital leaders that tobacco interventions were not a fit with the mandate of an acute care institution; technical and privacy issues related to the installation of an automated telephone follow-up system; data entry related to the follow-up system; the cost of hospital staff time to support the program; perceived time pressures on frontline staff; and demands from other, competing quality improvement initiatives.

Key informants identified that the OMSC training, education, and research updates provided by the outreach facilitators were key components to an inpatient tobacco cessation program's sustainability and that continuous training was necessary given staff turnover in nursing units. Training and education provide the skills necessary to administer the program, and an opportunity to change stakeholder awareness and attitudes about hospital-based cessation programs. Education about the effectiveness of patient follow-up on smoking cessation impacted the hospital's decision to continue with that component of the program.

Program champions appear to be needed at various levels within an organization, and their message needs to be tailored to different stakeholder expectations.[22–24] Further research is needed to define the role of program champions, to understand what characteristics successful champions have, and what actions they take to enhance the sustainability processes.

The OMSC uses the automated telephone follow-up system to track patients after discharge and to collect, store, and report performance data. Because information on program effectiveness and impact can enhance stakeholders' perceptions of the program's value, or prompt actions to improve performance, it is important to recognize barriers (e.g. staff time and actual costs) identified by some hospitals. Lack of performance feedback and data on cessation rates may jeopardize the sustainability of the hospital-based smoking cessation interventions.

SUMMARY AND FUTURE DIRECTIONS

Individuals who smoke are frequently hospitalized and their hospitalization affords an important opportunity to engage them in smoking cessation interventions. Effective interventions for treating tobacco dependence in hospitalized patients who smoke exist and key elements of these interventions are reflected in existing clinical practice guidelines. These elements include processes to ascertain smoking status, provision of in-hospital counselling and smoking cessation medications, and follow-up after hospital discharge. Organizational change processes are designed to help hospitals create an environment where healthcare professionals and other hospital staff can easily and routinely meet hospitalized smokers' needs related to the management of acute nicotine withdrawal and/or long-term smoking cessation.

Using program "champions," incorporating relevant performance feedback, conducting ongoing education, training, and promotion, designating a hospital-based coordinator role, and demonstrating program impact are important factors for sustainability. Sustained program funding, obtained either from external sources or reallocated from within existing funding envelopes, is necessary to support ongoing program operation. Future research is needed to determine the type and amount of external support that is beneficial in sustaining hospital participation while being affordable and feasible for the supporting organization. Hospital-initiated interventions typically require centralized support in the form of outreach facilitation, training, shared learning opportunities, program monitoring, and performance feedback.

Future innovations are required to streamline the transfer of patients from hospital interventions to community-based and primary care follow-up. Additional research is required to: understand the effectiveness of smoking cessation medications initiated during hospitalization and continued after discharge; the health, healthcare, and cost consequences of hospital-initiated cessation interventions; and the effectiveness of different models of care.

REFERENCES

1   Reid RD, Mullen KA, Pipe AL. Systematic approaches to smoking cessation in the cardiac setting. Curr Opin Cardiol. 26(5):443-8. Epub 2011/07/07.

2   Wilkins K, Shields M, Rotermann M. Smokers' use of acute care hospitals–a prospective study. Health Rep. 2009;20(4):75-83. Epub 2010/01/30.

3   US Department of Health and Human Services. The health consequences of smoking: a report of the Surgeon General. In: US Department of Health and Human Services CfDCaP, Office on Smoking and Health. Atlanta: Author; 2004.

4   Mohiuddin SM, Mooss AN, Hunter CB, Grollmes TL, Cloutier DA, Hilleman DE. Intensive smoking cessation intervention reduces mortality in high-risk smokers with cardiovascular disease. Chest. 2007;131(2):446-52. Epub 2007/02/14.

5   Parsons A, Daley A, Begh R, Aveyard P. Influence of smoking cessation after diagnosis of early stage lung cancer on prognosis: systematic review of observational studies with meta-analysis. BMJ. 2010;340:b5569. Epub 2010/01/23.

6   Godtfredsen NS, Prescott E. Benefits of smoking cessation with focus on cardiovascular and respiratory comorbidities. Clinical Respiratory J. 2011;5(4):187-94. Epub 2011/06/22.

7   Moller A, Villebro N. Interventions for preoperative smoking cessation. Cochrane Database Syst Rev 2005(3):CD002294. Epub 2005/07/22.

8   Thomsen T, Tonnesen H, Moller AM. Effect of preoperative smoking cessation interventions on postoperative complications and smoking cessation. Br J Surg. 2009;96(5):451-61. Epub 2009/04/10.

9   Myers K, Hajek P, Hinds C, McRobbie H. Stopping smoking shortly before surgery and postoperative complications: a systematic review and meta-analysis. Arch Intern Med. 2011;171(11):983-9. Epub 2011/03/16.

10 Reid RD, Pipe AL, Quinlan B. Promoting smoking cessation during hospitalization for coronary artery disease. Can J Cardiol. 2006;22(9):775-80. Epub 2006/07/13.

11   Reid RD, Mullen KA, Slovinec D'Angelo ME, Aitken DA, Papadakis S, Haley PM, et al. Smoking cessation for hospitalized smokers: an evaluation of the "Ottawa Model". Nicotine Tob Res. 2010;12(1):11-18. Epub 2009/11/12.

12   Benowitz NL. Neurobiology of nicotine addiction: implications for smoking cessation treatment. Am J Med. 2008;121(4 Suppl 1):S3-10. Epub 2008/03/26.

13   Hughes JR. Effects of abstinence from tobacco: valid symptoms and time course. Nicotine Tob Res. 2007;9(3):315-27. Epub 2007/03/17.

14   Rigotti NA, Munafo MR, Stead LF. Interventions for smoking cessation in hospitalised patients. Cochrane Database Syst Rev 2007(3):CD001837. Epub 2007/07/20.

15   Fiore MC, Jaen CR, Baker TB, Bailey WC, Benowitz N, Curry SJ, et al. Treating tobacco use and dependence: 2008 update. Rockville MD: US Department of Health and Human Services; 2008 [accessed 2012 May 19]. Available from: http://www.surgeongeneral.gov/initiatives/tobacco/index.html.

16   New Zealand Ministry of Health. New Zealand smoking cessation guidelines. In: Health Mo, editor. Wellington: Ministry of Health; 2007.

17   Registered Nurses Association of Ontario. Integrating smoking cessation into daily nursing practice. Toronto: Registered Nurses Association of Ontario; 2007.

18   CAN-ADAPTT's Clinical Practice Guideline Development Group. Hospital-Based Populations. Toronto: Centre for Addiction and Mental Health; 2011. Available from: http://www.can-adaptt.net/English/Guideline/Introduction.aspx.

19   Reid RD, Pipe AL, Quinlan B, Oda J. Interactive voice response telephony to promote smoking cessation in patients with heart disease: a pilot study. Patient Educ Couns. 2007;66(3):319-26. Epub 2007/03/06.

20   Taylor CB, Miller NH, Cameron RP, Fagans EW, Das S. Dissemination of an effective inpatient tobacco use cessation program. Nicotine Tob Res. 2005;7(1):129-37. Epub 2005/04/05.

21   Campbell S, Pieters K, Mullen KA, Reece R, Reid RD. Examining sustainability in a hospital setting: case of smoking cessation. Implement Sci. 2011;6:108. Epub 2011/09/16.

22   Greenhalgh T, Robert G, Macfarlane F, Bate P, Kyriakidou O. Diffusion of innovations in service organizations: systematic review and recommendations. Milbank Q. 2004;82(4):581-629. Epub 2004/12/15.

23   Gruen RL, Elliott JH, Nolan ML, Lawton PD, Parkhill A, McLaren CJ, et al. Sustainability science: an integrated approach for health-programme planning. Lancet. 2008;372(9649):1579-89. Epub 2008/11/06.

24   O'Loughlin J, Renaud L, Richard L, Gomez LS, Paradis G. Correlates of the sustainability of community-based heart health promotion interventions. Prev Med. 1998;27(5 Pt 1):702-12. Epub 1998/11/11.

12

Tobacco Use and Addiction Management in Primary Care Settings

DIANE KUNYK, SOPHIA PAPADAKIS, CHARL ELS AND EMILENE REISDORFER

AS MOST INDIVIDUALS ACCESS PRIMARY CARE SERVICES FOR THEIR HEALTH NEEDS throughout their lifespan, the primary care setting is arguably the most ideal location for treating all stages of tobacco use and addiction. This includes stopping the progression from tobacco use experimentation to regular tobacco use, the advancement to tobacco addiction, and the subsequent development of tobacco-related chronic diseases. Tobacco addiction, as with other chronic diseases, requires management on a longitudinal paradigm that takes into account the individuals' readiness for change, response to treatment, recovery support, and relapse to tobacco use. Given the experience of primary care professionals in providing both disease prevention and chronic illness care, often to the same patient and sometimes in the same visit, tobacco management can be, and has been, successfully integrated into primary care settings. For those settings that have not yet done so, incorporating tobacco management into primary care settings appears to be a most logical step. Although many different groups of health professionals and practice settings occur in primary care, this chapter will place a particular focus on physicians and their settings as this is the area with the predominance of research in the field.

OPPORTUNITY

Many individuals and their families who regularly access services in primary care settings are either directly or indirectly affected by the use of tobacco products.

Approximately 80% of individuals that smoke visited their physicians at least once in the last calendar year.[1] When compared with their colleagues, family physicians are uniquely positioned to intervene because they see their patients more frequently and for longer periods of time than do specialists, and may develop a strong rapport with their patients. Moreover many individuals with high rates of tobacco use and tobacco addiction access primary care services on a regular basis, for example, women in their childbearing years, individuals with psychiatric or other substance use disorders, those with other chronic diseases (e.g. heart disease, cancer, diabetes), and others presenting with multiple combinations of risk factors. The magnitude of the health consequences induced by tobacco warrants the prioritization of tobacco use and addiction treatment as a standard of care in the primary care setting.[2] If a patient uses tobacco, there is no other clinical intervention as powerful in reducing their burden of disease, disability, and death as tobacco cessation[3,4]

There is great potential for healthcare professionals in primary care settings to positively intervene with their patients that are experimenting with tobacco, currently smoking or using other forms of tobacco, at risk of relapse to tobacco use or having returned to smoking. Thirty percent of people who are currently smoking report their intention to quit within the next 30 days, and almost half of individuals that smoke had tried to quit within the last year.[1] With this level of interest in changing tobacco use patterns, healthcare professionals have tremendous opportunities to be major positive contributors to the efforts of their patients to reduce or quit.

Primary care settings offer an opportunity to routinely and regularly offer treatment for all stages of tobacco use and addiction. In 1985, Chapman concluded that smoking cessation initiatives are inconsequential "if they are incapable of being incorporated into a delivery system involving significant numbers of the smoking community." When considering the contributions of smoking cessation on whole populations, specialty smoking cessation clinics are inconsequential in contributing to reducing smoking in whole populations.[5] His observation draws attention to the importance, and the prevalence of tobacco use speaks to the immediacy of routinely incorporating tobacco management into primary care practices.

TOBACCO USE SCREENING AND TREATMENT BY HEALTHCARE PROFESSIONALS

The integration of tobacco screening and treatment into the everyday practices of all the healthcare disciplines is important for positive change. Even brief intervention by a healthcare professional can significantly increase cessation rates, and the likelihood of quitting increases when the patient hears the message from a number of healthcare professionals from a variety of disciplines.[6]

There are several well-established interventions for increasing the motivation of an individual who uses tobacco to quit (see Table 1.0). A healthcare professional's advice to quit has been shown to increase both motivation to quit and long term success with quitting.[6] A study by Ossip-Klein (2000) documented that patients who quit smoking report their practitioners' advice to quit as having influenced their decision to quit "extremely" or "quite a lot".[7] Two meta-analyses have been published that summarize the evidence regarding the efficacy of practitioner advice and counselling on smoking abstinence. The United States Department of Human Health Service (USD-HHS) Clinical Practice Guidelines for Treating Tobacco Use and Dependence reported the pooled odds ratio (OR) of long-term cessation (6 to 12 months) for physician advice to quit compared to no advice was 1.3 [95% CI 1.01, 1.6] for brief counselling (< 3 minutes); 1.6 [95% CI 1.2-2.0] for low intensity counselling (3 to 10 minutes); and 2.3 [95% CI 2.0-2.7] for higher intensity counselling (>10 minutes).[6] This is the equivalent of an increase in the rate of cessation of approximately 2.5%, 5%, and 11.2%, respectively, compared to controls.

A second meta-analysis published by the Cochrane Collaboration, comparing physician advice to controls, reported on the efficacy of *minimal advice* and intensive cessation interventions delivered by physicians.[8] Within the review, *minimal advice* was defined as advice provided during a single consultation lasting less than 20 minutes with up to one follow-up visit. *Intensive intervention* was considered to involve a greater time commitment at the initial consultation, the use of additional materials other than a leaflet, or more than one follow-up visit. Similar to the USDHHS guideline, the review found a significant increase in the rate of quitting relative risk (RR) 1.66 [95% CI 1.42-1.94] for *minimal advice* and RR 1.84 [95% CI 1.60-2.13] for *intensive intervention*.[8]

A healthcare professional's advice is most impactful when it is personally relevant to the patient's clinical situation, and is delivered clearly and unambiguously in a non-judgmental manner.[6] A recent meta-analysis revealed that providing advice *along with an offer of assistance and support* will be substantially more effective in increasing a patient's motivation to quit than simply providing advice.[9]

TABLE 1. Summary of Best Practice Smoking Cessation
Interventions

Intervention	Increase in quit rate
Price (taxation)[a]	
10%	7.1%
15	10.6%
20%	14.0%
Mass Media & Targeted Promotional Campaigns[a-c]	2.5%
Health Professional Advice to Quit[a,d]	
Advice (< 3 mins)	2.5%
Brief Intervention (3-10 mins)	5.0%
Intervention (> 10 mins)	11.0%
Availability of Cost Free Pharmacotherapy[d,e]	8.9%

Sources: [a]National Institutes of Health, National Cancer Institute. Population based smoking cessation; 2000. [b]Flay BR. Mass media and smoking cessation: a critical review. Am. J. Public Health 1987 Feb; 77(2):153-160. [c]Friend K, Levy DT. Reductions in smoking prevalence and cigarette consumption associated with mass media campaigns. Health Educ. Res. 2002 Feb; 17(1):85-98. [d]Fiore MC, Jaen C, Baker T, Bailey W, Benowitz N, et al. (2008). Clinical Practice Guideline: Treating Tobacco Use and Dependence, 2008 Update. USDHHS. [e]Reda AA, Kotz D, Evers SMAA, van Schayck CP. Healthcare financing systems for increasing the use of tobacco dependence treatment. Cochrane Database of Systematic Reviews 2012, Issue 6. Art. No.:CD004305. DOI: 10.1002/14651858.CD004305.pub4.

    In a joint statement developed by the Canadian Associations of occupational therapists, social workers, dentists, physicians, nurses, physiotherapists, pharmacists, respiratory therapists, and psychologists, it was identified that tobacco cessation is one of the most important interventions a care provider can offer, that a comprehensive and multidisciplinary approach is important, each health profession offers its own knowledge and skills to advance the strategy, and that health professionals should take advantage of opportunities to reduce tobacco use.[10] Aveyard and Raw (2012) observed that in the case of tobacco addiction and hypertension, it is possible to stop smoking and reduce blood pressure by lifestyle changes alone. In both cases, there is also good evidence that medication interventions increase the success rates. Therefore, they conclude that it seems reasonable to identify and to offer medical intervention often for both tobacco addiction and hypertension in primary care.[9]

RATES OF TOBACCO TREATMENT DELIVERY IN PRIMARY CARE SETTINGS

The interventions of tobacco use screening and treatment have been summarized into a "5A" strategy mnemonic in the USDHHS Guidelines. These are to "Ask" and record the smoking status of all patients at each visit; "Advise" all individuals currently smoking to quit; "Assess" readiness of those currently smoking to make a quit attempt; "Assist" with decreasing or quitting tobacco use (e.g. psycho-social and/or pharmaceutical support), and "Arranging" for follow-up.[6] When provided by health care professionals, these are considered highly effective interventions in terms of their relative health impact, health effectiveness, and cost-effectiveness.[6]

Tobacco use screening and treatment are not implemented as widely or comprehensively as could be in primary care settings. Busy healthcare professionals sometimes miss opportunities for interventions. The Canadian Tobacco Use Monitoring Survey found fifty-six percent of smokers who saw a physician in the previous 12-month received advice to quit smoking. The rate a which cessation advice is delivered to patients has increased over the last decade (See Figure 1).[1] However, in a multi-country review, it was determined that although many may question new patients, few physicians routinely ask their regular patients regarding their smoking status (thereby not identifying new users or their patients having relapsed).[11]

FIGURE 1: Percentage of visitors to doctor who received advice to quit in the past 12 months, 2013-2010

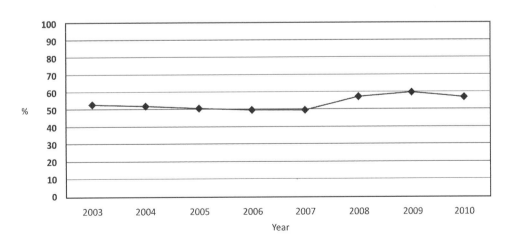

Adapted from Reid 2012; Original Source CTUMS 2003-2010.

FIGURE 2: Percentage of current smokers who received advice to quit and information on quitting assistance from health professionals in the past 12 months, 2010

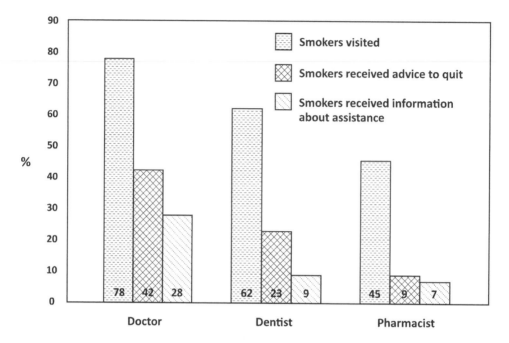

Adapted from Reid 2012; Original Source CTUMS, 2010.

The rates at which assistance with quitting and arranging follow-up support are recorded at lower numbers.[1] Published studies conducted in the primary care setting have documented that between 15-49% of smokers are offered assistance with quitting, 3-8% prescribed a quit smoking medication, and 3-9 % arranged follow-up contact.[12,13,14,15] This stands in stark contrast to the treatment of other chronic conditions such as hypertensionwhere 80% of Canadians receive evidence-based interventions and 66% are successfully treated for high blood pressure.[16] In terms of enhancing the potential of primary care, the critical next steps appear to be to continue to support and enhance tobacco use screening but to emphasize further extension of healthcare providers' involvement into tobacco addiction treatment interventions.

BARRIERS TO IMPLEMENTATION

Multiple barriers have been cited to account for the evidence-practice gap in tobacco use and addiction treatment such as competing priorities, inadequate time, insufficient training, perceived lack of knowledge and skills, limited practice supports, lack of organizational leadership and perceived patient reluctance.[11,18,19] One study documented that only one quarter to one third of family physicians have received smoking cessation training.[20] Some authors have concluded that guidelines on tobacco cessation are pushing physicians to intervene in a way that they do not feel comfortable with and are asking for more time than considered reasonable.[20] Healthcare professional groups have been examined to determine their correlates for tobacco cessation intervention. In a study of general practitioners, pharmacists, dentists, dental hygienists, nurses and respiratory therapists, similar findings appeared. Improved performance of counseling across these health disciplines included having interventions that addressed beliefs that cessation counseling is the role of health professionals, self-efficacy for performing interventions, and knowledge of resources.[21] Proposed solutions have been to develop tools to help physicians to support this work, exploring the use of briefer interventions, sharing the intervention responsibility across the healthcare delivery team, and creating system level supports for tobacco use and addiction management.[22]

SYSTEMS LEVEL SUPPORTS FOR INTERVENTION

For primary care health professionals to positively intervene, it appears critical to develop a mechanism that empowers, motivates, and supports the development of necessary knowledge, skills, and confidence for treating tobacco addiction. To increase this capacity, both individual care providers and the organization/system in which they work are considered focal points for intervention. In terms of organizational capacity for supporting practitioners and patients to change their behaviours, seven critical functions have been identified. These include professional development, priming and prompting, identification of risk and related complications, continuing care opportunities, linkages and networks for support, options for assistance as well as information management.[23]

The specific integration of a comprehensive, evidence-based system level intervention for tobacco addiction management into healthcare systems and practices has been specifically addressed in the USDHHS Guidelines.[22] These have been identified as having the potential to increase rates of tobacco-user identification and intervention, and subsequently to improve the health of patients through facilitating quit attempts. The identified key elements that are relevant to primary care settings include:

1. The implementation of a tobacco-use identification system in every clinic to ensure tobacco-use status is queried and documented at

every visit. Prompting of the healthcare professional increase the rate of asking about tobacco use and has been demonstrated to increase the rate at which intervention occurs.

2. Healthcare systems should ensure that healthcare professionals have: a) sufficient training to treat tobacco addiction; b) healthcare professionals and their patients have the necessary resources for assistance with tobacco cessation, and; c) healthcare professionals are given feedback about their tobacco addiction treatment practices.

3. Dedicating staff to provide tobacco-dependent treatment and assessing the delivery of this treatment in staff performance evaluations. Clinical sites should communicate to all staff members about the importance of intervening with individuals who are addicted to tobacco. Having a designated core staff member in the lead role for providing treatment or ensuring that treatment is provided has been demonstrated to improve treatment delivery. Non-physician personnel may also serve as effective providers of tobacco addiction interventions.

4. Provide comprehensive coverage for effective tobacco addiction treatments as these reduce barriers for accessing care.

5. Reimburse healthcare professionals for delivering effective tobacco addiction treatments and include these interventions among their defined dutes.[22]

EFFICACY OF INTERVENTIONS IN PRIMARY CARE

Papadakis (2010) performed a systematic review 37 trials and meta-analysis of evidence-based strategies for increasing the delivery of smoking cessation treatments in primary care clinics supported to efficacy of interventions in increasing the delivery of the '5As' (See table 2). Components which contributed to positive outcomes included provider training, checklists, screeners, Electronic Medical Record prompts, academic detailing, provider performance feedback, increased length of physician consultation, and adjunct counselling. The review also found when delivered in isolation, provider training, tailored print patient education materials, screeners/vital sign stamps, and provider incentives did not affect provider treatment rates or smoking abstinence.[24]

TABLE 2: Pooled odds ratio of 5As delivery for patient-level, physician-level, practice-level, system-level and multi-component intervention strategies delivered in primary care settings

Intervention	Smoking Abstinence		Ask		Advise		Assess		Assist Meds		Assist Quit Date		Assist		Arrange	
	k	OR [95%CI]	k	OR [95%CI]	k	OR [95%CI]	k	OR [95%CI]	k	OR [95%CI]	k	OR [95%CI]	k	OR [95%CI]	k	OR [95%CI]
Patient-Level																
Adjunct Counselling	7	1.7 [1.5, 2.0]	1	2.0 [1.7, 2.3]	1	1.6 [0.9, 2.8]	-	-	2	6.3 [4.5, 8.8]	-	-	-	-	3	13.8 [9.9, 19]
Tailored Print	2	1.5 [1.1, 2.1]	-	-	-	-	-	-	-	-	-	-	-	-	-	-
Practitioner-Level																
Training	2	0.9 [0.62, 1.3]	1	1.3 [1.0, 1.7]	-	-	-	-	-	-	-	-	-	-	-	-
Performance Feedback	-	-	2	2.9 [0.8, 11.2]	2	1.4 [0.8, 2.3]	1	2.9 [1.4, 5.9]	-	-	-	-	2	9.4 [5.2, 17.2]	1	47.4 [2.8, 795]
Practice-Level																
Screeners/Vital Stamp	2	0.9 [0.8, 1.0]	3	1.4 [1.3, 1.6]	3	0.6 [0.5, 0.6]	-	-	1	0.6 [0.5, 0.8]	1	0.6 [0.4, 0.7]	-	-	1	0.3 [0.2, 0.4]
Checklist	-	-	-	-	-	-	-	-	-	-	-	-	1	6.9 [3.8, 12.6]	-	-
Electronic Prompts	-	-	4	1.7 [1.4, 1.9]	1	1.4 [1.2, 1.6]	2	2.3 [2.0, 2.6]	-	-	-	-	2	1.2 [1.0, 1.3]	1	2.3 [1.9, 2.8]
Academic Detailing	1	1.0 [0.63, 1.5]	-	-	1	1.3 [1.0, 1.6]	-	-	-	-	-	-	-	-	1	0.7 [0.6, 0.9]
System-Level																
Provider Incentives	1	1.2 [1.0, 1.5]	1	1.4 [1.2, 1.6]	1	1.1 [0.8, 1.5]	-	-	-	-	-	-	-	-	1	2.9 [2.6, 3.3]
Multi-Component	7	2.2 [1.7, 2.8]	6	1.8 [1.6, 2.1]	7	1.6 [1.4, 1.8]	3	1.9 [1.4, 2.7]	5	3.5 [2.8, 4.2]	4	9.3 [6.8, 12.8]	1	1.2 [0.8, 1.9]	1	8.5 [5.1, 14.2]

Source: Papadakis, S., et al. 2010. Strategies to increase the delivery of smoking cessation treatments in primary care settings: A systematic review and meta-analysis. Preventive Medicine 51, no. 3-4:199-213. Includes studies published before January 1, 2009. k=number of studies. Odds ratios (OR) and 95% CI have been adjusted to reflect clustering for all trials who reported ICC values within the publication. Reproduced with permission of Elsevier.

Multi-component interventions that combine two or more intervention strategies have been shown to be the most effective method for increasing healthcare provider performance in the delivery of tobacco cessation treatments and have been shown to improve cessation rates among patients.[22,24,25,26] Multiple large-scale controlled trials have demonstrated a significant impact of multi-component interventions in increasing the rates at which primary care providers deliver evidence-based smoking cessation treatments to patients as well as patient cessation rates. One study, exploring the influence of system interventions on tobacco use and addiction treatment in 60 primary care clinics, found that healthcare providers were significantly more likely (2.04 to 5.62 fold) to perform all 5 A interventions when they were working in a setting that incorporated enhanced delivery system designs, clinical information systems, and patient self-management supports for smoking cessation.[27] This included the use of proactive, planned chronic care visits (rather than reactive responses to acute illness episodes) in addition to the use of self-care strategies which provided patients with information, skills and confidence in meeting their health goals.[27]

MODELS OF INTERVENTION

With almost 1 in 5 adults smoking, the responsibility for the burden of care cannot be limited to physicians or to specialty referral services. A shared care model recognizes that healthcare professional groups all have unique contributions and can play a key role in tobacco use and addiction management. Systematic reviews and clinical experience have demonstrated that practices with comprehensive interventions that incorporate all members of the healthcare team are more likely to promote healthy change than those with isolated interventions. The effectiveness of the interventions are probably maximized when practices have systems in place to support the entire counselling sequence—all of the 5 A's—rather than simply components of the process.[22,24,28,29]

According to treatment guidelines, more intensive support is more effective and the best support is to offer, when appropriate, a combination of therapies including a comprehensive psychosocial intervention. For some primary care settings without the necessary capacity, and for treatment resistant patients, referrals or linkages with other resources may be initiated. Models of care delivery in these situations may include referrals to a tobacco treatment specialist service, a telephone quitline service, or to group classes, among other options (see Chapter 8).

The appropriateness and convenience of these services as referral sources may be limited by, for example, availability, accessibility, expense, patient resistance and utilization, and communication strategies. Bidirectional communication between practices and referral sources is a critical component for safe healthcare delivery is critical for primary care. As with any consulting relationship, it is necessary for these resources to work with primary care professionals in a team approach, reporting to and consulting with clinicians as counselling progresses, and integrating follow-up into ongoing healthcare.[32]

Considerable systemic challenges exist for this to occur. A national study on fax referral systems linking patients to quitlines noted that for success, there was the necessity for knowledge of existing patterns of care and tailored organizational changes to ensure new systems are prioritized, ease of integration into current office routines, formal assignment to specific staff members, and support by internal systems to ensure adequate tracing and follow-up of patients.[33] The complexity of appropriate communication is a substantial barrier for the referral process.

CONCLUSIONS

Healthcare professionals in primary care settings are uniquely positioned to intervene with their patients as they cycle from tobacco experimentation to addiction, quit attempts, and relapse. There is an opportunity to increase the rates and scope of intervention, and system level supports can positively support this to occur. The integration of tobacco management into routine primary care practice provides opportunities to significantly improve the quality and duration of patients' lives. Improving the implementation of tobacco management into primary care settings is an important public health goal.

REFERENCES

1   Reid JL, Hammond D, Burkhalter R, Ahmed R. Tobacco Use in Canada: Patterns and Trends, 2012 Edition. Waterloo, ON: Propel Centre for Population Health Impact, University of Waterloo. www.tobaccoreport.ca.

2   WHO Report on the Global Tobacco Epidemic, 2008: The MPOWER package. Geneva: World Health Organization; 2008.

3   Woolf SH. The need for perspective in evidence-based medicine. JAMA. 1999 Dec 22-29;282(24):2358-65.

4   Gaziano TA, Galea G, Reddy KS. Scaling up interventions for chronic disease prevention: the evidence. Lancet. 2007 Dec 8;370(9603):1939-46.

5   Chapman S. Stop smoking clinics: a case for their abandonment. Lancet. 1985;1:918-20.

6   Fiore MC, Jaén CR, Baker TB, Bailey, WC, Benowitz, NL, Curry, SJ, et al. Treating tobacco use and dependence: 2008 update. Clinical practice guideline. Rockville MD: U.S. Department of Health and Human Services. Public Health Service; 2008 May [cited 2012 Mar 16]. Available from: http://www.surgeongeneral.gov/tobacco/treating_tobacco_use08.pdf.

7   Ossip-Klein DJ, McIntosh S, Utman C, Burton K, Spada J, Guido J. Smokers ages 50+: who gets physician advice to quit? Prev Med. 2000 Oct;31(4):364-9.

8   Stead LF, Bergson G, Lancaster T. Physician advice for smoking cessation. Cochrane Database Syst Rev. 2008(2):CD000165.

9   Aveyard P, Begh R, Parsons A, West R. Brief opportunistic smoking cessation interventions: a systematic review and meta-analysis to compare advice to quit and offer of assistance. Addiction. 2012 Jun;107(6):1066-73.

10   Joint statement: tobacco: the role of health professionals. Issued by: Canadian Association of Occupational Therapists, Canadian Association of Social Workers, Canadian Dental, Association, Canadian Medical Association, Canadian Nurses Association, Canadian Pharmacists Association, Canadian Physiotherapy Association, Canadian Psychological Association, and Canadian Society of Respiratory Therapists; Jan 2001.

11   Stead M, Angus K, Holme I, et al. Factors influencing European GPs' engagement in smoking cessation: a multi-country review. Br J Gen Pract. 2009;5(566):682-90.

12   Canadian Tobacco Use Monitoring Survey (CTUMS). (2005). Smoking-cessation advice from health-care providers---Canada, 2005. Retrieved from http://www.cdc.gov/mmwr/preview/mmwrhtml/mm5628a3.htm

13   Goldstein MG, Niaura R, Willey-Lessne C. DePue J, Eaton C, Rakowski W, Dube C. (1997). Physicians counseling smokers. A population-based survey of patients' perceptions of health care provider-delivered smoking cessation interventions. Archives of Internal Medicine 2007;157(12), 1313-19.

14   Gottlieb NH, Huang PP, Blozis SA, Guo J, Smith MM. The impact of put prevention into practice on selected clinical preventive services in five Texas sites. American Journal of Preventive Medicine. 2001;21(1), 35-40.

15   Quinn VP Stevens VJ, Hollis JF, Rigotti NA, Solberg LI, Gordon N, . . . Zapka J. Tobacco-cessation services and patient satisfaction in nine nonprofit HMOs. American Journal of Preventive Medicine, 2005;29(2), 77-84. doi:DOI: 10.1016/j.amepre.2005.04.006.

16   Canadian Health Measure Survey (CMHS). Canadian Health Measures Survey: Blood Pressure in Adults 2007-2009. Retrieved from http://www.statcan.gc.ca/daily-quotidien/100217/dq100217b-eng.htm

18   Vogt F, Hall S, Marteau T. General practitioners' and family physicians' negative beliefs and attitudes towards discussing smoking cessation with patients: a systematic review. Addiction. 2005;100:1423-31.

19   Association of American Medical Colleges. Physician behavior and practice patterns related to smoking cessation; 2007 [accessed 2012 May 19]. Available from: https://www.aamc.org/download/55438/data/smokingcessationsummary.pdf.

20   Tremblay M, Cournoyer D, O'Loughlin J. Do the correlates of smoking cessation counseling differ across health professional groups? Nicotine Tob Res. 2009;11(11):1330-8.

21   Coleman T, Murphy E, Cheater F. Factors influencing discussion of smoking between general practitioners and patients who smoke: a qualitative study. Br J Gen Pract. 2000; 50:207-10.

22   Fiore MC, Keller PS, Curry SJ (2007). Health system changes to facilitate the delivery of tobacco-dependence treatment. Am J Prev Med. 33(6 Suppl); S349-56.

23   Skinner H. Promoting Health Through Organizational Change. 2002. San Francisco: Benjamin Cummings.

24   Papadakis S, McDonald P, Mullen KA, et al. Strategies to increase the delivery of smoking cessation treatments in primary care settings: a systematic review and meta-analysis. Prev Med. 2010;51(3-4):199-213.

25   Grimshaw JM et al. Changing provider behavior: an overview of systematic reviews of interventions. Medical Care 2001 39, no. 8 Suppl 2:II2-45.

26   Anderson P, Jane-Llopis E. How can we increase the involvement of primary health care in the treatment of tobacco dependence? A meta-analysis. Addiction. 2004;99, 299–312.

27   Hung D, Shelley D, Multilevel analysis of the chronic care model and 5A services for treating tobacco use in urban primary care clinic. Health Services Research. 2009; 44(1).103-27.

28   An LC, Foldes SS, Alesci NL, Bluhm JH, Bland PC, Davern ME, . . . Manley MW (2008). The impact of smoking-cessation intervention by multiple health professionals. American Journal of Preventive Medicine. 2008;34(1), 54-60. doi:DOI: 10.1016/j.amepre.2007.09.019

29   Gorin SS, Heck JE. Meta-analysis of the efficacy of tobacco counseling by health care providers. Cancer Epidemiology, Biomarkers & Prevention, 2004;13(12), 2012-2022.

30   Hollis JF, Lichtenstein E, Vogt TM, Stevens, V. J., & Biglan, A. (1993). Nurse-assisted counseling for smokers in primary care. Annals of Internal Medicine, 118(7), 521-525.

31   Kottke, T. E., Battista, R. N., DeFriese, G. H., & Brekke, M. L. (1988). Attributes of successful smoking cessation interventions in medical practice. A meta-analysis of 39 controlled trials. Journal of the American Medical Association, 259, 2882-2889

32   Woolf S, Grasgow R, Krist A et al. Putting it together: finding success in behavior change through integration of services. Ann Fam Med 2004;3(Suppl 2): 520-7.

33   Cantrell J, Shelly D. Implementing a fax referral program for quitline smoking cessation services in urban health centers: a qualitative study. BMC Fam Pract. 2009;10:81.

13

Cessation and the Workplace

DIANE KUNYK, CHARL ELS AND DAVID VAN DRIESUM

This chapter has been adapted from the original article: Kunyk D, Els C, Selby P. Smoking cessation and the workplace: what physicians need to know. Smoking Cessation Rounds. 2008; 2(5): The Minto Prevention and Rehabilitation Centre, University of Ottawa Heart Institute and the Addiction Medicine Service, Centre for Addiction and Mental Health, University of Toronto, used with permission.

THE WORKPLACE IS RECOGNIZED AS AN IDEAL SETTING FOR HEALTH PROMOTION activities given the large number of adults who spend several hours each day at work, the opportunity to deliver uniquely tailored programs, and the benefits that accrue to both participants and employers. Tobacco cessation is no exception. Successful workplace cessation programs often follow the introduction of smoke-free policies in a corporate setting. Both can enhance employee health, business performance, and community wellbeing.

SMOKING AS A CAUSE OF ABSENTEEISM AND "PRESENTEEISM"

Many employers understand the significant costs incurred in the workplace by their tobacco-addicted employees. Employees who smoke take more days of sick leave and tend to be more prone to workplace injuries when compared with their non-smoking counterparts.[1] In a review of 30 studies of employee absenteeism conducted between 1960 and 1998, all but one found higher rates of absenteeism among individuals who smoke, and 17 studies reported absenteeism at least 20% higher than among non-smokers.[2] Data from the Canadian Community Health Survey (2004) revealed that individuals who smoke are absent from work two more days annually than non-smoking colleagues.[3] The Conference Board of Canada (2006) translates this absenteeism into an average of $323 per smoker per year in lost revenue to the employer.[b, 4]

The cost of breaks taken for smoking during the workday has also been quantified. On average, 5 cigarettes are smoked during the workday[c] and 89% of employees who smoke will have a cigarette every 1–2 hours. At least 2 of these cigarettes (requiring an average time consumption of 20 minutes each[d]) will occur outside sanctioned break periods, and thus at the direct expense of the employer. These typically unauthorized breaks are considered lost productive time and have negative repercussions on work performance and the organization's bottom line. The phenomenon of "presenteeism" was estimated to cost an employer $13.45 daily or $3,053 annually for each employee who smokes (based on a mean salary of $38,978 as reported by Statistics Canada).[4]

There are other intangible costs associated with smoking. One is that the professional image of the corporation may be negatively impacted when employees smoke, particularly in highly visible public areas where smoking is perceived by society in a negative light. This has obvious implications for hospitals and other healthcare practice settings, as the public may be sensitive to what may be seen as hypocritical behavior by those having a fundamental commitment to health and well-being.

TOWARDS A TOBACCO-FREE WORKFORCE

Some employers who are aware of the impact of tobacco use on their bottom line are taking steps to encourage their employees who smoke to quit. There are some that are refusing to employ applicants who smoke,[5] and others that require new employees to commit to being non-smokers by a certain date; dismissal may follow for those who are unsuccessful.[6]

---

[b] The average daily per-employee payroll cost is made up of the average daily wages for Canadian workers, and taxes and benefits paid by the employer. This includes legislated payroll taxes as well as supplementary health insurance premiums.

[c] The daily number of cigarettes consumed at the time of the report was 15.2 per day. To determine loss of productivity to smoking breaks, a day was assumed to be 16 hours (with the other 8 allocated for sleep). The model assumed that the most cigarettes would be consumed outside of working time, with only 5 cigarettes being consumed in an 8-hour workday. Of these 5 cigarettes, 3 would be consumed during employer-sanctioned breaks taken by all staff: lunch, one mid-morning and one mid-afternoon break.

[d] Broken down into 10 minutes to smoke and 10 to travel to a designated site. This estimate assumes that smoking is lost productive time, but it could be argued that this time could be spent discussing, contemplating, or reading about business matters.

These policies raise questions about discriminatory practices towards individuals with a medical condition.[7] Such approaches would be most effective when combined with policies designed to sensitively, strategically, and effectively assist cessation. It is worth noting that in addition to the improvement in workforce health and productivity, tobacco-free workforce policies send strong signals to students and young adults about the increasing unacceptability of smoking—a disincentive to starting smoking.[8]

Tobacco-free workforce policies also raise questions regarding respect of personal privacy by an employer. It has been argued that off-duty conduct—even if dangerous or unhealthy—is not the concern of an employer. Maltby (2008) notes that junk food, red meat, lack of exercise or sleep, multiple sex partners, and recreational activities all increase medical costs for the employer. The recommendation is that employment decisions should be based on job performance rather than focusing on so-called private lifestyle choices.[9] Personal privacy concerns may be lessened when the employer is willing to provide the cessation assistance that is necessary to help the employee quit using tobacco. Berman and Crane (2008) posit that if the employer demonstrates an appropriate understanding of the difficulty of tobacco cessation (and the multiple attempts that may be involved in the process), the requirement to attempt quitting does not infringe on personal privacy more than other employer conditions. Employees are often required to move, upgrade their skills, relinquish other outside employment, refrain from using or endorsing competitors' products, and rearrange their personal schedules.[8] Tobacco-free workforce policies are best placed within workforce-wellness agendas that may include healthier foods in cafeterias, opportunities for physical activity, and access to fitness programs.

NICOTINE WITHDRAWAL

Addiction to nicotine influences tobacco dependent employees through the manifestation of withdrawal symptoms during the working day. Nicotine is delivered rapidly to the brain with each inhalation but the effect is usually short-acting. When unable to smoke, the individual may, and will likely, experience both physical and psychological withdrawal from nicotine, commonly manifested by symptoms such as anxiety, restlessness, irritability, impaired task performance, and diminished concentration. The ongoing, repetitive, and prolonged withdrawals from nicotine that smoking employees suffer each day in the workplace may diminish both productivity and affability. As a measure to reduce this discomfort, and to reduce the need for unsanctioned breaks, the employer could provide nicotine replacement products as a measure to remedy the impact of withdrawal symptoms. However, it has to be established whether the employer takes on any potential excess risk by supplying these products, in case of any putative adverse events.

WORKPLACE TOBACCO CESSATION

Investments in employee health and wellness are considered sound investments. Lowe (2003) examined the economic case and the return on investment for programs that improve health outcomes for employees, reduce employer healthcare insurance costs, and improve productivity. It was calculated that within 5 years there is a return of between $3 and $8 for every $1 invested in health promotion programs; most of this 'dividend' accrues as a result of reduced absenteeism.[10]

Addressing tobacco reduction in the workplace provides access to a large number of people, has the potential for higher participation rates than might be the case in other, non-workplace environments, can encourage sustained peer group support and positive peer pressure, and the employee is not required to travel to participate. This may also be a particularly good opportunity to target young men who often do not access medical care and have high rates of smoking. A systematic review of 33 research studies on tobacco cessation in the workplace revealed strong evidence that these interventions increase the likelihood of quitting smoking. Critical elements for program success include: advice from a health professional regarding the importance of cessation, individual and group counselling, as well as the provision of pharmacotherapy to aid in the control of withdrawal symptoms and cravings. Self-help interventions were found to be less effective.[11]

The workplace environment can support employees in their attempts to reduce or quit smoking. Workplace tobacco policies and bans can significantly decrease cigarette consumption during the working day and the exposure of non-smoking employees to environmental tobacco smoke at work.[12] These encourage employees to make a quit attempt and improve their ability to remain abstinent from smoking. Employers may wish to enhance the quality of smoking cessation programs and improve the chances their employees will successfully quit smoking by extending benefits to their employees' family members. Individuals who make a quit attempt are more likely to succeed, and less likely to relapse, when there is no smoking in their home.[13]

The most salient barriers currently faced by individuals for quitting pertain to the accessibility, affordability, and availability of evidence-based interventions for smoking cessation. State-of-the-art smoking cessation programs incorporate both education and the provision of specific assistance with cessation. Ironically, many workplace drug-benefit plans do not cover the cost of cessation pharmacotherapies, despite evidence of significance in enhancing the likelihood of successful cessation. Tobacco dependence treatments are both clinically effective and highly cost-effective relative to interventions for other clinical disorders, and providing coverage (on par with other chronic disease interventions) increases quit rates, improves health outcomes, limits excess healthcare spending, and improves productivity.

CONCLUSION

Tobacco addiction profoundly impacts the workplace and the health of employees that smoke. Addressing the use of tobacco products by employees is a key area for employers to consider when their goal is to reduce overall expenditures and improve corporate yield while, at the same time, recognizing that both employee and community health will benefit. Progressive and enlightened workplace policies will increase the likelihood of quitting smoking thereby producing personal health and economic benefits while, at the same time, contributing to enhanced workplace productivity and safety. Organizations have identified that addressing key employee health issues can boost productivity and positively impact their bottom line.

REFERENCES

1   Wilkins K, Mackenzie SG. Work injuries. Health Reports. Statistics Canada, catalogue 82-003;2007;18:3.

2   US Centers for Disease Control and Prevention. Annual smoking attributable mortality, years of potential life lost and economic costs – United States, 1995-1999. Morbidity and Mortality Weekly Report. 2002;51(14):303.

3   Statistics Canada. Canadian Tobacco Use Monitoring Survey. Ottawa: Author; 2004. Public use micro-data files.

4   Conference Board of Canada. Smoking and the bottom line: updating the costs of smoking in the workplace. Ottawa: Author; 2006.

5   Colliver V. Employers ponder tough tactics to halt smoking. San Francisco Chronicle, June 18, 2008 [accessed 2012 May 19]. Available from: http://www.sfgate.com/cgi-bin/article.cgi?f=/c/a/2008/06/16/BUKG11A2VO.DTL.

6   Curet M, Stammen K. Your smokes or your job. Columbus Dispatch, Dec 9, 2005.

7   Pierotti J. Comment: the "bottom line" a smokescreen for the reality that antitobacco employment practices are hazardous to minority health and equality. J Contemp Health Law Pol. 2010:26(2):441-71.

8   Berman M, Crane R. Mandating a tobacco-free workforce: a convergence of business and public health interests. William Mitchell Law Rev. 2008;34(4):1651-74.

9   Maltby L. Whose life is it anyway? Employer control of off-duty smoking and individual autonomy. William Mitchell Law Rev. 2008;34(4):1639-49.

10   Lowe G. Healthy workplaces and productivity: a discussion paper. Ottawa: Economic Analysis and Evaluation Division, Health Canada; 2003.

11   Moher M, Hey K, Lancaster T. Workplace interventions for smoking cessation. Cochrane Database Syst Rev. 2008.

12   Fichtenberg C, Glantz S. Effect of smoke-free workplaces on smoking behavior: systematic review. BMJ. 2002;325:188-91.

13   Farkas A, Gilpin A, Distefan J, Pierce J. The effects of household and workplace smoking restrictions

14

Nontraditional Tobacco Use among Aboriginal Canadians

DENNIS WARDMAN, ROD MCCORMICK, DANIEL MCKENNITT AND PAMELA O'DONAGHEY

This chapter is dedicated to co-author Dr. Dennis Wardman's brother, Lance O'Soup, who died of lung cancer during its writing. Lance was 47 years old and was a smoker.

CANADA'S ABORIGINAL PEOPLES' HIGH SMOKING RATE WARRANTS SPECIAL ATTENTION for many reasons. First, and most critically, is the large number of preventable deaths. Especially alarming are First Nations infant deaths, at a rate of up to 8.3% from smoking-attributable illnesses such as respiratory distress syndrome and sudden infant death syndrome.[1] Another reason concerns the particular history of Canada's 1.2 million Aboriginal people—30% of which are First Nations (Status Indian) living on-reserve, 30% First Nations living off-reserve, 33% Métis, 4% Inuit, and 3% Multiple and Other Aboriginal groups.[2] The trauma arising from colonization, policies of assimilation, and loss of culture through residential schools and other means have been described as "collective emotional and psychological injury over the lifespan and across generations ... with the effects being psychological, behavioural, and medical."[3] This troubled history has to be taken into account in considering the incidence, causes, and impacts of smoking among Aboriginal people as well as the methods and approaches that will be most successful in its prevention or elimination.

For thousands of years prior to European contact, Aboriginal people's traditional relationship with tobacco was not recreational but medicinal and spiritual. Tobacco served as an analgesic to alleviate childbirth pains, toothaches, headaches, and earaches. It was applied as an antiseptic to treat open wounds. It was also used to treat ailments such as asthma, cough, rheumatism, convulsions, and intestinal disorders. Considered to be a sacred intermediary between the individual and Creator, tobacco was offered as a sacrifice to the Great Spirit, as a gift when welcoming guests to the community, and as an offering to those asked to pray or share wisdom.[4] Tobacco was also presented to the spirits for reasons such as encouraging rain in times of drought or ensuring the safe passage of travellers. The most powerful way to communicate with the spirit world was to smoke tobacco in a sacred pipe. The arrival of Europeans resulted in the widespread, nonreligious use of tobacco in trade meetings and as a substance for trade.[5] This ultimately led to its widespread misuse as a commercially produced substance that imperils the health, quality of life, and life expectancy of so many Aboriginal people.

In this chapter we will begin to weave the tapestry of tobacco and its impact on Canada's Aboriginal people; a tapestry that includes an examination of smoking rates, risk factors, causal connections, quit rates, intervention options, and programming issues; and a tapestry that reveals the importance of personal, community, and cultural empowerment in reducing the deadly effects of non-traditional tobacco use. Along with an overview and discussion of the research findings and their implications and applications arising from the authors' clinical practice with Aboriginal people, this chapter will provide practical suggestions for other healthcare providers working with Aboriginal adults and youth to help them address addiction to commercial tobacco and to discover ways to live healthier lives. Recognizing that for many of our people, healing is viewed in holistic terms and embraces the mental, physical, emotional, and spiritual realms, we will attempt to embrace all of these dimensions and their role in reversing tobacco misuse and reclaiming the health of Aboriginal people.

A NOTE ON TERMINOLOGY

Karina Czyzewski

We wish to recognize the debate surrounding appropriate terminology for this chapter. There is no consensus for a number of reasons. Although accepted as a global identifier and in academic circles, some feel the term Indigenous refers to people who were not displaced from their traditional lands and is therefore not specific to Canada. Others prefer the use of Aboriginal as it is specific to Canada and includes First Nations, Métis and Inuit; however, others dislike the term in part because it is an externally-imposed identifier. Many still use Native or Indian, although usage is limited and generally only accepted among community members. The use of peoples versus people is also significant: peoples refer to groups of people (of different Nations and cultures), whereas people implies less heterogeneity. Capitalization, as well as consistency, is also precarious: Indigenous, Aboriginal and First Peoples are used synonymously in many texts —often without stating as such.

There are those that feel the debate be put to rest and energies expended on more pressing matters; on the other hand, how the colonial government dictated and continues to impose or deny labels reveals the impact of politically-charged semantics and the significance of self-determining Indigenous identify.

The identifiers used in this text reflect their use by several authors, organizations and by a wider audience. There is no pan-Aboriginal or Indigenous person, traditions or values though, and the terms themselves encompass different political and legal implications. We also acknowledge that there are truer terms for the First Peoples of Turtle Island—terms that denote specific Nations, terms in Blackfoot or Cree, for instance, that mean the "original", "real" or "true" peoples. This caveat is not a solution but rather an acknowledgement of this debate and journey.

LITERATURE REVIEW

This literature review explores the prevalence of nontraditional tobacco use among Aboriginal people, risk factors that contribute to smoking, protective factors that prevent smoking, reasons for quitting, issues impacting quit attempts, as well as effective interventions. It examines studies featuring Canadian Aboriginal people as well as Indigenous peoples in the United States, Australia, and New Zealand. Aboriginal people in all 4 countries experience the harmful impacts of colonization and low socioeconomic status, higher smoking rates including among pregnant women, a younger average smoking initiation age, and elevated levels of secondhand smoke in the home.[6] These parallels, coupled with shared health impacts such as disproportionately higher rates of tobacco-related illnesses such as cancer, coronary heart disease, diabetes, and chronic lung disease indicate that the results of studies of Indigenous peoples in these countries would also shed light on some of issues related to tobacco use among Canadian Aboriginal people.

Prevalence of tobacco use among Aboriginal Canadians Less than half (43%) of First Nations adults smoke daily with an additional 13.7% self-identifying as smoking occasionally. This rate is more than double that of the general Canadian population (19%). As education levels increase, the proportion of daily smoking decreases, with a smoking rate of 47.8% in those with less than a high school education compared with 30.9% of those with graduate studies.[7] Women's smoking rates tend to be higher among those who are single, divorced, and unemployed.[8] High levels of dual tobacco use (cigarettes and smokeless tobacco) are associated with low levels of education and few social contacts.[9]

Younger First Nations adults, aged 18 to 29 years, have the highest proportion of daily smoking (51.5%), with smoking rates much higher among teenage girls than teenage boys. Sixty-one percent of Aboriginal girls aged 15 to 17 years smoke, a rate that is 4 times that of the 15% of 15- to 17-year-old girls in the general population.[10]

Smoking rates during pregnancy are also significant, with pre-pregnancy prevalence between 46.9% and 55.6% among younger Native women.[11] As pregnancies among young Aboriginal women occur at more than double the rate of the general population,[2] and many infants are considered to be at risk. Increased education is associated with dramatically less smoking during pregnancy, with a 53.5% smoking rate among mothers with less than a high school education contrasted with an 18% smoking rate among mothers with a university degree.[7]

Risk factors that contribute to high smoking rates The following risk factors contribute to high smoking rates among Canada's Aboriginal people.

High proportion of youth In Aboriginal communities, 48% of the population is 24 years of age and under as compared with 31% of the general population.[2] The average age of smoking initiation is 12 years old. Current smoking rates among Aboriginal youth are more than double that of non-Aboriginal youth (24.9% versus 10.4%). Aboriginal youth are also more likely to be regularly exposed to secondhand smoke at home (37.3% versus 19.7%) and in cars (51.0% versus 30.3%). In addition, they are less likely than non-Aboriginal youth to have tried to quit smoking.[10]

While more girls smoke than boys, girls smoke fewer cigarettes. Having a best friend who smokes is the most powerful predictor that a young person would start smoking as well, and young people with high depression scores have increased odds of smoking.[12] The co-use of smoking and alcohol consumption is also a salient issue among youth, and increased tobacco use is associated with increased levels of alcohol consumption.[13] This is a concern, given that Aboriginal youth are 2 to 6 times more likely to have alcohol-related problems than their non-Aboriginal peers.[14] Smoking is also directly related to other addictive behaviour including problem gambling.[15] Aboriginal youth are more likely than non-Aboriginal youth to experience gambling problems, and problem gamblers are more likely to be smokers than those who are not.[16]

Lone Parent Homes   Being brought up in a lone parent home is a risk factor for numerous dangerous behaviors, including tobacco misuse. Thirty-five percent of Aboriginal children are being raised in lone parent homes, a rate that is more than double the 17% of such children in the general population.[2]

Low education level   The proportion of the Aboriginal population aged 25 to 64 years without a high school diploma (34%) is 19 percentage points higher than the 15% in the non-Aboriginal population.[7]

Low employment and income levels   Smoking levels increase as employment and income levels decrease. The employment rate for Aboriginal people living on-reserve is 47.2%,[17] as compared with 61.8% for non-Aboriginal people. The unemployment rate for Aboriginal people aged 15 and over increased from 10.4% in 2008 to 13.9% in 2009, while the rate for non-Aboriginal people rose from 6.0% to 8.1%. During that same period, the employment rate for off-reserve Aboriginal youth 15–24 years old fell by 6.8%, compared with a decline of 4.2% among non-Aboriginal youth.[2] Further, there is a 30% median income gap between Aboriginal people ($18,962), and that of the rest of Canadians ($27,097).[18]

Preventing Aboriginal youth from starting to smoke   A supportive home environment and a balanced life are significant in preventing youth from smoking.[10] Factors such as not using drugs, college aspirations, and playing music are also preventative in nature,[19] as is involvement in sporting activities.[20]

Reasons Aboriginal individuals quit smoking   On average, First Nations smokers quit by age 32. The main reason by far is a desire for a healthier lifestyle. Other reasons include a health condition, respect for loved ones, and pregnancy.[10] Additional motivators to quit include perceived adverse health effects of tobacco, improved self-image and appearance, and the potential to be a role model for family and friends as a non-tobacco user.[21]

Issues that impact quit attempts   Aboriginal people who are 65–74 years of age or older, smoke fewer than 6 cigarettes daily, smoke infrequently, have smoked for fewer years, start smoking at 17 years or older, and have a history of diabetes[22] are more likely to quit smoking. Additional promising circumstances for quitting smoking include having a smoking ban in the home and being educated on the benefits of nicotine replacement therapy.[23]

The availability of lower priced cigarettes, as is the case in many First Nations communities, is associated with lower rates of quit attempts and cessation when compared with those who purchased from full-priced outlets.[24] Other factors that discourage quitting include feelings of mistrust and negative experiences with doctors; low knowledge and poor understanding of the benefits of pharmacotherapy; and historic and continuing racism.[25] Current alcohol use is another deterrent to stopping smoking.[26] Given that First Nations alcohol users are more than twice as likely to smoke (81.2 % versus 31.4%), this is a concern.[10]

Barriers preventing youth from quitting smoking include addiction and cravings, boredom, widespread tobacco use among peers and other community members, and lack of availability of effective resources to quit in their home communities.[21] Barriers notwithstanding, motivation among Aboriginal youth to quit smoking is high,[12] and in fact may be higher than among non-Aboriginal youth.[27]

Smoking cessation interventions and their effectiveness   Many Aboriginal people are interested in quitting smoking and nicotine replacement therapy (NRT), specifically nicotine patch, is one of the favoured options by which former smokers have stopped along with cold turkey, the use of spirituality, and family support[10] However, many smokers are disinclined to consult with a physician and to use medication therapy. Lack of awareness of the pharmacotherapy subsidy to which First Nations people are entitled along with the requirement for a physician prescription are additional barriers to using pharmacotherapy.[28]

Combining pharmacotherapy with individual or group behavioural counselling has proven effective.[29,30] Despite mistrust and lack of information about tobacco dependence treatment and its benefits, Aboriginal smokers are willing to try pharmacotherapy if it is made accessible in their community, and if community members offer testimonials.[25]

The literature indicates an urgent need for culturally sensitive smoking cessation interventions.[31] This includes increasing use of Native imagery and addressing the traditional/sacred/ceremonial meaning of tobacco.[32] There is no need to discourage use of tobacco for ceremonial purposes and in fact using traditional tobacco can increase abstinence from commercial tobacco use.[33] Ojibwe traditional healers and spiritual leaders have cautioned health professionals to "recognize, be amenable to learn, and to understand that sacred tobacco use and smoking commercial cigarette tobacco have separate purposes and functions."[34]

All Nations Breath of Life, comprised of weekly in-person group support sessions with individual telephone calls using motivational interviewing; discussion of sacred tobacco, and information about health, addiction, and the process of quitting, appears to be a successful example of culturally sensitive programming.[33]

Cultural sensitivity, along with the need to address peer smoking, is also at the centre of successful interventions for Aboriginal youth:

> "Peer-organized community-wide initiatives may represent a particularly potent approach to cigarette use, especially if these initiatives are part of a broad plan for cultural rejuvenation in communities to promote resilience and cultural continuity … because youth who are grounded in their culture and have strong family relationships have a solid basis for constructing their future self … [and are] … less likely to experience depression and engage in risk-taking behaviours". (Hutchinson et al, 2008 p.421)[12]

Aboriginal youth indicate that parent and family support is important in motivating them to quit tobacco, irrespective of parental tobacco use. They also favour talking circles or group counselling, along with personal stories of smokers who have quit and/or have experienced adverse health effects[21]

In the American Lung Association's *Not on Tobacco* (N-O-T) program for youth, Native young people meet weekly for hour-long, same-sex group sessions of up to 12 teens, led by a same-sex facilitator. The content includes the history of tobacco and its evolution from traditional to commercial use; culturally tailored graphics, print materials, audio media, and activities; and an emphasis on group identity and cohesion rather than individual efforts. This is an effective intervention, particularly with male youths.[35]

Elders in First Nations communities are seen to be another culturally relevant resource, whether as models for non-smoking or for teaching cultural traditions such as the ceremonial use of tobacco.[36] Training Aboriginal health workers in brief smoking cessation intervention with patients is likely to contribute to increased quit rates.[30]

Interventions that tap into the online community are also showing promise. Such interventions include sending supportive text messages to youth wanting to quit smoking, an initiative that "offers potential for a new way to help young smokers to quit, being affordable, personalized, age appropriate, and not location dependent."[37] Native youth are also receptive to a web-based Zine-style intervention tool, provided its look and feel is oriented toward their cultural images.[38]

Quitlines are another promising intervention for all age groups, with higher quit rates for Aboriginals than for non-Aboriginals, particularly for men.

Concern about future health and current health problems are the most common reasons Aboriginal participants call the quitline.[39]

Although youth respond favourably to incentives such as door prizes to encourage them to enroll and remain in a smoking cessation program,[21] within the broader community incentives (usually cash) may only attract smokers already motivated to quit, and would likely result in only 1% of smokers quitting smoking. Quit rates may be initially high but are likely to decrease over time.[40]

IMPLICATIONS AND KEY LEARNINGS FROM EMPIRICAL RESEARCH

Given the high incidence of tobacco use and its dangers, smoking is an important focus for all healthcare providers working with Aboriginal people. Healthcare providers must be prepared to play an educational role regarding tobacco use. Physicians need to educate their patients on the impact of smoking on their particular health issues and to be ready to address possible fear, mistrust, and misinformation concerning NRT. It is essential to educate pregnant women, their partners, and families about the effects of smoking and of secondhand smoke during pregnancy. Females in their childbearing years need to become aware of the dangers of smoking, not just for them, but for any children they might have. Physicians may also need to address alcohol use as this often exacerbates smoking.

Physicians need to be aware of historic mistrust toward conventional medicine and doctors, to be mindful of ways to address these concerns, and to be willing to be learners as well as educators. If they are to be effective in urging others to stop, they may need to address their own tobacco use if that is an issue. They also need to be willing to partner with clinicians in other disciplines in efforts to help patents stop smoking, particularly given that NRT is significantly more effective in conjunction with other modalities such as counselling, group therapy, Aboriginal healing practices, etc. It is essential to be aware of culturally sensitive services and resources in the community and on the web and to be ready to refer clients/patients to them. It can also be helpful to contribute to, partner with, and encourage community anti-smoking initiatives such as cessation groups, quitlines, etc.

Given the high incidence of risk factors, social determinants, and commercial tobacco use among Aboriginal communities, it is vitally important to provide as much positive support and feedback and to marshal as many resources as possible to those with the courage to quit.

CAN-ADAPTT SUMMARY STATEMENTS FOR ABORIGINAL PEOPLES

1. Tobacco misuse status should be updated for all Aboriginal peoples by all healthcare providers on a regular basis.
2. All healthcare providers should offer assistance to Aboriginal peoples who misuse tobacco, with specific emphasis on culturally appropriate methods.
3. All healthcare providers should be familiar with available cessation support services for Aboriginal peoples.
4. All individuals working with Aboriginal peoples should seek appropriate training in providing evidence-based smoking cessation support.

Source: CAN-ADAPTT. Canadian smoking cessation clinical practice guideline. Toronto: Canadian Action Network for the Advancement, Dissemination and Adoption of Practice-informed Tobacco Treatment, Centre for Addiction and Mental Health; 2011. Available from: www.can-adaptt.net. Reprinted with permission.

APPLICATIONS FOR HEALTHCARE PROVIDERS

Building positive healthcare relationships Healthcare providers who create respectful, supportive relationships with the Aboriginal people in their care are making a strong contribution toward assisting them in ending their tobacco dependency. Below are some of the elements of such relationships.

- **Valuing the person's opinion and experience.** Many Aboriginal communities are nonhierarchical and there is a common tendency to resent "experts." Also, as indicated earlier, there is historic mistrust, particularly toward physicians. Share relevant and appropriate information about yourself and be willing to learn about the person, his or her family, community, etc. Ask about cultural practices to address addictions, including addiction to commercial tobacco, and encourage the use of those that are personally meaningful. Many cultural practices include behavioural interventions that support healing in the spiritual, emotional, and mental dimensions.

247

- **Seeking training in Aboriginal culture and traditions.** Cultural training may be available through the community or the Health Authority. In some jurisdictions, online cultural training may also available through provincial health authorities. A fundamental realization to bear in mind is Aboriginal people's sense of interconnectedness with family, community, nation, and creation. Within that worldview, tobacco is a relation, not a thing apart. Being educated about traditional tobacco use and having access to people/sources that can elaborate on it is essential.

- **Allowing people to choose whether they want Aboriginal-specific programming.** Not all Aboriginal people do. Ask those who do if they would like to talk with an elder about stopping smoking. An elder can offer cultural support, can identify treatment strategies, and can provide context about social and historical issues that Aboriginal people have faced and the role that commercial tobacco use may have played in dealing with them. Most health and social programs have access to elders.

- **Addressing concerns about medications.** There may be a reluctance to use medications due to misinformation, concerns about becoming addicted to NRT, etc. Health providers should be ready to address such concerns and to provide accurate information about what medications are available, how they work, how to obtain them, etc. Inform them about medications covered by non-insured health benefits (NIHB), and, if necessary, assist them in accessing these. It may also be necessary to ensure that NRT is available in the patient's community.

- **Playing an advocacy role for policies that discourage commercial tobacco use**. Such policies include taxing cigarettes and providing smoke-free spaces at venues such as bingo halls and restaurants. Educating people about these issues supports them in addressing addiction to commercial tobacco at a personal and at a community level. Lobbying policy-makers to eliminate the need for a doctor's prescription to obtain NRT would help remove one deterrent to quitting smoking.

- **Supporting smoking cessation groups**. Make it widely known that individuals who combine behavioural interventions with medications tend to be more likely to quit than those who just use medications on their own. Seek the on-going support of community members who have stopped smoking and who might be willing to provide testimonials, to be role models for those attempting to quit, and to speak to youth and adult smoking cessation groups. Success stories about people who have used cessation medications and other means to stop are very effective, especially if they're people that group members know. Since stories of people experiencing negative health outcomes from smoking are effective with youth, there may be patients or clients in that situation who would be willing to talk to them.

- **Involving the community and building on community strengths in developing smoking cessation programs**. Consult with elders, elected leaders, addiction workers, health directors, healthcare providers, etc. to determine what smoking cessation resources (e.g. a support group) are already available in the community. Integrate with other programming such as diabetes and other addictions, which is desirable both practically and clinically. If it's warranted, partner with community leaders to get their perspective on developing a smoking cessation program that meets the needs of their community. Their involvement and buy-in is essential for obtaining referrals and ensuring the program's success, especially if it didn't originate in the community. Training community workers to facilitate cessation groups and to provide services such as brief smoking cessation interventions can be very effective. Offering training in peer-led smoking cessation groups is also important.

Addressing tobacco cessation with adults   In light of the above considerations about forging positive relationships, here are some specific guidelines in supporting Aboriginal clients address their tobacco use:

- Ask the person if s/he smokes and how it has affected him/her. Ask if s/he is interested in stopping. Educate the person about health effects that are specific to his/her medical profile. Discuss concurrent addictions such as alcohol and the need to address these as well. Discuss the impact of social determinant stresses such as housing, spousal abuse, addiction issues in the family, etc.

- Discuss intervention options. Take a holistic approach which embraces the physical, emotional, mental, and spiritual dimensions of his/her life—e.g. combining pharmacological approaches with individual counselling (e.g. to address anxiety), participation in a smoking cessation group, consulting with an elder, and getting involved in traditional spiritual practices (bearing in mind that not everyone will choose Aboriginal-specific programming).
- Offer practical tips, such as creating a smoke-free home or smoke-free spaces in the home if other family members smoke. Emphasize the positive effects of stopping, not just the negatives of continuing to smoke.
- Discuss resources that may be available in the community such as smoking cessation groups, elders, and spiritual/cultural practices. Other possibilities include telephone counselling, quitlines, websites, telehealth smoking cessation groups, and other such interventions.
- If needed, create a smoking cessation group. Involve an elder to educate clients regarding the role and function of traditional tobacco. Be prepared for clients to discuss social issues such as housing and spousal abuse. It may be helpful to encourage participants to explore the deeper reasons for smoking—e.g. to defy authority, or to cope with grief or survivor guilt from having lost relatives or friends to tragic events such as accidents, illness, or suicide. Significant mental health issues may surface and mental health and counselling resources may need to be available.
- Patients/clients interested in stopping may want to consider what specific needs nontraditional tobacco use is currently fulfilling in their lives. The need to belong could be a factor, whether it's to the adult world or to a particular circle of friends. Discovering ways in which such needs can be met in a healthy manner can make successful quitting more likely. They may also need help to identify formal and informal supports and healthy role models and to address those areas in their life that are not supportive of their intention to stop smoking.
- Aftercare support is essential as a follow-up from a group or clinical encounter. Peer-led support groups can be invaluable. Workshops delivered via technology are another option.

Addressing tobacco cessation with Aboriginal youth   Many of the preceding points about supporting adults also apply to working with youth, in addition to the following:

- Since young Aboriginal people start smoking as early as age 12, and sometimes younger, intervention needs to begin at as young an age as possible.
- Let youth know that free NRT is available to help them quit. This message can be conveyed through educational material, class presentations, workshops in the community, etc.
- Engage their family. Anecdotal evidence shows that it is often very difficult for Aboriginal youth to stop if their parents or siblings are smoking. Encouraging the whole family to attend a so-called Tobacco Cessation Day, or other cessation initiative on a community health level could be helpful. Some topics could include NRT and relapse prevention strategies.
- With school and community input and involvement, set up a youth smoking cessation group. Offering incentives such as lunch or prizes improves attendance. Additionally, making it more formalized and giving school credit could increase participation rates. Having ready access to NRT for those wanting to quit is also important.
- Try text messaging youth group members regularly with inspirational messages and educational information to support stopping. This has the potential to improve patient–provider relationships and can lead to better outcomes.
- Educate youth as to the distinction between traditional and commercial tobacco. Encouraging traditional use, which is culturally relevant, will not increase recreational use.
- Inform youth about holistic healing (spiritual, mental, emotional, physical) and discuss with them how this applies to their lives. Talk about the social/emotional/spiritual origins of smoking among Aboriginal people. Encourage them to share their emotions and support them (perhaps with elder, mental health and/or counselling support) in healing the underlying trauma.

THE TRADITIONAL PLACE OF TOBACCO

Karina Czyzewski

Commercial tobacco as a globalized and quotidian commodity is still a fairly recent phenomenon. Trade systems were already present when the first Europeans arrived, but only through the exploitation of Turtle Island's resources at the hands of Europeans did trade and commercialization of tobacco on a global scale begin. There are many stories as to how semaa* came to be. The archaeological record shares a story that traces the trade of plants from South America up to more Northern communities. The Haudenosaunee's creation story differs slightly with one's teachings but tells of pregnant Skywoman falling from the Spirit World onto the back of the Great Turtle. One version tells of Skywoman's daughter who dies in childbirth, her body becoming Mother Earth and from the many plants that are born from her, tobacco grows from her heart.

Historically, tobacco was used as an appetite suppressant, mild analgesic and stimulant. Today, numerous Nations and the communities therein still treat tobacco as a traditional medicine: it is used for offerings of prayer and thanks, when making a request to an Elder, for purification, and in ceremony (such as a pipe ceremony where it is not inhaled). Although there is a growing movement to use sacred tobacco (Nicotiana rustica) for the traditional purposes just mentioned, most still use commercial or non-traditional (Nicotiana tabacum) for these purposes because of access and normalization. The sacred and traditional place of tobacco among many First Peoples in Canada is not a given though: generally the Inuit do not practice the traditional use of tobacco, neither do some First Nations, such as some communities in British Columbia. Other communities would have used willow bark in the same way that tobacco is used today. These examples are in part due to culture, climate, geography and the capacity to cultivate tobacco. As with any teaching, protocol or practice, there is no one-size-fits-all approach.

*Tobacco in Anishnaabemowin

REVERSING NONTRADITIONAL TOBACCO USE AND RESTORING TOBACCO'S RIGHTFUL ROLE IN ABORIGINAL COMMUNITIES

In general, the most successful smoking interventions are integrated, flexible, community-based, culturally relevant approaches that increase service access, address negative perceptions and experiences with medications, and are tailored and targeted to local Aboriginal populations. Aboriginal peoples' holistic perception of health means that smoking cessation cannot just involve the medical or psychological realm in isolation from other aspects of the person's being. Engaging the mental realm could mean engaging with sources of meaning such as community, culture, spirituality, and the land. This is already occurring among Aboriginal people, despite 150 years of residential schools, separation from traditional lands, and prohibitions against language, traditional ceremonies, and so on. This demonstrates profound strength as a people, and needs to be honoured by healthcare providers.

Because of tobacco's traditional sacred role, portraying it as negative or evil, as is often the case in mainstream smoking cessation programs, is neither helpful nor accurate. Many Aboriginal healers, elders, and leaders view the reconsecration of tobacco as not just a means of restoring the health of individuals but also of helping to reclaim spiritual wholeness as a people. Having used tobacco in ceremonies, rituals, and prayer for thousands of years, traditional tobacco can be used in a sacred manner in the present day to seek guidance from and to communicate thoughts and feelings to the spirit world and to the Creator. In so doing, toxin-laden commercial tobacco, which is widely seen as disrespectful to the Creator and to the spirit world, can begin to lose its power in this context. Tobacco can then claim its rightful place as a messenger to and from the spirit world and as a great source of empowerment for Aboriginal individuals and communities.

REFERENCES

1   Wardman D, Khan N. Smoking-attributable mortality among British Columbia's First Nations populations. International Journal of Circumpolar Health 2004;63(1):81-92.

2   Statistics Canada. Census of Canada, 2006: Aboriginal Ancestry (14), Area of Residence (6), Age Groups (8), Sex (3) and Selected Demographic. Ottawa: Author [producer and distributor], 2008/12/02 (Special interest profiles; 97-564-xcb2006001).

3   Mitchell TL, Maracle DT. Healing the generations: post-traumatic stress and the health status of Aboriginal populations in Canada. Journal of Aboriginal Health 2005;Mar;14-23.

4   Bacchus Network. American Indians and tobacco. [Cited 2012 Mar 30.] Available from: www.tobaccofreeu.org/your_state/documents/NAFactsheet.pdf.

5   National Indian & Inuit Community Health Representatives Organization. Traditional and nontraditional use of tobacco. [Cited 2012 Mar 30.] Available from: http://www.niichro.com/Tobacco%202002/tob02_4.html.

6   Centre for Excellence in Indigenous Tobacco Control (CEITC). Smoking in Indigenous communities around the world. Melbourne AU: University of Melbourne [cited 2012 Jan 9]. Available from: http://www.ceitc.org.au/ceitc-publications-and-resources.

7   Human Resources and Skills Development Canada. Indicators of well-being in Canada: learning – educational attainment, 2008–2010 [cited 2012 Mar 30]. Available from: http://www4.hrsdc.gc.ca/.3ndic.1t.4r@-eng.jsp?iid=29#M_4.

8   Hodge FS, Casken J. Characteristics of American Indian women cigarette smokers: prevalence and cessation status. Health Care Women Int 1999;20(5):455-69.

9   Spangler JG, Michielutte R, Bell RA, Knick S, Dignan MB, Summerson JH. Dual tobacco use among Native American adults in southeastern North Carolina. Prev Med 2001 Jun;32(6):521-28.

10   Assembly of First Nations/First Nations Information Governance Committee. First Nations regional longitudinal health survey (RHS) 2002–2003. Revised 2nd Edition; 2007 [cited 2012 Mar 30]. Available from: http://www.rhs-ers.ca/sites/default/files/ENpdf/RHS_2002/rhs2002-03-the_peoples_report_afn.pdf.

11   Tong VT, Dietz PM, England LJ, Farr SL, Kim SY, D'Angelo D, Bombard JM. Age and racial/ethnic disparities in prepregnancy smoking among women who delivered live births. Prev Chronic Dis 2011;8(6):A121.

12   Hutchinson PJ, Richardson CG, Bottorff JL. Emergent cigarette smoking, correlates with depression and interest in cessation among Aboriginal adolescents in British Columbia. Can J Public Health 2008;99(5):418-22.

13   Falk DE, Yi HY, Hiller-Sturmhofel S. An epidemiologic analysis of co-occurring alcohol and tobacco use and disorders: findings from the National Epidemiologic Survey on Alcohol and Related Conditions. Alcohol Res Health 2006;29(3):162-71.

14   Health Canada. Treatment and rehabilitation for youth with substance use problems [accessed 2012 Mar 30]. Available from http://www.hc-sc.gc.ca/hc-ps/pubs/adp-apd/youth-jeunes/ii-7-eng.php.

15   Petry N, Oncken C. Cigarette smoking is associated with increased severity of gambling problems in treatment-seeking gamblers. Addiction 2002;97;745-53.

16   McKennitt D. A smoking prevention program for Aboriginal youth. First Peoples Child & Family Review 2007;3(2);52-55.

17   The First Nations Information Governance Centre. First Nations regional health survey: RHS Phase 2 (2008–2010) Preliminary Results; 2011 [cited 2012 Mar 30]. Available from: http://www.rhs-ers.ca/sites/default/files/RHSPreliminaryReport.pdf.

18   Wilson D, Macdonald D. The income gap between Aboriginal peoples and the rest of Canada. Ottawa: Canadian Centre for Policy Alternatives; 2010.

19   Osilla KC, Lonczak, HS, Mall PD, Larimer ME, Marlatt GA. Regular tobacco use among American Indian and Alaska native adolescents: an examination of protective mechanisms. J Ethn Subst Abuse 2007;6(3-4):143-53.

20   Yakiwchuk C, Stasiuk H, Wiltshire W, Brothwell D. Tobacco use among young North American Aboriginal athletes. Journal Canadian Dental Association 2005;71:403a-403d.

21   Patten CA, Enoch C, Renner CC, Offord KP, Nevak C, Kelley SF, Thomas J, Decker PA, Hurt RD, Lanier A, Kaur JS. Focus groups of Alaska Native adolescent tobacco users: preferences for tobacco cessation interventions and barriers to participation. Health Educ Behav 2009;36(4):711-23. Epub 2007 Nov 29.

22   Henderson PN, Rhoades PN, Henderson JA, Welty TK, Buchwald D. Smoking cessation and its determinants among older American Indians: the strong heart study. Ethn Dis 2004 Spring;4(2):274-79.

23   Fu SS, Burgess DJ, van Ryn M, Rhodes K, Widome R, Ricards JJ, Noorbaloochi S, Clothier B, Su J, Joseph AM. Smoking-cessation strategies for American Indians: should smoking-cessation treatment include a prescription for a complete home smoking ban? J Prev Med 2010 Dec;39(6 Suppl 1):S56-65.

24   Hyland A, Higbee C, Li Q, Bauer JE, Giovino GA, Alford T, Cummings KM. Access to low-taxed cigarettes deters smoking cessation attempts. Am J Public Health 2005 Jun;95(6):994-5.

25   Burgess D, Fu SS, Joseph AM, Hatsukami DK, Solomon, J, van Ryn M. Beliefs and experiences regarding smoking cessation among American Indians. Nicotine Tobacco Res 2007 Jan;9 Suppl 1:S19-28.

26   Drobes DJ. Concurrent alcohol and tobacco dependence: mechanisms and treatment. Bethesda MD: National Institute on Alcohol Abuse and Alcoholism, 2002. Available from: http://pubs.niaaa.nih.gov/publications/arh26-2/136-142.htm

27   Horn K, Noerachmanto N, Dino G, Manzo K, Brayboy M. Who wants to quit? characteristics of American Indian youth. J Community Health 2009 Apr;34(2):153-63.

28   Wardman D, Quantz D, Tootoosis J, Khan N. Tobacco cessation drug therapy among Canada's Aboriginal people. Nicotine Tob Res 2007 May;9(5):607-11.

29   D'Silva J, Schillo, BA, Sandman NR, Leonard TL, Boyle RG. Evaluation of a tailored approach for tobacco dependence treatment for American Indians. Am J Health Promot 2011 May-Jun;25(5 Suppl):S66-9.

30   Power J, Grealy C, Rintoul D. Tobacco interventions for Indigenous Australians: a review of current evidence. Health Promot J Austral 2009 Dec;20(3):186-94.

31   Gohdes D, Harwell TS, Cummings S, Moore KR, Smilie KG, Helgerson SD. Smoking cessation and prevention: an urgent public health priority for American Indians in the Northern Plains. Public Health Rep 2002 May-Jun;117(3):281-90.

32   Choi WS, Daley CM, James A, Thomas J, Schupbach R, Segraves M, Barnoskie R, Ahluwalia JS. Beliefs and attitudes regarding smoking cessation among American Indians: a pilot study. Ethn Dis 2006 Winter;16(1):35-40.

33   Daley, CM, Greiner KA, Nazir N, Solomon CL, Braiuca SL, Smith TE, Choi WS. All Nations Breath of Life: using community-based participatory research to address health disparities in cigarette smoking among American Indians. Ethn Dis 2010 Autumn; 20(4):334-8.

34   Struthers R, Hodge FS. Sacred tobacco use in Ojibwe communities. J Holist Nurs 2004 Sep;22(3):209-25.

35   Horn K, McGloin T, Dino G, Manzo K, McCracken L, Shorty L, Lowry-Chavis L, Noerach-manto N. Quit and reduction rates for a pilot study of the American Indian Not on Tobacco (N-O-T) program. Prev Chronic Dis 2005 Oct;2(4):A13. Epub 2005 Sep 15.

36   Varcoe, C, Bottorff JL, Carey J, Sullivan D, Williams W. Wisdom and influence of elders: Possibilities for health promotion and decreasing tobacco exposure in First Nations communities. Can J Public Health 2010 Mar-Apr;101(2):154-8.

37   Rodgers RA, Corbett T, Bramley D, Riddell T, Wills M, Lin RB, Jones M. Do u smoke after txt? Results of a randomised trial of smoking cessation using mobile phone text messaging. Tob Control 2005 Aug;14(4):255-61.

38   Taualii M, Bush N, Bowen DJ, Forquera R. Adaptation of a smoking cessation and preven-tion website for urban American Indian/Alaska Native youth. J Cancer Educ 2010 Mar;25(1):23-31.

39   Hayward LM, Campbell HS, Sutherland-Brown C. Aboriginal users of Canadian quitlines: an exploratory analysis. Tob Control 2007 Dec;16 Suppl 1:i60-4.

40   Bains N, Pickett W, Hoey J. The use and impact of incentives in population-based smoking cessation programs: a review. Am J Health Promot 1998 May-Jun;12(5):307-20.

15

Treatment of Tobacco Dependence in Mental Health and Addictive Disorders

MARLEEN FILIMON AND TONY GEORGE

WHEN COMPARED WITH THE GENERAL POPULATION THE PREVALENCE OF SMOKING IS higher among individuals with psychiatric and substance use disorders, and they have lower success rates with quitting tobacco smoking. There have been several reports in the literature suggesting that people with schizophrenia and other serious mental illness including injection drug abuse have a strong desire to quit smoking. Treatments for tobacco dependence have achieved substantial progress during the past decade, especially among individuals with mental health and addictive disorders. However, despite an increase in the efficacy of these treatments over the past 20 years, long-term quit rates remain disappointingly low among the psychiatric population (e.g. less than 5% at 6 months). The effectiveness of tobacco dependence treatment among individuals with psychiatric disorders may require targeted treatments based on a better understanding of the pathophysiology of these disorders.

This chapter reviews approaches to treatment of tobacco use and dependence for individuals with mental health and addictive disorders: specifically, the clinical assessment of tobacco use, and behavioural and pharmacological treatments for this population, including the first line medications for smoking cessation, nicotine replacement therapies (NRTs), sustained-release bupropion, and varenicline are reviewed. Finally, the integration of tobacco dependence treatments into mental health and addictions settings is discussed.

THE EPIDEMIOLOGY OF TOBACCO DEPENDENCE IN MENTAL HEALTH AND ADDICTIVE DISORDERS

There is a higher prevalence of cigarette smoking in individuals with mental health and addictive disorders when compared with the general population.[1,2] Individuals with mental health and addiction disorders who also smoke consume approximately 34.2% of all cigarettes sold and have a higher rate of nicotine dependence compared with the general population.[3] The prevalence of smoking among those with mental health and addictive disorders exceeds the general population by two- to fourfold.[4,5] For example, McClave and colleagues analyzed data from the National Health Interview Survey on 23,393 adults with lifetime mental illnesses to obtain estimates on smoking prevalence and frequency.[2] They found that the smoking prevalence of adults with mental illnesses ranged from 34.3% (phobias) to 59.1% (schizophrenia) compared with only 18.3% of adults with no such illnesses. In a population-based study analyzing the data of 4,411 respondents, Lasser et al. found that lifetime smoking prevalence among people with psychiatric disorders (55.3%) and substance use disorders (72.2%) were significantly higher compared with the general population (39.1%).[4]

Although cessation attempts among people with and without mental illness are comparable, lower success rates with quitting have been observed in individuals with mental illness diagnoses.[2] In the same study by Lasser et al., the quit rate for the population without any mental illness was 42.5%, whereas the quit rate for people with a diagnosis of social phobia (33.4%), antisocial or conduct disorder (27.8%) posttraumatic stress disorder (28.4%), generalized anxiety disorder (32.7%), or drug abuse disorder (32.1%) were significantly lower. In accordance with these results, studies have found that people with mental health disorders are at increased risk for developing tobacco-related diseases.[6,7]

Among patients with mental health and addictive disorders, smoking prevalence seems to be highest among those with a diagnosis of schizophrenia and substance use disorders, with prevalence rates of 70–90%.[8] For example, in a study by Poirier et al., the prevalence of tobacco smoking and of nicotine dependence was examined among 711 French psychiatric in- and outpatients.[9] The results suggested that diagnoses of substance-related disorders and schizophrenia were most commonly associated among individuals who smoked. Furthermore, smokers with schizophrenia seem to smoke more heavily, extract more nicotine from each cigarette, and have higher nicotine dependence when compared with the general population.[10] Similarly, tobacco quit rates in a Veterans Affairs smoking cessation clinic in West Los Angeles were lowest among smokers with comorbid schizophrenia and alcoholism.[11] A more recent clinic-based study in Canada has also supported these findings.[12]

NEUROBIOLOGY OF TOBACCO USE AND COMORBIDITY WITH MENTAL HEALTH AND ADDICTION DISORDERS

In tobacco, nicotine is the major toxic compound with psychoactive properties.[13,14] The psychoactive properties of nicotine include decreased anxiety, elevated states of mood, decreased appetite, improved attentiveness, and cognitive enhancements.[13] For a full discussion on nicotine properties, see chapter 5.

Once nicotine enters the brain, it binds to its primary site of action, the nicotine acetylcholine receptor (nAChR).[13] In general, activation of nAChRs causes membrane depolarization of the presynaptic and postsynaptic terminal of neurons. This depolarization can directly or indirectly activate the calcium (Ca^{2+}) channels which triggers the release of several neurotransmitters, mainly dopamine in the mesolimbic system.[15] Nicotine AChRs also regulate the release of neurotransmitters such as acetylcholine (ACh), endogenous opioid peptides (EOPs), γ-aminobutyric acid (GABA), glutamate (Glu), norepinephrine (NE), and serotonin (5-HT),[5,16] all of which are involved in the pathogenesis of mental health and addiction disorders.[17,18]

Together, the presynaptic and postsynaptic nAChRs effects generate long-term changes in synaptic transmission[15,16] and in doing so play a big part in synaptic plasticity which is involved in cognitive processes such as attention, learning, memory, and development.[16] Several studies have been conducted focusing on the neurocognitive effects smoking has in humans. For example, Durazzo et al. had 57 participants complete a neurocognitive test battery to study neurocognitive dysfunction associated with chronic cigarette smoking.[19] Their results showed that chronic smoking was associated with inferior performance on measures of general intelligence, visuospatial learning and memory, and fine motor dexterity. In another study by Weiser et al., 20,221 military recruits completed an IQ questionnaire; compared with their non-smoking colleagues, those who smoked had lower IQ scores.[20]

There is evidence that nicotine may have different effects in patients with a mental health and/or addiction disorder compared with the general population.[14] Evidence from multiple studies suggests that certain neurocognitive impairments associated with schizophrenia are less severe in those with the disorder who smoke compared with those who do not.[18,21,22] Interestingly, nicotine administration through cigarette smoking may have positive effects on neurocognitive function in people with schizophrenia,[21,23] and such cognitive enhancement appears to be mediated by nAChR stimulation.[21,24,25]

Many studies indicate a link between tobacco smoking and depression. For example, Mineur and Picciotto have shown that nicotine compounds are effective antidepressants.[26] In another study, Salin-Pascual and colleagues studied the effects of open-label transdernal nicotine patch on patients with a diagnosis of major depression and found that improvements of depressive mood was observed within 2–3 days.[27] As a proof of concept that modulation of central nAChRs could have antidepressant effects, a clinical study by George et al. examined the effects of the non-competitive nicotinic receptor antagonist mecamylamine (MEC) in a placebo-controlled trial in N=21 patients with major depression unresponsive to SSRI therapy. It was found that active MEC significantly reduced depressive symptoms versus placebo, suggesting that nAChR antagonism may be a novel method for antidepressant augmentation, and that nicotinic cholinergic mechanisms are involved in the pathophysiology of depression.[28]

CLINICAL ASSESSMENT OF TOBACCO DEPENDENCE IN THE MENTAL HEALTH AND ADDICTIVE DISORDER POPULATION

The accurate assessment of tobacco use, craving, and withdrawal has received a fair amount of attention during the last few years. For research on tobacco and nicotine dependence in a mental health and addiction population, it is important to know the reliability and validity of the different clinical assessment tools to test for these values. Several measures exist to clinically assess tobacco dependence and nicotine dependence.

Similar to assessment in the general population (covered in Chapter 6), all clinical assessments of tobacco use should include a detailed evaluation of tobacco consumption. Most tobacco use (>98%) is by cigarette smoking, and the most common method in clinical research is through the use of timeline followback (TLFB) methods.[29] These entail a retrospective recall of daily cigarette use for typical periods of 1–2 weeks. The test-retest reliability of the TLFB methods for quantifying cigarette consumption is very high in smokers with schizophrenia (0.95) and comparable to non-psychiatric control smokers (0.91).[30]

The most commonly used test of nicotine dependence is the Fagerström Tolerance Questionnaire (FTQ)[31] and its revised version known as the Fagerström Test for Nicotine Dependence (FTND).[32] The FTND is a 6-item scale (scored 0–10) that assesses the different aspects of smoking behaviour, including the number of cigarettes smoked per day, finding the first cigarette of the day most satisfying, and the time of the first cigarette after waking up. Scores of ≥5 or higher are consistent with physiological nicotine dependence.[32] Both measures were developed for use as a clinical assessment tool to provide short self-report measures of nicotine dependence[33] and have both been found reliable and valid in several different contexts, including measuring in the general population,[34-36] in schizophrenia,[30] and in posttraumatic stress disorder.[37] Critics of the FTND claim that the test is a weak predictor of smoking cessation and is low in its comprehensiveness.[35,38,39]

As an alternative measure to the FTND, Etter and colleagues developed a new self-administered measure of cigarette dependence; the Cigarette Dependence Scale (CDS).[38] This test was designed to assess the *DSM-IV-TR* and ICD-10 criteria of addiction to cigarettes and has been shown to be a reliable and valid measure for cigarette dependence in the general population.[35,36,38] The reliability and validity of the CDS has been tested among psychiatric populations including psychotic disorders, depression, bipolar disorders, personality disorders, and substance abuse disorders.[40]

Because the length of the FTND is not an ideal tool for population-based surveys, the Heaviness of Smoking Index (HSI) was developed as an alternative. The HSI includes two questions from the FTQ and the FTND, namely the time for the first cigarette in the morning and the number of cigarettes per day, to measure the same construct.[41] However, several studies have shown that the HSI does not have high rates of reliability or validity, and seems to measure only the number of cigarettes per day.[33,41,42] No data could be found on the reliability and validity of the HSI in populations with a diagnosis of mental health and addiction disorders.

The Minnesota Nicotine Withdrawal Scale (MNWS) is another commonly used test. The test has 8 items measuring for withdrawal symptoms such as craving, irritability, anxiety, difficulty concentrating, restlessness, increased appetite or weight gain, depression, and insomnia.[43] Several studies show this scale to be reliable and valid among the general population,[44] in schizophrenia,[30] and attention-deficit/hyperactivity disorder.[45]

A frequently used measure to assess tobacco craving is the Tiffany Questionnaire of Smoking Urges (TQSU). The statements presented to patients in this scale are "My desire to smoke seems overpowering," "I would be less irritable now if I could smoke," and "I could control things better right now if I could smoke."[46] This test has been found to be quite reliable and valid, and has been tested among individuals who smoke in the general population,[46] and with schizophrenia.[30]

TREATMENT OPTIONS FOR TOBACCO DEPENDENCE IN MENTAL HEALTH AND ADDICTION DISORDERS

In the latest practice guidelines published by the US Department of Health and Human Services, clinicians who treat this population group are encouraged to use the same smoking cessation strategies as with the general population.[47] An important note made in the American Psychiatric Association Clinical Practice Guidelines regarding smoking cessation treatments within a mental health and addiction population is that "the primary aims of treatment include motivating the patient to change and helping the patient learn, practice, and internalize changes in attitudes and behaviour conducive to relapse prevention."[48] Studies on smoking, tobacco dependence, and comorbidity with mental health and addiction disorders also emphasize the importance of motivating cessation attempts by supporting patients in their attempts to quit smoking, providing more behaviourally oriented interventions,[49] more information about the negative consequences of smoking,[50] providing a combination of pharmacotherapy and counselling,[51] and administering evidence-based cessation treatment interventions.[52]

Studies indicate that although the quit attempt rates for patients with mental health and addiction disorders are low, the motivation to quit smoking is present. Solty and colleagues developed a study to evaluate the motivation for smoking cessation in psychiatric inpatients.[53] Their results showed that among the total number of inpatients participating in the study (n = 342), 12.7% were actively thinking about ways to quit and 36.2% were ready to quit smoking. Duffy and colleagues analyzed a group of 146 veterans with a psychiatric disorder diagnosis on self-reported motivation to quit smoking.[49] They concluded that veterans with a psychiatric disorder compared with veterans without a psychiatric disorder were 2.6 times more likely to think that quitting would have a positive influence on their health, and were 4.4 times more likely of thinking to quit smoking within the next 30 days.

To date, there are few studies analyzing the effects of smoking cessation treatments on the course and prognosis of mental health and addictive disorders. An important theoretical consideration is the validity of the "self-medication" versus the "addiction vulnerability" hypotheses to explain the astonishing high levels of cigarette smoking in mental health and addiction disorder. Proponents of the self-medication hypothesis state that patients smoke cigarettes in an attempt to reduce their cognitive deficits, reduce schizophrenia symptoms, produce antidepressant effects, or reduce the motor side effects of antipsychotics.[54-57] Proponents of the addiction vulnerability hypothesis suggest that people with a diagnosis of schizophrenia have an increased vulnerability to addictive behaviour due to altered dopaminergic neurotransmission in the mesolimbic systems that may enhance drug craving and reward mechanisms, and dopaminergic deficits in the prefrontal cortex, which may explain negative symptoms and executive cognitive dysfunction.[18,58] This theory posits that the neurochemical dysfunction associated with schizophrenia neuropathology is a common vulnerability factor for both psychotic symptoms and the initiation and maintenance of drug addiction.[58-60]

In the following sections, we briefly review studies of smoking cessation treatments for mental health and addiction disorders, and summarize data from controlled clinical trials in Tables for various mental health/addictive disorders.

Smoking cessation treatments in schizophrenia A combination of behavioural therapies and pharmacological therapies appears to produce the best results for smoking cessation in schizophrenia. George and colleagues designed a study to determine the feasibility and efficacy of sustained-release bupropion versus placebo in combination with transdermal nicotine patch (21 mg/24 h) and group behavioural therapy (which included motivational interviewing, coping skills therapy, and psychoeducation) to assist patients with schizophrenia and schizoaffective disorder to quit smoking during a 10-week randomized trial, with a follow-up at 26 weeks.[61] Fifty-eight individuals with a diagnosis of schizophrenia or schizoaffective disorder who were currently smoking were randomized in this trial. The results show that the combination of bupropion SR versus placebo, and NRT with behavioural support, lead to significantly higher short- (10-week; 35 versus 10%) and long- (26 week; 15 versus 0%) week cessation outcomes. A study by Tidey and colleagues examined the efficacy of combining a contingency management intervention with bupropion to reduce smoking in people with schizophrenia.[62] Together, the contingency management with the administration of bupropion proved to be an effective intervention for reducing smoking in individuals with a diagnosis of schizophrenia. Table 1 presents an overview of the different smoking cessation treatments studied for use for individuals with schizophrenia.

TABLE 1: Smoking cessation treatments in schizophrenia

Study	Results
George TP, Ziedonis DM, Feingold A, Pepper WT, Satterburg CA, Winkel J, et al. Nicotine transdermal patch and atypical antipsychotic medications for smoking cessation in schizophrenia. Am J Psychiatry. 2000;157(11):1835-42.	This study compared subjects treated with atypical (n=18) versus typical (n=27) antipsychotics in combination with TNP and group behavioural therapy during a 12-week trial. Treatment with atypical antipsychotic drugs was found to be associated with a 2.5-fold increase in biochemically-verified quit rates at the end of the trial.
Evins AE, Mays VK, Rigotti NA, Tisdale T, Cather C, Goff DC. A pilot trial of bupropion added to cognitive behavioral therapy for smoking cessation in schizophrenia. Nicotine Tob Res. 2001;3:397-403.	18 subjects participated in this study to investigate the effect of adding sustained-release bupropion to CBT on smoking behaviour and stability of psychiatric symptoms. The results suggest that bupropion combined with CBT may lead to a reduction in smoking in schizophrenia.
George TP, Vessicchio JC, Termine A, Bregartner TA, Feingold A, Rounsaville BJ, et al. (2002). A placebo controlled trial of bupropion for smoking cessation in schizophrenia. Biol Psychiatry. 2002;52(1):53-61.	In a study with 32 subjects diagnosed with either schizophrenia or schizoaffective disorder, smoking cessation was investigated by administering sustained-release bupropion or a placebo. Furthermore, it was found that atypical antipsychotic medication treatment was associated with better smoking cessation outcomes with bupropion.

Gallagher SM, Penn PE, Schindler E, Layne W. A comparison of smoking cessation treatments for persons with schizophrenia and other serious mental illnesses. J Psychoactive Drugs. 2007;39(4):487-97.	181 individuals with a diagnosis of schizophrenia or a serious mental illness were given <u>CR</u>, <u>CR + nicotine patch</u>, or self-control quit group. Results show very small differences between interventions.
Evins AE, Cather C, Deckersbach T, et al. (2005): A double-blind placebo-controlled trial of bupropion sustained-release for smoking cessation in schizophrenia. J Clin Psychopharmacol. 25: 218-225.	12 week study of Bupropion SR versus Placebo in N=53 smokers with schizophrenia. Findings suggested the safety and superiority of Bupropion SR for smoking cessation in this population.
George TP, Vessicchio JC, Sacco KA, Weinberger AH, Dudas MM, Allen TM, et al. A placebo-controlled trial of bupropion combined with nicotine patch for smoking cessation in schizophrenia. Biol Psychiatry. 2008;63:1092-96.	10-week study in which 58 schizophrenia patients were randomized to either in a placebo + TNP group or in the bupropion + TNP group. The combination of <u>bupropion</u> with <u>TNP</u> significantly improved smoking abstinence at trial endpoint (Week 10).
Tidey JW, Rohsenow DJ, Kaplan GB, Swift RM, Reid N. Effects of contingency management and bupropion on cigarette smoking in smokers with schizophrenia. Psychopharmacology. 2011;217:279-87.	To study the effectiveness of a combination of <u>CM</u> and <u>bupropion</u> in smoking cessation in individuals with schizophrenia. The results show that this combination if more effective than either CM or bupropion alone.
Williams JM, Anthenelli RM, Morris C, Tredow J, Thompson JR, Yunis C, George TP. A double-blind, placebo-controlled study evaluating the safety and efficacy of varenicline tartarate for smoking cessation in schizophrenia and schizoaffective disorder. J Clin Psychiatry. 2012; forthcoming.	Multi-centre trial of <u>varenicline</u> versus placebo for smoking cessation in schizophrenia and schizoaffective disorder (N=127) found that varenicline (up to 2 mg/day) significantly improved short-term smoking cessation outcomes, and was not associated with changes in psychotic symptoms or an increase in suicidal thinking.

Abbreviations: CBT: Cognitive Behavioural Therapy; CM: Contingency Management; CR: Contingent Reinforcement; TNP: Transdermal Nicotine Patch

Smoking cessation treatments in mood disorders There have been few studies of smoking cessation in individuals with a diagnosis of mood disorders. Most studies found seem to focus on a combination of behavioural therapies with pharmacological treatment. For example, Chengappa et al. asked 25 adults with a diagnosis of either Major Depressive Disorder or Depressive Disorder NOS to participate in their 9-week study.[63] Bupropion sustained-release (SR) was given in addition to their SSRI treatment, starting with 150 mg per day up to 300 mg per day. Furthermore, participants received smoking cessation counselling and chose a quit date after the initiation of bupropion SR. Thirty-two percent of the participants were abstinent after the 9-week trial, and at a 3-month follow-up 3 participants remained abstinent. As a conclusion, it was found that the addition of bupropion SR to SSRI treatment had a modest effect on smoking cessation.

Evins and colleagues studied the effects of bupropion, transdermal nicotine replacement therapy (NRT) and cognitive behavioural therapy (CBT) on abstinence rates in smokers with Major Depressive Disorder (MDD).[64] Ninety adults with current MDD and 109 adults with a past diagnosis of MDD were randomly assigned to receive either bupropion, NRT and CBT or a placebo, NRT and CBT for 13 weeks. Due to a 50% drop-out rate caused by a high prevalence of comorbid anxiety disorder, an intent-to-treat analysis with last observation of abstinence status was performed. The data obtained showed a significant result whereby 56% of the bupropion group and 41% of the placebo group met the criteria for abstinence. Bupropion, NRT, and CBT seemed to provide high abstinence rates, given that there was no comorbid anxiety disorder. Table 2 presents an overview of the different smoking cessation treatments studied for use for individuals with mood disorders.

Smoking cessation treatments in anxiety disorders Few studies could be found assessing pharmacological or behavioural treatments for smoking cessation among individuals with anxiety disorders. Most studies regarding this topic are on the integration of smoking cessation interventions and health care for posttraumatic stress disorder (PTSD). McFall and colleagues found that the integration of smoking cessation treatment into mental health care for veterans with PTSD improved smoking abstinence rates and remained significant at an 18-month follow-up.[65] In another study by McFall and colleagues, similar results were obtained among veterans with a diagnosis of PSTD and combining mental health care with an evidence-based smoking cessation treatment.[66] Clearly, more research needs to be done regarding this topic. Table 3 presents an overview of the different smoking cessation treatments studied to date for use for individuals with anxiety disorders.

TABLE 2: Smoking cessation treatments in mood disorders

Study	Results
Chengappa KN, Kambhampati RK, Perkins K, Nigam R, Anderson T, Brar JS, et al. Bupropion sustained release as a smoking cessation treatment in remitted depressed patients maintained on treatment with selective serotonin reuptake inhibitor antidepressants. J Clin Psychiatry. 2001;62(7):503-8.	In this study, 25 adults with a *DSM-IV* diagnosis of major depressive disorder or depressive disorder NOS received bupropion sustained release (150mg/day up to 300mg/day) in addition to their SSRI treatment. In addition, participants received smoking cessation counselling and chose a target quit date. The results suggest a modest effectiveness for the use of bupropion SR as a smoking cessation agent in individuals with depression on SSRI treatment.
Brown RA, Niaura R, Lloyd-Richardson EE, Strong DR, Kahler CW, Abrantes AM, et al. Bupropion and cognitive-behavioral treatment for depression in smoking cessation. Nicotine Tob Res. 2007;9(7):721-30.	524 smokers were randomized to either CBT + bupropion, CBT + placebo, or standard cessation treatment + CBT + bupropion. Bupropion resulted in better smoking cessation outcomes. Adding CBT did not result in improved smoking cessation outcomes.
Evins AE, Culhane MA, Alpert JE, Pava J, Liese BS, Farabaugh A, et al. A controlled trial of bupropion added to nicotine patch and behavioral therapy for smoking cessation in adults with unipolar depressive disorders. J Clin Psychopharmacol. 2008;28:660-6.	A study to determine whether bupropion + NRT + CBT improve abstinence rates in smokers with unipolar depressive disorder. Bupropion neither increased the efficacy of CBT and NRT for smoking cessation, but did provide an advantage for smoking cessation.
Philip NS, Carpenter LL, Tyrka AR, Whiteley LB, Price LH. Varenicline augmentation in depressed smokers: an 8-week, open-label study. J Clin Psychiatry. 2009;70(7):1026-31.	18 patients were assessed for possible antidepressant effects of varenicline augmentation. Results showed improvements of depressive symptoms in correlation to smoking cessation.

TABLE 3: Smoking cessation treatments in anxiety disorders

Study	Results
Hertzberg MA, Moore SD, Feldman ME, Beckham JC. A preliminary study of bupropion sustained-release for smoking cessation in patients with chronic posttraumatic stress disorder. J Clin Psychopharmacol. 2001;21(1):94-8.	15 individuals with chronic PTSD were randomly assigned to receiving either bupropion or a placebo. Results showed that bupropion seemed to be an effective treatment for smoking cessation in this population.
McFall M, Saxon AJ, Thompson CE, Yoshimoto D, Malte C, Straits-Troster K, et al. Improving the rates of quitting smoking for veterans with posttraumatic stress disorder. Am J Psychiatry. 2005;162(7):1311-9.	66 veterans undergoing treatment for PTSD and currently smoking were assigned to either receiving tobacco use treatment integrated in their psychiatric health care, or receiving tobacco use treatment separately given by specialists. The individuals receiving cessation treatment integrated in the standard health care were five times more likely to abstain from smoking at follow ups.
McFall M, Saxon AJ, Thaneemit-Chen S, Smith MW, Joseph AM, Carmody TP, et al. Integrating smoking cessation into mental health care for posttraumatic stress disorder. Clinical Trials. 2007;4(2):178-89.	This study assessed the effectiveness of integrating smoking cessation treatment into mental health care. A total of 1,400 veterans with a diagnosis of PTSD were followed for up to four years and tested for smoking abstinence and measures of depression, PTSD, and economic value. The results showed an improvement in smoking abstinence rates.
McFall M, Saxon AJ, Malte CA, Chow B, Bailey S, Baker DG, et al. Integrating tobacco cessation into mental health care for posttraumatic stress disorder: a randomized controlled trial. JAMA. 2010;304(22):2485-93.	This study also assessed the effectiveness of integrating smoking cessation treatment into mental health care and analysed the long term smoking abstinence rates. 943 smokers with military-related PTSD were recruited to participate in this study. Integrated smoking cessation care was observed to be better than treatment in smoking cessation clinics (8.9% vs. 4.5%) and resulted in greater prolonged abstinence.

TABLE 4: Smoking cessation treatments in substance use disorders

Study	Results
Ait-Daoud N, Lynch WJ, Penberthy JK, Breland AB, Marzani-Nissen GR, Johnson BA. Treating smoking dependence in depressed alcoholics. Alcohol Res Health. 2006;29(3):213-20.	Topiramate showed potential for promoting smoking cessation in alcoholics.
Stein MD, Weinstock MC, Herman DS, Anderson BJ, Anthony JL, Niaura R. A smoking cessation intervention for the methadone-maintained. Addiction. 2006;101:599-607.	383 methadone-maintained smokers were randomly assigned to receive a nicotine patch + motivational intervention + a quit date behavioral skills counselling session + a relapse prevention follow-up session or a nicotine patch + brief advice using the National Cancer Institute's 4 A's model. Results showed that behavioural intervention did not increase quit rates over the nicotine patch and using the advice model.
Kalman D, Herz L, Monti P, Kahler CW, Mooney M, Rodrigues S, et al. Incremental efficacy of adding bupropion to the nicotine patch for smoking cessation in smokers with a recent history of alcohol dependence: results from a randomized, double-blind, placebo-controlled study. Drug Alcohol Depend. 2011;118(2–3):111-8.	148 smokers participated in this study to compare the efficacy of smoking cessation treatment using either nicotine patch and bupropion vs. nicotine patch and placebo bupropion. Findings do not support the combination of nicotine patch and bupropion for smoking cessation treatments in smokers with a history of alcohol dependence.

Smoking cessation treatments in substance use disorders Recent studies have investigated the different smoking cessation treatment options for individuals with substance use disorders. For example, Kalman and colleagues investigated the efficacy of either nicotine patch and bupropion or nicotine patch and placebo on smoking cessation in alcoholic smokers.[67] A sample of 148 smokers with 2–12 months of alcohol abstinence were assigned to a smoking cessation treatment program. In addition to receiving nicotine patch plus bupropion or a placebo, all participants received counselling cessation. Unfortunately, the findings did not point to the effectiveness of nicotine patch and bupropion in smoking cessation. However, the researchers did notice the importance of providing smokers with comorbid substance use disorder a combination of behavioural and pharmacological treatments. Table 4 presents an overview of the different smoking cessation treatments studied for use for individuals with substance use disorders.

CONCLUSIONS AND RECOMMENDATIONS

It is evident from the preceding review that addressing tobacco dependence in people with mental health and addictive disorders should be a priority for clinicians who work with these patients. However, it is well-appreciated that this segment of the smoking population may not have easy access to treatment. Knowledge of mechanisms to engage these individuals in treatment, as well as the erroneous belief that quitting smoking may be harmful to symptoms and recovery, is unfortunately widespread and adversely impacts access to care. Moreover, development of tobacco-free treatment and residential settings, despite considerable evidence that they make a significant difference insofar as motivating patients to seek tobacco treatment and lead to better patient outcomes[68,69] has shown little uptake and implementation in community settings. This is particularly unfortunate given that the leading cause of death in persons with comorbid psychiatric and substance use disorders appears to be tobacco-related medical illness.[13,69,70–72]

Fortunately, there is increasing evidence that standard pharmacological and behavioural treatments, with modest adaptations, can be used safely and effectively in mental health and addictions populations. One important challenge from a services perspective is that there is rarely an integration of psychiatric/addiction care with tobacco treatment services. The studies by McFall and colleagues in smokers with PTSD have clearly demonstrated the importance of cross-training of staff to deliver integrated tobacco and mental health care, and that this leads to better tobacco cessation and mental health treatment outcomes than when such treatments are delivered separately.[65,73] The recent availability of non-nicotine pharmacotherapies (e.g. sustained-release bupropion, varenicine) in some jurisdictions as part of scheduled benefits is a fine example of how the science of tobacco addiction and tobacco control in collaboration with public policy makers can lead to the more broad coverage of smoking cessation treatments, and more widespread dissemination of these effective treatments. In parallel, it will be important to ensure that while progress is being made in the general population, special populations who are known to be vulnerable to the initiation and maintenance of tobacco addiction are targeted, given the higher prevalence of tobacco use and dependence, less ability to quit smoking, and higher risk of morbidity and mortality. Needless to say, clinicians need to become more proficient at asking about smoking behaviours in mental health and addictions populations[74] and use stepped care approaches[13,75] to ensure that the identification and treatment of tobacco smokers with mental illness and substance abuse is being addressed.

ACKNOWLEDGEMENTS

This work was supported in part by the Chair in Addiction Psychiatry at the University of Toronto (to TPG), an operating grant from the National Institute on Drug Abuse (NIDA; 2U01-DA-020830-07, to Caryn Lerman, Rachel Tyndale and TPG) and Canadian Institutes of Health Research (CIHR MOP#115145, to TPG), and the Ontario Mental Health Foundation (to TPG).

REFERENCES

1   Stein MD, Weinstock MC, Herman DS, Anderson BJ, Anthony JL, Niaura R. A smoking cessation intervention for the methadone-maintained. Addiction. 2006;101:599-607.

2   McClave AK, McKnight-Eily LR, Davis SP, Dube SR. Smoking characteristics of adults with selected lifetime mental illnesses: results from the 2007 National Health Interview Survey. Am J Public Health. 2010;100(12):2462-72.

3   Grant BF, Hasin DS, Chou P, Stinson FS, Dawson DA. Nicotine dependence and psychiatric disorders in the United States: results from the National Epidemiologic Survey on Alcohol and Related Conditions. Arch Gen Psychiatry. 2004;61:1107-15.

4   Lasser K, Boyd JW, Woolhandler S, Himmelstein DU, McCormick D, Bor DH. Smoking and mental illness: a population-based prevalence study. JAMA. 2000;284(20):2606-10.

5   Allen TM, Sacco KA, Weinberger AH, George TP. Medication treatments for nicotine dependence in psychiatric and substance use disorders. In: George TP, editor. Medication treatments for nicotine dependence. New Haven CT: CRC Press; 2007. p. 245-62.

6   Hennekens CH, Hennekens AR, Hollar D, Casey DE. (2005). Schizophrenia and increased risks of cardiovascular disease. Am Heart J. 2005;150(6):1115-21.

7   Brown S, Kim M, Mitchell C, Inskip H. Twenty-five year mortality of a community cohort with schizophrenia. Br J Psychiatry. 2010;196:116-21.

8   Morisano D, Bacher I, Audrain-McGovern J, George TP. Mechanisms underlying the co-morbidity of tobacco use in mental health and addictive disorders. Can J Psychiatr. 2009;54(6):356-67.

9   Poirier M, Canceil O, Bayle F, Millet B, Bourdel M, Moatti C, et al. Prevalence of smoking in psychiatric patients. Prog Neuropsychopharmacol Biol Psychiatry. 2002;26:529-37.

10   de Leon J, Diaz FJ. A meta-analysis of worldwide studies demonstrates an association between schizophrenia and tobacco smoking behaviors. Schizophrenia Res. 2005;76:135-57.

11   Gershon-Grand RB, Hwang S, Han J, George TP, Brody AL. Short-term naturalistic treatment outcomes in cigarette smokers with substance abuse and/or mental illness. J Clin Psychiatry. 2007;68(6):892-8.

12   Selby P, Voci SC, Zawertailo LA, George TP, Brands B. Individualized smoking cessation treatment in an outpatient setting: predictors of outcome in a sample with psychiatric and addictions co-morbidity. Addict Behav. 2010;35:811-7.

13   George TP. (2011). Nicotine and tobacco. In: Goldman L, Schafer AI, editors. Goldman's cecil medicine. 24th ed. Elsevier – Health Sciences Div. p.142-6.

14   Aubin H, Rollema H, Svensson TH, Winterer G. (2012). Smoking, quitting, and psychiatric disease: a review. Neurosci Biobehav Rev. 2012;36:271-84.

15   McKay BE, Placzek AN, Dani JA. Regulation of synaptic transmission and plasticity by neuronal nicotinic acetylcholine receptors. Biochem Pharmacol. 2007;74:1120-33.

16   Dani JA, Betrand D. Nicotinic acetylcholine receptors and nicotinic cholinergic mechanisms of the central nervous system. Annu Rev Pharmacol Toxicol. 2007;47:699-729.

17   Picciotto MR. Nicotine as a modulator of behavior: beyond the inverted U. Trends Pharmacol Sci. 2003;24(9):493-9.

18   Wing VC, Bacher I, Sacco KA, George TP. Neuropsychological performance in patients with schizophrenia and controls as a function of cigarette smoking status. Psychiatry Res. 2011;188:320-6.

19   Durazzo TC, Meyerhoff DJ, Nixon S. A comprehensive assessment of neurocognition in middle-aged chronic cigarette smokers. Drug Alcohol Depend. 2011;doi:10.1016/j.drugalcdep.2011.09.019.

20   Weiser M, Zarka S, Werbeloff N, Kravitz E, Lubin G. Cognitive test scores in male adolescent cigarette smokers compared to non-smokers: a population-based study. Addiction. 2009;105:358-63.

21   Sacco KA, Bannon KL, George TP. Nicotinic receptor mechanisms and cognition in normal states and in neuropsychiatric disorders. J Psychopharmacol. 2004;18: 457-74.

22   Wing VC, Moss TG, Rabin RA, George TP. Effects of cigarette smoking status on delay discounting in schizophrenia and healthy controls. Addict Behav. 2012;37:67-72.

23   Wing VC, Wass CE, Soh DW, George TP A review of neurobiological vulnerability factors and treatment implications for comorbid tobacco dependence in schizophrenia. Ann NY Acad Sci. 2012;1248:Addiction Reviews 89-106.

24   George TP, Termine A, Sacco KA, Seyal AA, Dudas MM, Allen TM, Vessicchio JC, Duncan EJ. A preliminary study of the effects of cigarette smoking on prepulse inhibition in schizophrenia: involvement of nicotinic receptor mechanisms. Schizophr Res. 2006;87:307-15.

25   Hong LE, Thaker GK, McMahon RP, Summerfelt A, Rachbeisel J, Fuller RL, et al. Effects of moderate-dose treatment with varenicline on neurobiological and cognitive biomarkers in smokers and non-smokers with schizophrenia or schizoaffective disorder. Arch Gen Psychiatry. 2011;68:1195-1206.

26   Mineur YS, Picciotto MR (2010). Nicotine receptors and depression: revisiting and revising the cholinergic hypothesis. Trends Pharmacol Sci. 2010;31(12):580-6.

27   Salín-Pascual RJ, Rosas M, Jimenez-Genchi A, Rivera-Meza BL, Delgado-Parra V. Antidepressant effect of transdermal nicotine patches in nonsmoking patients with major depression. J Clin Psychiatry. 1996;57(9):387-9.

28   George TP, Sacco KA, Vessicchio JC, Weinberger AH, Shytle RD. Nicotinic antagonist augmentation of selective serotonin reuptake inhibitor-refractory major depressive disorder: a preliminary study. J Clin Psychopharmacol. 2008;28(3):340-4.

29   Sobell LC, Sobell MB, Leo GI, Cancilla A. Reliability of a time-line method: assessing drinkers' reports of recent drinking and a comparative evaluation across several populations. Br J Addict. 1988;83:393-402.

30   Weinberger AH, Reutenauer EL, Allen TM, Termine A, Vessicchio JC, Sacco KA, et al. Reliability of the Fagerström Test for Nicotine Dependence, Minnesota Nicotine Withdrawal Scale, and Tiffany Questionnaire for Smoking Urges in smokers with and without schizophrenia. Drug Alcohol Depend. 2007;86:278-82.

31   Fagerström KO. Measuring degree of physical dependence to tobacco smoking with reference to individualization of treatment. Addict Behav. 1978;3:235-41.

32   Heatherton TF, Kozlowski LT, Frecker RC, Fagerström KO. The Fagerström Test for Nicotine Dependence: a revision of the Fagerström Tolerance Questionnaire. Br J Addict. 1991;86(9):1119-27.

33   Courvoisier DS, Etter JF. (2009). Comparing the predictive validity of five cigarette dependence questionnaires. Drug Alcohol Depend. 2009;107(2–3):128-33.

34   Dijkstra A, Tromp D. Is the FTND a measure of physical as well as psychological tobacco dependence? J Subst Abuse Treat. 2002;23:367-74.

35   Etter J. A comparison of the content-, construct- and predictive validity of the cigarette dependence scale and the Fagerström test for nicotine dependence. Drug Alcohol Depend. 2005;77:259-68.

36   Stavem K, Røgeberg OJ, Olsen JA, Boe J. (2008). Properties of the Cigarette Dependence Scale and the Fagerström Test of Nicotine Dependence in a representative sample of smokers in Norway. Addiction. 2008;103(9):1141-9.

37   Buckley TC, Mozley SL, Holohan DR, Walsh K, Beckham JC, Kassel JD. A psychometric evaluation of the Fagerström Test for Nicotine Dependence in PTSD smokers. Addict Behav. 2005;30:1029-33.

38   Etter J, Le Houezec J, Perneger TV. A self-administered questionnaire to measure dependence on cigarettes: the Cigarette Dependence Scale. Neuropsychopharmacology. 2003;28:359-70.

39   Sledjeski EM, Dierker LC, Costello D, Shiffman S, Donny E, Flay BR. Predictive validity of four nicotine dependence measures in a college sample. Drug Alcohol Depend. 2007;87:10-9.

40   Etter J, Le Houezec J, Huguelet P, Etter M. Testing the Cigarette Dependence Scale in 4 samples of daily smokers: psychiatric clinics, smoking cessation clinics, a smoking cessation website and in the general population. Addict Behav. 2009;34: 446-50.

41   Kozlowski LT, Porter CQ, Orleans CT, Pope MA, Heatherton T. Predicting smoking cessation with self-reported measures of nicotine dependence: FTQ, FTND, and HSI. Drug Alcohol Depend. 1994;34:211-6.

42   Etter JF, Duc TV, Perneger TV. Validity of the Fagerstrom test for nicotine dependence and of the Heaviness of Smoking Index among relatively light smokers. Addiction. 1991;94(2):269-81.

43   Toll BA, O'Malley SS, McKee SA, Salovey P, Krishnan-Sarin S. Confirmatory factor analysis of the Minnesota Nicotine Withdrawal Scale. Psychology Addict Behav. 2007;21(2):216-25.

44   Cappelleri JC, Bushmakin AG, Baker CL, Merikle E, Olufade AO, Gilbert DG. Revealing the multidimensional framework of the Minnesota nicotine withdrawal scale. Curr Med Res Opin. 2005;21(5):749-60.

45   Gray KM, Baker NL, Carpenter MJ, Lewis AL, Upadhyaya HP. Attention-Deficit/Hyperactivity Disorder confounds nicotine withdrawal self-report in adolescent smokers. Am J Addict. 2012;19:325-31.

46   Toll BA, McKee SA, Krishnan-Sarin S, O'Malley SS. Revisiting the factor structure of the questionnaire on smoking urges. Psychological Assessment. 2004;6(4):391-5.

47   Fiore MC, Jaen CR, Baker TB, Bailey WC, Benowitz NL, Curry SJ, et al. (2008 May). Treating tobacco use and dependence: 2008 update. Clinical Practice Guideline. Executive Summary [cited 2011 Dec 9]. Available from: http://www.ahrq.gov/path/tobacco.htm#clinic.

48   Kleber HD, Weiss RD, Anton RF, Rounsaville BJ, George TP, Strain EC, et al. Treatment of patients with substance use disorders, second edition. American Psychiatic Association. Am J Psychiatry. 2006;163(8 Suppl):5-82.

49   Duffy SA, Essenmacher C, Karvonen-Gutierrez C, Ewing LA. Motivation to quit smoking among veterans diagnosed with psychiatric and substance abuse disorders. J Addictions Nurs. 2010;21:105-13.

50   Tidey JW, Rohsenow DJ. Smoking expectancies and intention to quit in smokers with schizophrenia, schizoaffective disorder and non-psychiatric controls. Schizophr Res. 2009;115(2-3):310-6.

51   Fagerström K, Aubin H. Management of smoking cessation in patients with psychiatric disorders. Curr Med Res Opin. 2009;25(2):511-8.

52   Ferron JC, Brunette MF, He X, Xie H, McHugo GJ, Drake RE. Course of smoking and quit attempts among clients with co-occurring severe mental illness and substance use disorders. Psychiatr Serv. 2011;62(4):353-9.

53   Solty H, Crockford D, White WD, Currie S. Cigarette smoking, nicotine dependence, and motivation for smoking cessation in psychiatric inpatients. Can J Psychiatry. 2009;54(1):36-45.

54   de Leon J, Diaz FJ, Aguilar MC, Jurado D, Gurpegui M. Does smoking reduce akathisia? Testing a narrow version of the self-medication hypothesis. Schizophr Res. 2006;86:256-68.

55   Wilhelm K, Wedgwood L, Niven H, Kay-Lambkin F. Smoking cessation and depression: current knowledge and future directions. Drug Alcohol Revue. 2006;25(1):97-107.

56   Tizabi Y, Getachew B, Rezvani AH, Hauser SR, Overstreet DH. Antidepressant-like effects of nicotine and reduced nicotinic receptor binding in the Fawn-Hooded rat, an animal model of co-morbid depression and alcoholism. Prog Neuropsychopharmacol Biol Psychiatry. 2009;33:398-402.

57   Segarra R, Zabala A, Eguiluz JI, Ojeda N, Elizagarate E, Sanchez P, et al. Cognitive performance and smoking in first-episode psychosis:the self-medication hypothesis. Eur Arch Psychiatry Clin Neurosci. 2011;261(4):241-50.

58   George TP. Neurobiological links between nicotine addiction and schizophrenia. J Dual Diagnosis. 2007;3(3-4):27-42.

59   Chambers RA, Krystal JH, Self DW. A neurobiological basis for substance abuse comorbidity in schizophrenia. Biol Psychiatry. 2001;50(2):71-83.

60   Chambers RA. A nicotine challenge to the self-medication hypothesis in a neurodevelopmental animal model of schizophrenia. J Dual Diagnosis. 2009;5:139-48.

61   George TP, Vessicchio JC, Sacco KA, Weinberger AH, Dudas MM, Allen TM, et al. A placebo-controlled trial of bupropion combined with nicotine patch for smoking cessation in schizophrenia. Biol Psychiatry. 2008;63:1092-6.

62   Tidey JW, Rohsenow DJ, Kaplan GB, Swift RM, Reid N. Effects of contingency management and bupropion on cigarette smoking in smokers with schizophrenia. Psychopharmacology. 2011;217:279-87.

63   Chengappa KN, Kambhampati RK, Perkins K, Nigam R, Anderson T, Brar JS, et al. Bupropion sustained release as a smoking cessation treatment in remitted depressed patients maintained on treatment with selective serotonin reuptake inhibitor antidepressants. J Clin Psychiatry. 2001;62(7):503-8.

64   Evins AE, Culhane MA, Alpert JE, Pava J, Liese BS, Farabaugh A, et al. (2008). A controlled trial of bupropion added to nicotine patch and behavioral therapy for smoking cessation in adults with unipolar depressive disorders. J Clin Psychopharmacol. 2008;28:660-6.

65   McFall M, Saxon AJ, Malte CA, Chow B, Bailey S, Baker DG, et al. Integrating tobacco cessation into mental health care for posttraumatic stress disorder: a randomized controlled trial. JAMA. 2010;304(22):2485-93.

66   McFall M, Saxon AJ, Thaneemit-Chen S, Smith MW, Joseph AM, Carmody TP, et al. Integrating smoking cessation into mental health care for post-traumatic stress disorder. Clinical Trials. 2007;4(2):178-89.

67   Kalman D, Herz L, Monti P, Kahler CW, Mooney M, Rodrigues S, et al. Incremental efficacy of adding bupropion to the nicotine patch for smoking cessation in smokers with a recent history of alcohol dependence: results from a randomized, double-blind, placebo-controlled study. Drug Alcohol Depend. 2011;118(2–3):111-8.

68   Lawn S, Pols R. (2005). Smoking bans in psychiatric inpatient settings? A review of the research. Aust N Z J Psychiatry. 2005;39(10):866-85.

69   Moss TG, Weinberger AH, Vessicchio JC, Mancuso V, Cushing SJ, Pett M, et al. A tobacco reconceptualization in psychiatry: toward the development of tobacco-free psychiatric facilities. Am J Addict. 2010;19(4):293-311.

70   Goff DC, Cather C, Evins AE, Henderson DC, Freudenreich O, Copeland PM, et al. Medical morbidity and mortality in schizophrenia: guidelines for psychiatrists. J Clin Psychiatry. 2005;66(2):183-94.

71   Ziedonis D, Hitsman B, Beckham JC, Zvolensky M, Adler LE, Audrain-McGovern J, et al. Tobacco use and cessation in psychiatric disorders: National Institute of Mental Health report. Nicotine Tob Res. 2008;10(12):1691-1715.

72   George TP, Ziedonis DM. Addressing tobacco dependence in psychiatric practice: promises and pitfalls. Can J Psychiatry. 2009;54(6):353-5.

73   McFall M, Saxon AJ, Thompson CE, Yoshimoto D, Malte C, Straits-Troster K, et al. Improving the rates of quitting smoking for veterans with posttraumatic stress disorder. Am J Psychiatry. 2005;162(7):1311-9.

74   Hitsman B, Moss TG, Montoya ID, George TP. Treatment of tobacco dependence in mental health and addictive disorders. Can J Psychiatry. 2009;54(6):368-78.

75   Tobacco use and dependence guideline panel. Treating tobacco use and dependence: 2008 update. Rockville MD: US Department of Health and Human Services; 2008 May.

16

Imagine: Gender-Specific Tobacco Reduction and Cessation Strategies in Pregnancy and the Postpartum

JOAN L. BOTTORFF, JOHN L. OLIFFE, LORRAINE GREAVES, NANCY POOLE, GAYL SARBIT AND NATALIE HEMSING

IN 1971, JOHN LENNON RELEASED A SEMINAL MELODY AND LYRIC OF HOPE FOR WORLD peace in an enduring song called "Imagine." Over the years, the lines, "Imagine all the people ... living life in peace" have arguably become even more relevant today. A slight change in Lennon's lyrics to "imagine all the parents ... living life smoke free ..." might also be understood as a seemingly simple yet challenging goal. Smoking during pregnancy and postpartum remains a serious public-health issue in Canada, despite declining overall smoking rates. National surveys indicate that 23% of women (20–24 years old) smoked regularly during their recent pregnancy and up to 24% of men continue to smoke during their childbearing years.[1]

The negative health effects of smoking on mother, fetus, infant, and child are well established. These include ectopic pregnancy (outside the uterus), spontaneous abortion (miscarriage), preterm labour, premature rupture of membranes, placental problems (previa and abruption), low birth weight, increased perinatal mortality, increased admissions to neonatal intensive care units, sudden

277

infant death syndrome (SIDS), decreased volume of breast milk and duration of breastfeeding, childhood respiratory illnesses (asthma, pneumonia, bronchitis), other childhood medical problems (e.g. ear infections), learning difficulties (reading, mathematics, general ability), behavioural problems, and attention deficit hyperactivity disorder.[2,3] Regardless of the mother's smoking status, when fathers smoke, it is associated with low birth weight, SIDS, as well as increased incidence of respiratory and middle-ear disease in infants and young children.[4] Moreover, exposure to secondhand smoke increases the likelihood of children becoming smokers themselves.

Women garner most of the attention in efforts to address smoking during pregnancy and the postpartum period. However, expectant and new fathers who smoke can also benefit from cessation interventions. Gendered roles and responsibilities enacted by women and men in their daily lives affect when, why, how, and how often tobacco is used in relation to reducing and stopping smoking. Women frequently experience less success than men on initial efforts to stop smoking, greater negativity during withdrawal, and less successful use of nicotine replacement therapy.[5,6] Women tend to relapse in situations involving conflict or stress, while men tend to relapse in positive situations such as social events.[7] Women are more likely to relapse or fail to quit smoking due to financial difficulties, while men are more likely to quit if they experience negative health events.[8] Pressure from family members and friends help men stop smoking, but not women,[9] and physicians provide smoking cessation advice more often to men than to women.[10] Pregnancy changes a couple's identities, roles, and lifestyle practices and thus disrupts existing tobacco-related interactions. In some situations, this change increases levels of conflict within relationships. With important gender influences at play, gender-specific approaches (rather than a one-size- fits-all) are needed to support women and men's smoking cessation during pregnancy and the postpartum period.

This chapter begins with a discussion of best practices for supporting women's tobacco reduction and cessation during pregnancy and the postpartum period. Following this, promising approaches for engaging expectant and new fathers in smoking cessation are presented. We argue that the use of "de-linked" interventions (i.e. separate tailored interventions for women and men), rather than couple interventions, are important in addressing gender influences related to tobacco use. In addition, a de-linked approach to supporting women's and men's cessation reduces the potential for aggravating heightened relationship tensions and conflict related to tobacco use during pregnancy that may place women at risk for partner abuse.[11]

PREGNANT AND POSTPARTUM WOMEN

While there has been a strong historical emphasis on intervening with pregnant women who smoke, there has been limited success in creating significant reduction or permanent cessation. Two systematic reviews of the intervention literature conducted in the past decade have identified the key components of successful interventions and led to recommended women-centred approaches aimed at fostering more permanent results.[12,13] Studies were systematically evaluated using a "better practices" methodology[12] for intervention studies published prior to 2003, and a systematic review methodology[13] for those studies published after 2003. Although there have been some modest shifts in intervention techniques, there is still a lack of effective interventions with sub-groups of women and girls that have higher than average rates of smoking during pregnancy (young women, women with trauma and mental health and substance use issues, Aboriginal women) and with pregnant women's partners. The evidence is presented here, focusing on promising intervention components and approaches.

Effective intervention components It is clear that multi-component approaches are the best in this field.[14] However, it remains impossible to assess the independent impact of these components, or glean from the evidence if certain components work best in a particular balance or combination, or with a particular population of pregnant smokers. The components that most often appeared in the effective interventions are:

1. Quit guides (printed material): Many interventions used some form of take-home, patient-focused guide to quitting, usually incorporating some skill building, tips on reduction and cessation, and advice.

2. Counselling: Many interventions included counselling, however brief, delivered by a range of practitioners from obstetricians to peers.

3. Buddy/peer support: Many interventions encouraged the identification and involvement of a "buddy" for the pregnant woman as social support during the cessation process.

4. Partner counselling/social context: Some interventions included identification of the smoking patterns of the partner/father, friends, and family as key aspects of the assessment process.

5. Information: Many interventions included some education about pregnancy and smoking in the form of pamphlets, videos, or other educational materials.

6. Nicotine replacement therapies: Pharmacological components existed in some interventions to complement other approaches.
7. Personal follow-up: Several interventions incorporated personal follow-up with a view to sustaining the impact of the other components and offering encouragement, including during the postpartum.
8. Other follow-up: Other forms of follow-up were a distinct component, including paper-based communications to assess the effect of the intervention.
9. Incentives: Both financial and symbolic rewards were incorporated into some interventions.
10. Feedback about biological changes: Ultrasound images, stress tests, or other biological data were delivered back to the pregnant woman to illustrate the effects of smoking on the fetus.
11. Groups: Some interventions included support groups or group counselling to deliver and/or sustain the intervention.

CAN-ADAPTT SUMMARY STATEMENTS FOR PREGNANT AND BREASTFEEDING WOMEN

1. Smoking cessation should be encouraged for all pregnant, breastfeeding, and postpartum women.
2. During pregnancy and breastfeeding, counselling is recommended as first-line treatment for smoking cessation.
3. If counselling is found ineffective, intermittent dosing nicotine replacement therapies (such as lozenges, gum) are preferred over continuous dosing of the patch after a risk–benefit analysis.
4. Partners, friends, and family members should also be offered smoking cessation interventions.
5. A smoke-free home environment should be encouraged for pregnant and breastfeeding women to avoid exposure to secondhand smoke.

Source: CAN-ADAPTT. Canadian smoking cessation clinical practice guideline. Toronto: Canadian Action Network for the Advancement, Dissemination and Adoption of Practice-informed Tobacco Treatment, Centre for Addiction and Mental Health; 2011. Available from: www.can-adaptt.net. Reprinted with permission.

The effectiveness of interventions varies for different groups of women. Smoking patterns among pregnant women are affected by poverty, socioeconomic status, education, and issues such as previous trauma. In addition, the degree of dependence and length of smoking career also affect the effectiveness and approach of interventions. While these vulnerabilities have been frequently identified, there is a clear lack of evidence examining the effectiveness of various interventions for specific sub-groups. For example, little is known about the best interventions for heavy smokers (smoking 10 or more cigarettes per day), the significant minority of women who spontaneously quit smoking during pregnancy (25% in a group of low-income pregnant women[15] and women who relapse during pregnancy.

Pregnant women who are young, who have partners who smoke, who are living on a low income, or who are Aboriginal or members of various ethnic groups all have specific smoking-related vulnerabilities and need to be differentiated in research and practice. While some interventions have been targeted to or tailored for women of low socioeconomic status, few interventions have been designed for pregnant teens, Aboriginal women, specific ethnocultural groups, women using substances, and women experiencing trauma and relationship violence, despite their higher rates of smoking.

Better practice approaches The wider literature in women's health, women-centred care, and teenaged girls' and women's smoking and substance use provides a basis for identifying promising approaches that could either be applied to the field of tobacco cessation with pregnant or postpartum women, or integrated into future intervention development and research. These approaches include:

Tailoring for specific sub-groups who experience difficulty stopping The development of more targeted/tailored approaches will allow for more effective matches between the interventions and pregnant smoking circumstances. This will require increased tracking of smoking patterns and experiences of other forms of substance use and/or mental health/violence issues along with smoking.

Women-centred care For pregnant women who smoke, a focus on *women's health* before and during pregnancy is required, and during and beyond the postpartum year. This would assist in shifting the motivation for tobacco cessation to the woman's own health, not solely for the benefits to fetal health. This shift in thinking and practice would de-emphasize the focus on cessation during pregnancy and support motivation for cessation over time for girls and women.

Reducing stigma Increasingly restrictive smoking policies coupled with goals of denormalization create an atmosphere where smoking, particularly by pregnant women, is increasingly noticed and stigmatized. If a woman is smoking while she is visibly pregnant or in the presence of infants or small children, she is often affected by public responses. In order to engage pregnant and new mothers to address smoking the effects of these increased pressures must be addressed and dealt with in clinical interventions.

Relapse prevention Relapse is a significant problem during pregnancy for those who have stopped but is often measured postpartum, not during pregnancy. While relapse prevention is emerging as a component of interventions designed for pregnant women, it is not generally applied to spontaneous quitters. After giving birth, women who have quit need to be re-engaged in conversations on how to deal well with new pressures to relapse.

Harm reduction This practice from the wider substance use field is less often applied to tobacco use. However, it is emerging as an element of the self-help guides and counselling approaches and effectively means that *all* measures would be taken to reduce the harm to the woman and the fetus during pregnancy. Specific to tobacco, an emphasis on smoking *reduction* during pregnancy and postpartum, along with nutritional counselling, folate supplementation, and encouraging physical activity and stress-reduction also reduce harm.

Partner/social support Both cessation and relapse are affected by the presence of others in the lives of pregnant smokers and the dynamics of those relationships that smoke. Emerging research on family, couple, and partner dynamics related to tobacco use and reduction during pregnancy and the postpartum[6,7,11] indicates that the effects of these dynamics are significant. This makes it imperative to separately address with the woman and her partner (male or female) and to create interventions that do the same. Critical to these dynamics are power, control, and abuse issues that surround tobacco reduction and cessation during pregnancy and the postpartum,[11] especially as interpersonal violence directed at pregnant women is one of the most significant sources of harm to both the woman and the fetus with or without tobacco reduction efforts.

Couples and Smoking

What You Need to Know When You are Pregnant

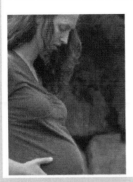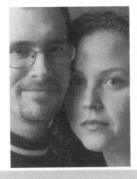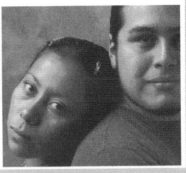

COUPLES AND SMOKING: WHAT YOU NEED TO KNOW WHEN YOU ARE PREGNANT

- Focuses on smoking in the context of women's lives and their relationships, rather than on fetal health.
- Illuminates women's experiences in reducing or stopping smoking, and how their partners influence this process.
- Provides suggestions about how to manage tensions related to tobacco use and appropriate support from their partner.

A booklet and guide for healthcare providers can be downloaded from www.facet.ubc.ca. Hard copies can be ordered from http://www. hcip-bc.org/resources-for-women/couplesandsmoking.htm.

Source: Bottorff, JL, Carey J, Poole N, Greaves L, Urquhart C. Couples and smoking: What you need to know when you are pregnant. Jointly published by the British Columbia Centre of Excellence for Women's Health, the Institute for Healthy Living and Chronic Disease Prevention, University of British Columbia Okanagan, and NEXUS, University of British Columbia Vancouver; 2008.

Social issues integration For many pregnant women, issues such as unemployment, violence, poverty, multiple roles, and stress are critical in and can overshadow the importance of tobacco cessation because smoking often serves multiple purposes, or "benefits" the woman in mediating her existence. For women who have multiple stressors and issues in their lives, it is important to acknowledge these difficulties and the factors that impede cessation. Clinical interventions should include steps through which women might gain awareness and acknowledgement of these issues, and offer mitigating strategies such as free cessation aids and nicotine replacement therapies (NRTs).

Approaches for healthcare providers In summary, there have been small improvements in effectiveness of interventions for pregnant women who smoke, supporting the 50% of pregnant women who either consider quitting or take steps towards quitting during pregnancy. Healthcare providers can support women by developing tailored approaches to smoking cessation that take into account both a woman's readiness to quit and her other life circumstances, such as socioeconomic status, cultural backgrounds, level of social support, vulnerability to partner abuse, level of nicotine addiction, and other substance-use issues.

In practice, healthcare providers can discuss a range of options for changing smoking behaviours with women such as decreasing the number of cigarettes smoked, instituting brief periods of cessation at any point in pregnancy and/or around delivery, and encouraging other health-promoting behaviours such as exercise and improved nutrition. Relapse prevention during and after pregnancy is an important area of engagement as many women continue to view quitting smoking during pregnancy as a temporary measure. In particular, "spontaneous quitters" who quit smoking during pregnancy without formal intervention require more direct practical and emotional support following birth.

Addressing the issue of smoking during pregnancy and postpartum continues to be a high priority for improving women's, maternal, fetal, and child health. However, intervention effectiveness has not improved markedly in the past decade, and requires more tailored and precise design and measurement in intervention research to achieve success with the most vulnerable groups of pregnant smokers.

Researchers at the BC Centre of Excellence for Women's Health (BCCEWH) are currently developing a brief, woman-centred tobacco intervention guide to provide practitioners with a tool to implement comprehensive tailored tobacco cessation support for women. As well, researchers are exploring how to support healthcare providers to engage in trauma-informed tobacco dependence treatment. More information on this work can be found at: http://www.bccewh.bc.ca/ and www.coalescing-vc.org.

EXPECTANT AND NEW FATHERS

The importance of developing effective interventions for expectant and new fathers who smoke is based on a growing body of research suggesting that men's smoking often impedes the ability of their pregnant partners to reduce and quit smoking,[18-22] influences fetal and infant health, and compromises men's own health. Findings from the *Families Controlling and Eliminating Tobacco* (FACET) program (www.facet.ubc.ca) of research carried out at the University of British Columbia indicated that many new and expectant fathers continue to smoke during their partners' pregnancy and the postpartum.[18] Yet despite the connectedness of fathers' smoking to family health, factors influencing their smoking were poorly understood, and as a result few men-centred, father-focussed smoking cessation interventions had been developed.

To address this shortcoming, FACET researchers began studying fathers who smoked during their partners' pregnancy and following the birth of their children.[18] These studies explored the linkages between masculinities, fatherhood and smoking—to garner insights into factors contributing to expectant and new fathers' smoking, including their resistance to quitting, their responses to tobacco control messages targeting men, and the influence of masculinities on their smoking and cessation experiences. The research findings indicate that the smoking issues faced by new fathers are distinctly different from those experienced by pregnant and postpartum mothers. In open-ended interviews conducted with men who smoked at 0–6 weeks following the birth of their newborns and again at 16–24 weeks postpartum, researchers found that smoking played an important role in men's masculine identities both at work and at home.[18] Smoking behaviours served to reinforce men's independence, physical resilience to harmful substances, and capacity to endure risk-taking. In their roles as fathers and partners, they viewed smoking as an ideal way to maintain emotional stability and manage stress. For many, smoking was explained as a deeply ingrained part of their lives, a longstanding source of enjoyment and reward, and they could not imagine their lives without cigarettes. Some men lamented the loss of some of their freedom to smoke once they became fathers as they modified their smoking behaviour to minimize the impact of their smoking on their infants. Few considered the impact of their continued smoking on their female partner's efforts to reduce and stop smoking, even though having a partner who smokes is a well-established risk factor for postpartum smoking relapse.[23] In the FACET interviews, although many men reported they were uncomfortable smoking now that they were fathers and expressed strong desires to reduce or quit, they were often unaware of helpful resources or reluctant to engage with healthcare providers to discuss their options for smoking cessation.[18]

Masculine ideals can emerge to both rationalize continued smoking and forge gender ideals about being a smoke-free father.[24] For example, many men asserted themselves as physically strong and invulnerable to the direct potential effects of smoking. At the same time, masculine protector and provider ideals drove many men's actions toward smoking cessation as means to ensuring their family's well-being. Feelings of guilt, embarrassment, regret, self-loathing, and shame associated with the stigma of being a father who smoked added to the pressures and strains they already faced in becoming a new parent.[25] Responding to this "punitive gaze," many men were deeply invested in adjusting their smoking. For example, smoking rituals aimed at keeping the smoke away from their families (washing themselves after smoking and before directly holding, touching, or directly caring for the baby) and smoking alone away from the house and sight of their partners and child.

Men's work and work commute often contributed to continued smoking in ways that challenge and counter cessation efforts. In one sub-study, fathers rationalized their smoking on the job as necessary in order to reduce stress, kill time, and reward achievement.[26] The jobsite separated men and their smoking from the domestic spaces where their child and female partner resided. As well, going to work released men from direct fathering duties and gave them the freedom to smoke without observation from or risk toward their child or partner. While many men smoked when travelling in their work vehicles to minimize the dangers of secondhand smoke, they made efforts to maintain the inside of the family home as a non-smoking area because of the presence of a baby. As they relocated their smoking to balconies, porches, yards, sheds, and parking lots, the men were also often forced to choose between smoking and direct fathering activities.

Men frequently link their continued smoking to masculine ideals and identities (e.g. freedom, confidence, independence and strength).[18,26,27] But when men became new fathers and engaged in direct care of their baby, these masculine ideals could shift to afford an array of legitimate options for tobacco reduction and cessation.[25,28] These findings support previous work[29] suggesting that in men's health promotion a focus on how masculine ideals contribute to, rather than work against, positive changes in health behaviour might best support the health of new fathers who smoke and their families. There was consensus among men that becoming a father was a positive and life-changing experience,[30] and coupled with this men wanted to be responsible parents and good role models for their child. They were aware of the social stigma surrounding their smoking and also recognized the significant added expense of continuing to smoke. Yet, for the most part, new fathers were not routinely asked by healthcare providers about their smoking status.[31] So despite an increased interest in reducing and quitting smoking, few new fathers were successful in becoming smoke free.[28]

During fathers' efforts to reduce or stop smoking during their partner's pregnancy and the postpartum period, self-reliance, willpower, and autonomy were valued manly virtues used to leverage their tobacco reduction and cessation efforts.[28] For example, men who tried to stop "cold turkey," constructed their attempt to quit around a snap decision reliant on willpower and strength rather than smoking cessation aids. Other men planned a gradual reduction in smoking beginning with developing lists of reasons to quit and detailed strategies to enhance the likelihood of success. Often, though, in their narratives the date or time by which they would be smoke-free was unclear. Some men's narratives of quitting smoking were centred on how the baby displaced their need to smoke, increased motivation to quit, and enhanced success. Finally, a story of forced reduction underscored the challenges of cessation for one highly tobacco addicted father and the tension and conflict this created in the relationship with his partner. These narratives of tobacco reduction and cessation suggest that fatherhood may be an opportune time to support men's quit attempts and that designing interventions that take into account men's challenges and desire to self-manage may be helpful. Supporting cessation at the time when men become new fathers has the potential to significantly improve men's well-being, support women's efforts to reduce and quit smoking, provide smoke-free environments for their children and strengthen the overall well-being of their families.

Approaches for healthcare providers The few studies that have evaluated approaches to supporting smoking cessation among expectant and new fathers have not generated effective approaches. A randomized control trial that included counselling and NRT by request found a significant decrease in men's smoking during pregnancy, but this was not sustained at 2, 6, or 12 months postpartum.[21] Although a study in which smoking cessation information and free NRT were provided to male partners yielded significant quit rates, these were only measured pre-birth.[32] Reliance on female partners to promote men's health also appears to be ineffective in engaging expectant and new fathers in smoking cessation. Having pregnant women provide a smoking cessation intervention to their male partners was found in 2 randomized control trials to be ineffective.[33,34] In FACET interviews, women reported they were deeply concerned about the effect of smoking on their partner's health and the health of their infants but were largely unsuccessful in getting their partners to stop smoking. Efforts to regulate their male partners' smoking often heightened potential for tension and conflict in their intimate relationships. As a result many women reduced potential relationship conflict and maintained their identity as supportive partners by positioning the decision to quit smoking as a man's personal choice.[27] These results suggest that healthcare providers need to intervene directly with men to relieve women of the responsibility of engaging expectant and new fathers in smoking cessation.

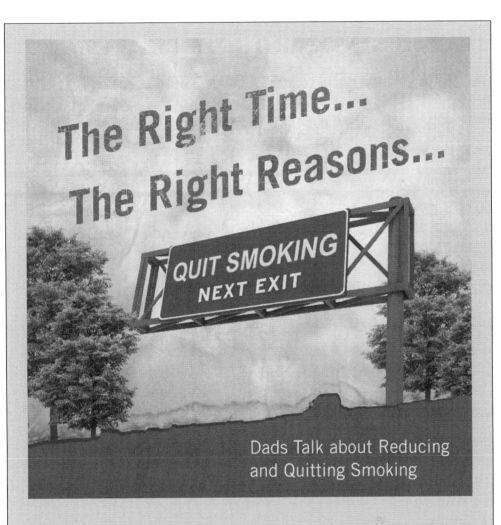

Dads Talk about Reducing and Quitting Smoking

Electronic copies of this booklet and a guide for healthcare providers can be downloaded from:

www.facet.ubc.ca

www.itag.ubc.ca

www.menshealthresearch.ubc.ca

Print copies can be ordered from the QuitNow website:

http://www.quitnow.ca/help_someone_quit/order_resources.php

Source: Oliffe JL, Bottorff JL, Sarbit G. The right time. The right reasons: dads talk about reducing and quitting smoking. Kelowna BC: Institute for Healthy Living and Chronic Disease Prevention, University of British Columbia Okanagan, Canada; 2010.

Promising approaches that are men-centred and father-focused are currently being developed and could assist healthcare providers to support cessation among expectant and new fathers. For example, based on the FACET research, a booklet has been developed to support and strengthen new and expectant fathers' motivation to take the first step to becoming smoke free: *The Right Time … The Right Reasons … Dads Talk about Reducing and Quitting Smoking*. The booklet is unique in that it has a masculine looking design, was written in a style that features "dads talking to dads" as opposed to "experts advising dads," and was based on the thoughts and experiences of fathers who have—or are currently trying to—quit smoking. Strategies fathers used to stop smoking are included so that men can make their own decisions about what method might work best for them. This booklet fills a gap in available resources to assist men in their cessation efforts.

In addition to this print-based resource, face-to-face programs can provide important opportunities for men to support each other as they reduce and stop smoking. The FACET team has developed and pilot tested an innovative program, *Dads in Gear* (DIG). The 8-week program design highlights men's masculine ideals to promote health, and talks directly with men about fathering, tobacco reduction, exercise, and health. Pilot study findings revealed the value of peer support and that the program was well received by participants. DIG is currently being refined to improve feasibility of the content and delivery. The program resources will be developed using Web 2.0 technologies to enable access for men regardless of their location. More information on this work can be found at: http://www.facet.ubc.ca

SUPPORTING CESSATION EFFORTS AMONG EXPECTANT AND NEW FATHERS

Underpinning the development of a suite of such resources have been some health promotion practice lessons that can be used to inform other approaches to support cessation among expectant and new fathers. These include:

Recognizing and mobilizing healthful masculine virtues Encouraging new fathers to become actively involved in the care of their infants and toddlers fosters an emotional connection with their children that has the potential to strengthen men's motivation to engage in smoking cessation. Using strength-based positive messaging to promote change without amplifying stigma, guilt, shame, and blame and helping men manage the stresses associated with being a new father demonstrates respect for men as good fathers and more positively encourages them to begin to reduce and stop smoking.

Respecting men's autonomy   Starting a conversation with expectant and new fathers about smoking, assessing their readiness to take the first step in reducing and quitting, and supporting men in their decisions about when and how to stop smoking supports the desires of men to be autonomous and decide their own path to being smoke free.

Quantifying the evidence   Many men show greater motivation to improve their health when presented with scientific evidence about risk factors or the benefits of specific lifestyle changes.[35-37] Providing current and meaningful information about the self and family health benefits of quitting smoking and reducing secondhand smoke has the potential to increase the likelihood that new fathers will begin to reduce and stop smoking.

Men at work   Worksites can be important venues to provide smoking cessation resources. Meeting fathers in the workplace can foster frank discussions dedicated to improving men's access to resources and opportunities to start to reduce and quit smoking.

The permission of other men to do health   Many men welcome health sessions with other men as a way to exchange health information and strategies to aid well-being.[38,39] Organizing group smoking cessation sessions garners peer permission and provides an opportunity for men to assist each other with cessation. Learning about the strategies used by other men can also help to normalize help-seeking for smoking cessation.

Men's role, identity and relationship changes can promote reappraisal   Fatherhood is a life-changing experience for many men as changes occur in family structure, gender roles, relationships, and the wider social milieu. Becoming a new father represents an ideal time in a man's life for smoking cessation to occur on his own terms.[4]

CONCLUSION

Pregnancy and postpartum provide important opportunities to influence both women and men's health by supporting efforts to reduce and stop smoking. All healthcare providers have a responsibility to intervene with women and men who smoke in ways that reduce stigma and guilt associated with smoking, recognize the influence of relationships and other social factors on smoking cessation efforts, and demonstrate a willingness to tailor approaches to address specific needs. Continuing efforts to develop effective gender-specific and gender-sensitive approaches are needed.

REFERENCES

1   Canadian Tobacco Use Monitoring Survey (CTUMS) 2010. Ottawa: Health Canada; 2010 [cited 2012 Mar 26] Available from: http://www.hc-sc.gc.ca/hc-ps/tobac-tabac/research-recher-che/stat/_ctums-esutc_2008/ann_summary-sommaire-eng.php

2   Health Canada. Second-hand smoke. Catalogue #H13-7/25-2006E-PDF. Ottawa: Author; 2006 [cited 2012 Mar 26]. Available from: http://www.hc-sc.gc.ca/hl-vs/iyh-vsv/life-vie/shs-fs-eng.php

3   Health Canada. Health concerns: Pregnancy; 2007 [cited 2012 Mar 26]. Available from: http://www.hc-sc.gc.ca/hc-ps/tobac-tabac/body-corps/preg-gros-eng.php.

4   Blackburn CM, Bonas S, Spencer NJ, Coe CJ, Dolan A, Moy R. Parental smoking and passive smoking in infants: Fathers matter too. Health Educ Res. 2005;20:185-94.

5   Perkins KA, Donny E, Caggiula AR. Sex differences in nicotine effects and self-administration: review of human and animal evidence. Nicotine Tob Res. 1999;1:301-15.

6   Wetter DW, Kenford SL, Smith SS, Fiore MC, Jorenby DE, Baker TB. Gender differences in smoking cessation. J Consult Clin Psychol. 1999;67:555-62.

7   Ortner R, Schindler D, Kraigher D, Mendelsohn A, Fischer G. Women addicted to nicotine. Arch Women's Mental Health. 2002;4:103-109.

8   McKee SA, Maciejewski PK, Falba T, Mazure CM. Sex differences in the effects of stressful life events on changes in smoking status. Addiction. 2003;98:847-55.

9   Westmaas JL, Wild TC, Ferrence R. Effects of gender in social control of smoking cessation. Health Psychology 2002;21:368–76.

10   Young JM, Ward JE. Influence of physician and patient gender on provision of smoking cessation advice in general practice. Tob Control. 1998;7:360-3.

11   Greaves L, Kalaw C, Bottorff JL. Case studies of power and control related to tobacco use during pregnancy. Womens Health Issues. 2007;17:325-32.

12   Moyer C, Garcia J, Cameron R, Maule C. Identifying promising solutions for complex health problems: model for a better practices process. Unpublished work, 2002 Nov.

13   National Institute for Health and Clinical Excellence (NICE). Methods for development of NICE public health guidance. London UK: National Institute for Health and Clinical Excellence; 2006.

14   Public Health Service and Office of the Surgeon General. Women and smoking: a report of the Surgeon General. Atlanta: Centers for Disease Control and Prevention; 2001.

15   Ockene JK, Ma Y, Zapka JG, Pbert LA, Valentine Goins K, Stoddard AM. Spontaneous cessation of smoking and alcohol use among low-income pregnant women. Am J Prev Med. 2002;23:150-9.

16   Bottorff JL, Kalaw C, Johnson JL, Stewart M, Greaves L, Carey J. Couple dynamics during women's tobacco reduction in pregnancy and postpartum. Nicotine Tob Res. 2006;8:499-509.

17   Bottorff JL, Carey J, Poole N, Greaves L, Urquhart C. Couples and smoking: what you need to know when you are pregnant. Jointly published by the British Columbia Centre of Excellence

for Women's Health, the Institute for Healthy Living and Chronic Disease Prevention, University of British Columbia Okanagan, and NEXUS, University of British Columbia; 2008 [cited 2012 Mar 26]. Available from: www.facet.ubc.ca and www.hcip-bc.org.

18   Bottorff JL, Oliffe J, Kalaw C, Carey J, Mroz L. Men's constructions of smoking in the context of women's tobacco reduction during pregnancy and postpartum. Soc Sci Med. 2006;62:3096-108.

19   Fang WL, Goldstein AO, Goldstein AO, Butzen AY, Hartsock SA, et al. Smoking cessation in pregnancy: a review of postpartum relapse prevention strategies. J Am Board Fam Pract. 2004;17:264-75.

20   Lu Y, Tong S, Oldenburg B. Determinants of smoking and cessation during and after pregnancy. Health Promot Int. 2001;16:355-65.

21   McBride CM, Baucom DH, Peterson BL, Pollak KI, Palmer C, Westman E, et al. Prenatal and postpartum smoking abstinence: a partner-assisted approach. Am J Prev Med. 2004;27:232-8.

22   Penn G, Owen L. Factors associated with continued smoking during pregnancy: analysis of socio-demographic, pregnancy and smoking-related factors. Drug Alcohol Rev. 2002;21(1):17-25.

23   Ashford KB, Hahn E, Hall L, Rayens MK, Noland M. Postpartum smoking relapse and secondhand smoke. Public Health Rep 2009;124:515-26.

24   Johnson JL, Oliffe JL, Kelly M, Bottorff JL, Le Beau K. The readings of smoking fathers: semiotics analyses of tobacco cesation images. Health Communication. 2009;24:532-47.

25   Greaves L, Oliffe JL, Ponic P, Kelly MT, Bottorff JL. Unclean fathers, responsible men: smoking, stigma and fatherhood. Health Sociology Rev. 2010;19:522-33.

26   Oliffe JL, Bottorff JL, Johnson JL, Kelly MT, LeBeau K. Fathers: locating smoking and masculinity in the postpartum. Qual Health Res. 2010;20:330-9.

27   Bottorff JL, Oliffe JL, Kelly MT, Greaves L, Johnson JL, Ponic P, et al. Men's business, women's work: gender influences and fathers' smoking. Sociol Health Illn. 2010;32:583-96.

28   Bottorff JL, Radsma J, Kelly M, Oliffe JL. Fathers' narratives of reducing and quitting smoking. Sociol Health Illn. 2009;31:185-200.

29   Sloan C, Gough B, Conner M. Healthy masculinities? how ostensibly healthy men talk about lifestyle, health and gender. Psychology & Health. 2010;25:783-803.

30   Fägerskiöld A. A change in life as experienced by first-time fathers. Scand J Caring Sci. 2008;22:64-71.

31   Fiore MC. US public health service clinical practice guideline: treating tobacco use and dependence. Respir Care. 2000;45:1200-62.

32   Stanton WR, Lowe JB, Moffatt J, Del Mar CB. Randomised control trial of a smoking cessation intervention directed at men whose partners are pregnant. Prev Med. 2004;38:6-9.

33   Loke AY, Lam TH. A randomized controlled trial of the simple advice given by obstetricians in Guangzhou, China, to non-smoking pregnant women to help their husbands quit smoking. Patient Educ Couns. 2005;59:31-7.

34   de Vries H, Bakker M, Mullen PD, van Breukelen G. The effects of smoking cessation counseling by midwives on Dutch pregnant women and their partners. Patient Educ Couns. 2006;63:177-87.

35   Aoun S, Johnson L. Men's health promotion by general practitioners in a workplace setting. Aust J Rural Health. 2002;10:268-72.

36   McMahon A, Hodgins M, Kelleher CC. Feasibility of a men's health promotion programme in Irish primary care. Ir J Med Sci. 2002;171:20-3.

37   Robertson LM, Douglas F, Ludbrook A, Reid G, van Teijlingen E. What works with men? a systematic review of health promoting interventions targeting men. BMC Health Serv Res. 2008;8:141.

38   Golding B., Foley A., Brown M. The international potential for men's shed-based learning. Adlib: Journal for Continuing Liberal Adult Education. 2007;34:9-13.

39   Evans J, Frank B, Oliffe JL, Gregory D. Health, illness, men, and masculinities (HIMM): a theoretical framework for understanding men and their health. J Men's Health. 2011;8(1):7-15.

40   Oliffe J, Bottorff JL, Sarbit G. Supporting fathers to be smoke free. Canadian J Nursing Res. 2012 (Forthcoming).

17

Young People and Smoking Cessation

BECKY FREEMAN

MOST PEOPLE FIRST START SMOKING WHEN THEY ARE YOUNG TEENAGERS. THAT FIRST cigarette might be stolen from a parent that smokes, bought by an older sibling or friend, or simply offered at a party. Regardless of the origins of that first, tentative, experimental puff, far too many teens go on to become tobacco-addicted as adults who struggle to stop, and suffer the devastating health consequences of chronic tobacco use. Naturally, it is rightly assumed that preventing young people from taking up smoking in the first place or helping those youth that have started to stop just makes good "common sense." What is less intuitive is how to best go about preventing yet another young generation addicted to tobacco. It is essential that evidence-based polices and interventions are given priority over programs that only appear appealing in reducing teen tobacco use. This can be a surprisingly difficult challenge when facing powerful opponents to such effective initiatives. It is telling that the tobacco industry is a creator and supporter of feel-good youth education programs that have no measurable impact on smoking rates.[1]

YOUTH SMOKING RATES

In 2010, according to the *Canadian Tobacco Use Monitoring Survey,* smoking among Canadian youth aged 15 to 19 years was 12%, the lowest rate of current smoking Health Canada has ever recorded for this age group.[2] Seven percent of youth reported smoking daily, and consumed an average of 11.6 cigarettes per day, while 5% of youth reported smoking occasionally. Contrary to popular belief, the proportion of smoking among young females had not increased and was reported to be at the same rate as their male counterparts. Encouragingly, among the younger age group of 15- to 17-year-olds, the smoking rate was even lower at 9%, with 5% reporting daily smoking. From the same survey, the prevalence of smoking among young adults aged 20 to 24 years was 22%, again with no statistical difference between males and females.

SUMMARY OF THE LIMITED EVIDENCE OF TAILORED YOUTH CESSATION INTERVENTIONS

While youth do report wanting to quit smoking, there is limited evidence to support the widespread implementation of youth-specific cessation programs. Cessation research involving youth is subject to the common challenges of recruitment, retention, and parental consent to participate.[3] This suggests that conventional cessation programs, even if they are proven to be successful in assisting cessation, will not attract or retain sufficient numbers of youth to make a significant impact on teen smoking rates.

Two 2009 reviews of experimental studies of youth smoking cessation agree that there is insufficient evidence for the effectiveness of any pharmacological treatments with youth smokers.[3,4] Additionally, these same review articles suggest that complex behavioural interventions that incorporate stages of change approaches, and using motivational enhancement and cognitive behavioural therapy, marginally increase the short-term chances of young people's successfully quitting smoking. But again, the issues of recruitment and retention of participants is an enormous hurdle. One of the few programs that has been evaluated and shown to have a very modest effect on increasing youth cessation is the American Lung Association's school and community based program *Not On Tobacco* or N-O-T as it is more commonly known.[4] *Not On Tobacco* is a resource- and time-intensive group-style cessation program.

While it has been well established that brief interventions and quit-smoking advice offered by health professionals to adult smokers is effective in promoting quit attempts and successful quitting among adults, less is known about the effect on adolescent smokers. A 2011 US study found that physician screening and advice regarding tobacco use with adolescent patients positively impacted on their attitudes, knowledge, intentions to smoke, and quitting behaviours.[5] Brief physician advice has the potential to reach much larger numbers of adolescents and be more cost effective than intensive youth cessation programs—if proven to be effective in increasing quitting.

WHAT WORKS BEST TO REDUCE YOUTH SMOKING?

While it is often remarked that smoking is an act of teenage rebellion, parental smoking is highly predictive of youth smoking.[6-8] Youth are role-modelling the behaviour of adults who are closest to them, not rebelling against it. Lowering smoking rates among adults is one of the best ways to reduce young people's smoking. When smoking is no longer viewed as a socially acceptable, adult behaviour, there is little attraction for young people to start.

Social norms around smoking are hugely influential in youth's stopping smoking. Five factors have been identified that robustly predict successful youth smoking cessation:[9]

1. Not having friends who smoke
2. Not having intentions to smoke in the future
3. Resisting peer pressure to smoke
4. Being older at first use of cigarette
5. Having negative beliefs about smoking

These factors clearly illustrate the importance of denormalizing smoking and tobacco use among friends, families, schools, communities, and the wider population.[10] Social denormalization strategies seek "to change the broad social norms around using tobacco—to push tobacco use out of the charmed circle of normal, desirable practice to being an abnormal practice."[11] Putting this advice into very practical terms means that child health providers should:

Serve as a role model for a tobacco-free lifestyle, routinely address tobacco issues with pediatric patients, and provide treatment and/or referrals for tobacco prevention and cessation resources. Beyond the clinic, pediatric professionals can support tobacco-free ordinances in their communities and participate in [provincial] and national tobacco control campaigns. Wherever possible, training of medical students, residents, fellows, and other pediatric professionals in tobacco counselling and advocacy would contribute to further resources for denormalization of tobacco. (Calabro et al. 2010)[12]

Strategies to positively impact youth cessation behaviours must provide a distal environment that supports positive changes, while acknowledging the tremendous influence that proximal factors, particularly peers and family, have on smoking uptake and quitting.[12] To this end, the World Health Organization (WHO), as part of the MPOWER initiative, outlines 6 key policy areas that have been shown to denormalize and reduce tobacco use:[13]

1. **M**onitor tobacco use and prevention policies
2. **P**rotect people from tobacco smoke
3. **O**ffer help to quit tobacco use
4. **W**arn about the dangers of tobacco
5. **E**nforce bans on tobacco advertising, promotion, and sponsorship
6. **R**aise taxes on tobacco

While all of these policy areas are part of implementing a successful, comprehensive tobacco control program, there are 4 that specifically target promoting cessation among young people and have the strongest available evidence base: protecting from tobacco smoke, warning about the health effects of smoking, enforcing tobacco advertising bans, and raising taxes.

CAN-ADAPTT SUMMARY STATEMENTS FOR YOUTH

1. Healthcare providers who work with youth (children and adolescents) should obtain information about tobacco use (cigarettes, cigarillos, waterpipe, etc.) on a regular basis.
2. Healthcare providers are encouraged to provide counselling that supports abstinence from tobacco and/or cessation to youth (children and adolescents) who use tobacco.
3. Healthcare providers in pediatric healthcare settings should counsel parents/guardians about the potentially harmful effects of secondhand smoke on the health of their children.

Source: CAN-ADAPTT. Canadian smoking cessation clinical practice guideline. Toronto: Canadian Action Network for the Advancement, Dissemination and Adoption of Practice-informed Tobacco Treatment, Centre for Addiction and Mental Health; 2011. Available from: www.can-adaptt.net. Reprinted with permission.

Protection from tobacco smoke While smoking bans in workplaces and public spaces have the primary intent of protecting employees and the public from harmful secondhand smoke, they have also been shown to reduce overall smoking rates.[14] Restrictions on smoking at home, more extensive bans on smoking in public places, and enforced bans on smoking at school may further reduce teenage smoking.[14] All parents, including smokers, should be encouraged to establish and maintain a completely smoke-free home, not only to protect their children from harmful tobacco smoke but to assist with the prevention and cessation of adolescent smoking.[15] Smoking bans in private cars carrying children are now required by most Canadian provinces and territories; this legislation may also help to reduce youth smoking rates.

Warning about the dangers of tobacco use   While there is limited evidence that standalone education programs have any measurable impact on youth smoking rates, hard-hitting mass media campaigns and graphic warnings on tobacco packages that focus on health effects have been shown to be effective.

Pictorial health warnings on tobacco packages lead young smokers to read and think about the health consequences of smoking and positively impact on cessation behaviour.[16] In experimental studies of plain packaging, where all tobacco brand elements on the pack are removed, and the size of pictorial health warnings is increased, tobacco brand appeal was reduced among those youth most susceptible to becoming established adult smokers.[17] In 2012 Australia and Canada both implemented tobacco packaging legislation to increase the size of health warning messages. On cigarettes and cigarillos sold in Canada the warning message now covers 75% of the front and back of packages. Other countries will no doubt follow with more stringent legislation of their own.

Mass media campaigns need not be designed specifically for a youth audience—campaigns aimed at adults have been shown to appeal to youth. For example, the Australian *Every Cigarette Is Doing You Damage* campaign was targeted at adult smokers but has been shown to be effective in changing youth attitudes and behaviours.[18] Given that government budgets for these types of campaigns are often limited, and that purchasing television airtime is also very expensive, the broader the reach of all tobacco cessation messages the better.

Enforcing bans on tobacco advertising, promotion and sponsorship [TAPS]   As a signatory to the global health treaty, the WHO Framework Convention on Tobacco Control, the Canadian government is obligated to ban all forms of TAPS. There is a large and diverse body of research evidence from multiple countries showing that tobacco advertising increases smoking prevalence and total tobacco consumption.[19] Nonsmoking adolescents who are more aware of or receptive to tobacco advertising are more likely to take up smoking.[20] Advertising bans must include not only traditional mass media channels, but also such promotional avenues as tobacco power walls at retail outlets and sponsorship of events. Additionally, the Internet is proving to be fertile ground for tobacco industry marketing efforts and governments are currently ill equipped to legis-late removal of pro-smoking content on this vast and dynamic medium.[21–23] It is essential that health professionals also make effective use of digital technology to counter these pro-smoking messages (this is discussed in-depth in the section below).

Raising taxes on tobacco It has long been established that cigarette price influences youth smoking rates. Encouragingly, such influence is not only in the uptake of tobacco, but also on smoking cessation behaviour among adoles-cents. Price has been shown to be the one of the strongest predictors of cessation behaviour among high school smokers.[24] Some health promotion stakeholders are concerned that high tobacco taxes further increase health inequalities, par-ticularly as most individuals that smoke are of lower socioeconomic status. Low income and young smokers are actually more likely to respond to price increases by reducing or quitting their tobacco use. High tobacco taxes then have the potential to benefit more disadvantaged groups and contribute to reducing health inequalities rather than exacerbating them.[23]

FUTURE OF YOUTH AND YOUNG ADULT SMOKING CESSATION: DIGITAL COMMUNICATIONS SHOW PROMISE

Mobile phone-based interventions for smoking cessation In a 2009 review of the effectiveness of mobile phones in helping individuals to quit smok-ing, it was found that mobile phone programs appear to be a useful option for those who want to stop smoking, but more trials were needed to assess the effect on long-term quit rates. The authors noted that mobile phones "have some advan-tages over most current treatment services: they can be delivered anywhere, at appropriate times, confidentially, and direct to the participant with minimal direct contact. These are characteristics which may be appreciated by some groups such as young people."[25]

In a study published in 2011, individuals who quit smoking with the assistance of a text messaging service were nearly twice as likely to be smoke-free 6 months later than those with no support.[26] Success rates for single strat-egy stop-smoking intervention are never high, and just over 10% of smokers in the text message group had successfully quit smoking. However, unlike more traditional cessation programs, text-messaging services are a low-cost option that could be used to reach a greater number of individuals as compared with intensive face-to-face counselling or traditional quitline telephone services. The explosive growth in people using web-enabled mobile phones and social media is a golden opportunity for public health agencies to make use of these same communication tools.[27] This is particularly true for young adults, for whom cessation support delivered through electronic media seems promising.[28]

Internet-based smoking cessation programs   A review of formal and intensive Internet-based interventions showed that such programs can assist with smoking cessation, especially if the information is appropriately tailored to the users and frequent automated contacts with users are ensured; however, not all trials showed consistent effects.[29] The results of this review suggest that different types of online support may be required as opposed to the typically prescriptive programs included in the review.

Social media and smoking cessation   A major advantage in favour of public health is that health information is one of the most commonly searched topics on the web. Yet it is no longer enough for health agencies to simply supply accurate information for health consumers on official organization websites. Health agencies routinely sink precious resources into revamping their websites with youth-oriented content in the hope of preventing youth from taking up smoking or helping smokers to quit.[30] Consumers, particularly young people, expect content to be interactive, shareable, multimedia in format, portable between mobile and other tech devices, and easily accessed through websites that they are most familiar with such as Facebook, YouTube and Twitter. Discouragingly, many public-health experts are actually banned from accessing these types of social media websites while at work and have received no formal training in how best to use these tools. One of the central tenets of any health promotion initiative is to go where your target audience is. Youth are online, they are on mobile phones, and no program, no matter how well-designed, will be able to impact on an audience that must be coerced to participate.

Of even greater advantage to tobacco control, "quit smoking" is itself a very popular online search term.[31] And as providing easy and free access to practical self-help materials is a cost effective way to help individuals to stop smoking,[32] online interventions need not be overly cumbersome or resource intensive. For example, while it appears there is a demand for quit-smoking applications on smart phones and there are dozens of quit apps available for the iPhone through the iTunes App store, the quality of these apps varies widely and overall is rated as very poor.[33] Evidence-based quit-smoking organizations partnered with experienced app developers could be well-placed to create useful and inexpensive smart phone applications for those who would prefer to use a digital self-help tool to help them with quitting.

Quit-smoking organizations could also follow the lead of pharmaceutical companies in creatively reaching out to tobacco consumers though social media. This is especially important given that pharmaceutical products have not been shown to be effective in assisting young people to quit smoking. In January 2011, the makers of Nicorette®, a nicotine replacement product, took advantage of New Year's resolutions to quit smoking and ran a promotional campaign on the social networking site Twitter. The promotion involved sponsoring the topic #QuittingSucks (referred to as a *hashtag*) so that it would appear in the Twitter "top trends" lists. Sponsored topics are a paid Twitter marketing method to stimulate and increase interest in a topic. While no data are publically available on the success of this campaign, on the days the Twitter campaign ran there was a mix of Twitter account holders using the tag to discuss their own quitting smoking, to draw people to their own tweets, to poke fun at the topic, and some for the intended purpose: to promote use of Nicorette®. People who shared ("reTweeted") the Nicorette® Twitter messages received coupons and vouchers for the product. Quit-smoking organisations could encourage similar message sharing by building an online community of former smokers who offer support and advice. Twitter "celebrities" with high numbers of followers could also be recruited to share quit-smoking stories and encourage followers to share their own.

The potential of online social media to accelerate smoking cessation among young people is exciting and warrants further investigation and experimentation by health agencies. The tobacco industry has already proven adept at exploiting these communication channels to promote tobacco use—it's time public health joined in.

CONCLUSION

While it is encouraging that smoking rates among young people are at their recorded lowest levels, failing to maintain momentum in implementing effective tobacco control polices will see these rates rise again. In addition to the adoption of high tobacco taxes and regulations endorsed by global health bodies, it is essential that health groups innovate how they reach and support young smokers. In the future, youth may well view smoking as outmoded as posting a handwritten letter or looking up information in a volume of an encyclopedia. The tobacco industry will do everything possible to keep smoking fashionable and youthful; without new teenage recruits, smokers are truly a dying breed.

REFERENCES

1   World Health Organization. Tobacco industry interference with tobacco control 2009 [cited 2012 Jan 1]. Available from: http://whqlibdoc.who.int/publications/2008/9789241597340_eng.pdf.

2   Health Canada. Canadian Tobacco Use Monitoring Survey (CTUMS) 2011 [cited 2012 Jan 1]. Available from: http://www.hc-sc.gc.ca/hc-ps/tobac-tabac/research-recherche/stat/_ctums-esutc_2010/ann_summary-sommaire-eng.php.

3   Curry SJ, Mermelstein RJ, Sporer AK. Therapy for specific problems: youth tobacco cessation. Annu Rev Psychol. 2009;60:229.

4   Grimshaw G, Stanton A. Tobacco cessation interventions for young people. Cochrane Database of Systematic Reviews; 2009 (4) [cited 2012 Jan 1]. Available from: http://summaries.cochrane.org/CD003289/are-there-any-smoking-cessation-programmes-which-can-help-adolescents-to-stop-smoking.

5   Hum AM, Robinson LA, Jackson AA, Ali KS. Physician communication regarding smoking and adolescent tobacco use. Pediatrics. 2011;127(6):e1368-74.

6   Farkas AJ, Distefan JM, Choi WS, Gilpin EA, Pierce JP. Does parental smoking cessation discourage adolescent smoking? Prev Med. 1999;28(3):213-8.

7   Bricker JB, Peterson AV, Jr., Leroux BG, Andersen MR, Rajan KB, Sarason IG. Prospective prediction of children's smoking transitions: role of parents' and older siblings' smoking. Addiction. 2006;101(1):128-36.

8   Bricker JB, Rajan KB, Andersen MR, Peterson AV, Jr. Does parental smoking cessation encourage their young adult children to quit smoking?: a prospective study. Addiction. 2005;100(3):379-86.

9   Cengelli S, O'Loughlin J, Lauzon B, Cornuz J. A systematic review of longitudinal population-based studies on the predictors of smoking cessation in adolescent and young adult smokers. Tobacco Control. 2011. doi: 10.1136/tc.2011.044149.

10   Chapman S, Freeman B. Markers of the denormalisation of smoking and the tobacco industry. Tob Control. 2008;17(1):25-31.

11   Hammond D, Fong GT, Zanna MP, Thrasher JF, Borland R. Tobacco denormalization and industry beliefs among smokers from four countries. Am J Prev Med. 2006;31(3):225-32.

12   Calabro KS, Costello TC, Prokhorov AV. Denormalization of tobacco use and the role of the pediatric health-care provider. Pediatr Allergy Immunol Pulmonol. 2010;23(4):273-8.

13   World Health Organization. Report on the global tobacco epidemic. The MPOWER package 2008 [cited 2012 Mar 13]. Available from: http://www.who.int/entity/tobacco/mpower/mpower_report_full_2008.pdf.

14   Fichtenberg CM, Glantz SA. Effect of smoke-free workplaces on smoking behaviour: systematic review. BMJ. 2002;325(7357):188.

15   Emory K, Saquib N, Gilpin EA, Pierce JP. The association between home smoking restrictions and youth smoking behaviour: a review. Tob Control. 2010;19(6):495-506.

16   Hammond D. Health warning messages on tobacco products: a review. Tob Control. 2011;20(5):327-37.

17   Germain D, Wakefield MA, Durkin SJ. Adolescents' perceptions of cigarette brand image: does plain packaging make a difference? J Adolesc Health. 2010;46(4):385-92.

18   White V, Tan N, Wakefield M, Hill D. Do adult focused anti-smoking campaigns have an impact on adolescents? the case of the Australian National Tobacco Campaign. Tob Control. 2003;12(suppl 2):ii23-9.

19   National Cancer Institute. Influence of tobacco marketing on smoking behavior. In: Monograph 19: The Role of the Media in Promoting and Reducing Tobacco Use. Bethesda MD: US Department of Health and Human Services, National Institutes of Health, National Cancer Institute; 2008 [cited 2012 Mar 27]. Available from: http://cancercontrol.cancer.gov/tcrb/monographs/19/monograph19.html.

20   Lovato C, Watts A, Stead L. Impact of tobacco advertising and promotion on increasing adolescent smoking behaviours. Cochrane Database Syst rev; 2011 (10) [cited 2012 Jan 1]. Available from: http://summaries.cochrane.org/CD003439/does-tobacco-advertising-and-promotion-make-it-more-likely-that-adolescents-will-start-to-smoke.

21   Freeman B, Chapman S. Is "YouTube" telling or selling you something? Tobacco content on the YouTube video-sharing website. Tob Control. 2007;16(3):207-10.

22   Freeman B, Chapman S. Gone viral? Heard the buzz? A guide for public health practitioners and researchers on how Web 2.0 can subvert advertising restrictions and spread health information. J Epidemiol Community Health. 2008;62(9):778-82.

23   Thomas S, Fayter D, Misso K, Ogilvie D, Petticrew M, Sowden A, et al. Population tobacco control interventions and their effects on social inequalities in smoking: systematic review. Tob Control. 2008;17(4):230-7.

24   Tworek C, Yamaguchi R, Kloska DD, Emery S, Barker DC, Giovino GA, et al. State-level tobacco control policies and youth smoking cessation measures. Health Policy. 2010;97(2-3):136-44.

25   Whittaker R, Borland R, Bullen C, Lin R, McRobbie H, Rodgers A. Mobile phone-based interventions for smoking cessation. Cochrane Database Syst rev; 2009 (4) [cited 2012 Jan 1]. Available from: http://www.thecochranelibrary.com/userfiles/ccoch/file/World%20No%20Tobacco%20Day/CD006611.pdf.

26   Free C, Knight R, Robertson S, Whittaker R, Edwards P, Zhou W, et al. Smoking cessation support delivered via mobile phone text messaging (txt2stop): a single-blind, randomised trial. Lancet. 2011;378(9785):49-55.

27   Freeman B. Quit-smoking texts send clear message to outdated health promoters. The Conversation; 2011 [cited 2012 Jan 1]. Available from: http://theconversation.edu.au/quit-smoking-texts-send-clear-message-to-outdated-health-promoters-2093.

28   Villanti AC, McKay HS, Abrams DB, Holtgrave DR, Bowie JV. Smoking-cessation interventions for US young adults: a systematic review. Am J Prev Med. 2010;39(6):564-74.

29   Civljak M, Sheikh A, Stead Lindsay F, Car J. Internet-based interventions for smoking cessation. Cochrane Database Syst rev; 2010 (9). Available from: http://www.mrw.interscience.wiley.com/cochrane/clsysrev/articles/CD007078/frame.htm.

30   Chapman S, Freeman B. Why has smoking in Australian youth never been lower? In: Bennett D, Towns S, Elliott E, Merrick J, editors. Challenges in adolescent health: an Australian perspective. New York: Nova Science; 2009. p. 153-61.

31   Google Insights for Search. Web search interest: quit smoking 2012 [cited 2012 Jan 1]. Available from: http://www.google.com/insights/search/#q=quit%20smoking&date=today%20 12-m&cmpt=q.

32   Lancaster T, Stead Lindsay F. Self-help interventions for smoking cessation. Cochrane Database Syst rev; 2005 (3) [cited 2012 Jan 1]. Available from: http://www.mrw.interscience.wiley. com/cochrane/clsysrev/articles/CD001118/frame.html

33   Abroms LC, Padmanabhan N, Thaweethai L, Phillips T. iPhone apps for smoking cessation: a content analysis. Am J Prev Med. 2011;40(3):279-85.

18

Ethical Contemplations

DIANE KUNYK, CHARL ELS AND PETER SELBY

FORMER US PRESIDENT GEORGE W. BUSH WAS RIDICULED FOR CHARACTERIZING other nations as an 'axis of evil.' Evil is a moral judgment determined by individuals, based on what is considered reprehensible behaviour, and it evokes feelings of discomfort and revulsion.[1] Is the term *evil* appropriately applied to an industry that knowingly profits from marketing and selling a highly addictive product known to inflict death and disease to its loyal customers? Can this term be used with a legal industry exercising its corporate responsibility of maximizing shareholder value? Where does the regulation of this industry tie into this equation? This example draws attention to the importance of ethical questions as they relate to the tobacco epidemic. It is also attentive to the heightened emotions evoked in this field confronted with often opposing goals of health and economic profit.

How ought we ethically contemplate the situation of tobacco in our societies? The magnitude and devastation of the tobacco epidemic demands the concerted attention of healthcare professionals and their students in these fields for the purposes of ameliorating its effect on the patients that we serve. This is a complex topic; certainly one with more questions than answers. Covering the spectrum of issues within this important subject in the course of a single chapter would not do it justice; rather the purpose of this chapter is to raise questions and uncertainties for the purpose of encouraging further contemplation and discussions as to the responsibilities and roles of the healthcare professions regarding tobacco.

The process of reviewing the contributions of almost 50 authors in this volume and our reflections on years of clinical practice and research provided a rich opportunity to contemplate and generate ethical questions in terms of tobacco reduction and cessation. The authors decided to pose a number of salient questions to help guide the reader to critically reflect on some of the complex issues that form part of our everyday lives and practices as these relate to tobacco. Contemplating dilemmas that are perplexing and appear, at least initially, to be insolvable may facilitate ethical contemplation. The reality is that in healthcare ethics, we can never be confident that we will ever know the 'right' thing to do and are often left with a sense of uncertainty.[2] Evoking this unease may continue to generate further questioning and allow for different contemplations regarding this important and complex field.

The purpose of generating ethical questions is not to provide answers (as these are not easily determined) but rather to allow the reader to have increased appreciation of the complexity of the tobacco pandemic and the challenges faced with enacting comprehensive tobacco control measures. The aim is to serve as a starting point in facilitating contemplation about the true nature of ethics in this field and to attempt to establish fundamental principles to guide discussions, to further alternative solutions, to defend particular directions taken, and to be open to other points of view. In the authors' experience, they are confident that this will yield valuable discourse but are also fairly certain that consensus will not always be reached. As with most ethical problems in health care, it is the engagement of individuals in these important discussions that are critical components of the process with advancing the field of study.[3] The following discussion does not address the scope of possible questions; rather these have been identified for the purposes of generating discussions and further questioning.

PUBLIC HEALTH MODEL

For the purposes of generating questions to stimulate ethical contemplation, the public health model (also called epidemiological homeostasis) provides a suitable framework for understanding the spread of the tobacco pandemic. It examines the interaction between the host, agent, vector, and environment.[4] Through consideration of the interaction between the host (i.e. the individual who uses or is addicted to tobacco), the agent (tobacco products), the vector (i.e. the tobacco industry and those propagating these products), and the broader environment in which the tobacco pandemic is expressed (i.e. government legislation and healthcare systems), new insights are generated. This framework incorporates biological, psychological, social, and spiritual theories as they pertain to the tobacco epidemic in a manner that can demonstrate their relationships. One advantage to the public health model is its ability to consider intervention at both the individual (i.e. clinical) and environmental (i.e. legislation and social marketing) levels. A number of questions have been arbitrarily raised within these key elements in the following discussions. These cannot be considered exhaustive; rather they ought to be considered as examples to provoke further questioning.

With this model, the host could be considered as the individual that experiments with tobacco products, uses these on a regular basis, or has become addicted to tobacco. It could also be the individual exposed to secondhand or thirdhand smoke, or the family suffering economic and/or social hardships due in part to one of their members' use of tobacco. In terms of personal agency, one has to wonder whether the person experimenting with tobacco truly understands its risks and what would constitute evidence of such understanding. This is a particularly relevant concept when it comes to the ability of children, youth, or those with cognitive disorders/symptoms (e.g. mental illnesses) to fully comprehend their risks when using tobacco. What would or could be considered a reasonable warning of these risks? This has yet to be determined. This uncertainty also raises questions regarding what may be the obligations of others (i.e. the manufacturer, governments, or healthcare professionals) to ensure that these risks are adequately understood. Where does the advancement of knowledge in the field of harm related to secondhand and thirdhand smoke fit in this equation? Further questions about autonomy are raised when individuals have become addicted to tobacco. Does the addictive nature of nicotine decrease an individual's ability to make autonomous decisions regarding continuing their use of tobacco? At what point does the use of tobacco products become an addiction with a possible loss of volitional control? What are the moral obligations for offering and ensuring access to opportunities for change? These are uncertain areas that beg to be addressed, and they have policy implications.

From the individual's perspective, most who use tobacco want to stop and repeatedly try to do so on their own. In order for individuals to seek out tobacco addiction treatment, it has been determined that there are 2 critical requirements.[5] These are to know about the existence of effective treatments and to have access to these. Are either of these critical conditions being attained, particularly amongst low-income and blue-collar populations where smoking rates remain the highest? Is it appropriate that treatment use is particularly limited among those with the highest smoking prevalence, such as those with comorbid psychiatric and substance abuse problems and lower levels of income and education, thereby contributing even more strongly to poor outcomes and to disparities in disease burden and mortality?[6]

Knowing the risks of tobacco on health and the existence of effective interventions, there are questions regarding the roles of healthcare professionals repeatedly asking about the use of tobacco, motivating quit attempts, offering interventions, and providing relapse prevention. One salient question is in regard to tobacco reduction as opposed to complete cessation given the known risks. In terms of assisting reduction and cessation, and given the current body of knowledge, does advice to try unassisted smoking cessation constitute sound public policy? And does this change whether considered from an individual or population level perspective? There are multiple questions regarding the offering of treatment interventions. For example, should pregnant women be encouraged to stop smoking of their own volition or offered medication to quit smoking? In light of the economic costs of treatment, should it be offered when the individual is considering reducing smoking or only when ready to quit? What is the role of off-label treatment if (based on the provider's judgment) it is likely to be effective and safe? Knowing that smokeless products contain more carcinogens than what is allowed in most consumer products but are known to be less harmful than forms of combustible tobacco, is it ethical to advise switching to smokeless products?[7]

As the World Health Organization has observed, everyone deserves the opportunity to obtain the highest level of one's own health.[7] One might examine the role of healthcare professionals, health systems, and funding agencies in this regard. There appears to be a confluence of debate regarding the relevance of appropriate cessation interventions to specific sub-populations. For example, it has been suggested that individuals be required to fail with multiple quit attempts before being offered more expensive cessation options.[8] When presenting with other more immediate health issues, is it appropriate to raise questions about tobacco use and addiction?[9] In light of limited healthcare resources, is it ethical to promote the use of cessation interventions and medications over population-based interventions? Smoking decisions (to start or not, to stop smoking once started, or to resume once discontinued) are personal and individual. The decision of how best to manage tobacco use and addiction is also personal and individual—and should not be dictated by healthcare providers, health systems, tobacco control advocates, or others. The principle of personal autonomy suggests that individuals ought to be informed of their menu of options to reduce or quit smoking in order for them to be able to make informed decisions on how best to proceed in their particular situations.

The agent in this model includes the multiple forms of tobacco products. Appreciating its toxicity and lethality and its contributions to human suffering, is it appropriate that tobacco remains a legal product? Would prohibition as a means to total abolition be an option? What would happen to currently addicted individuals if tobacco were to be banned in the near future? If nicotine products (i.e. pharmaceutical-grade nicotine and tobacco products) all deliver the same addictive psychoactive substance, nicotine, is it ethical that these products be regulated in the same fashion, with the most dangerous products (tobacco) under the least amount and the cleanest nicotine products (pharmaceutical grade) with the most? If tobacco products were held to the same standards and availability as other pharmaceutical products, would this include the requirement of prescriptions, childproof containers, and full-disclosure of contents?

When healthcare professionals and researchers collaborate with the pharmaceutical or tobacco industries, what constitutes arms-length relationship? Is it a conflict of interest when tobacco control advocates have financial relationships with the pharmaceutical industry? Can any level of collaboration between the tobacco industry and health professionals or health faculties be considered moral? Is it ethical for a health professional to testify in the interests of the tobacco industry?

The vector in the tobacco pandemic includes those individuals, organizations, and industries among others that made the product available, accessible, and desirable. There are many questions about the moral obligations of these groups in continuing to propagate the use of tobacco. As the tobacco industry has been known to target vulnerable groups in its marketing efforts, should their corporate social responsibility obligations be expanded?[11] At what point do restrictions on tobacco marketing and manufacturing become onerous and beyond those experienced by other corporate entities? Should the tobacco industry continue to be the focus of blame for the devastation as they are marketing a legal product and following their mandate and mission under the corporate laws, i.e. to maximize shareholder value? As tobacco has been demonstrated to be a lethal product, should governments be removing it from the market in a similar fashion to other formerly legal products such as DDT?[12] Can healthcare professionals justify owning stocks or shares in the tobacco industry? Are health professionals also tobacco agents/vectors if dispensing tobacco to patients, escorting patients to smoke, or smoking with patients while 'doing therapy'? What is the message when employers, particularly healthcare employers, expose their staff members to secondhand smoke in the course of their employed duties?

Our societies, cultures, healthcare organizations, and governments are just some of the agents that are influential in the tobacco pandemic in terms of our broader environment. The scope and health implications of the tobacco epidemic must raise questions regarding whether tobacco control is receiving an appropriate level of funding from governments and attention in healthcare systems. How should the relative priority each of the tobacco control pillars receives in funding and attention be decided? What is an appropriate balance between population- and individual-level interventions? Is it appropriate that most provincial governments provide little if any direct funding for smoking cessation?[13] These thoughts must also be considered by health professionals in terms of whether tobacco reduction and cessation is receiving an appropriate amount of attention in our daily practices.

Another disconcerting question is whether our current priorities and actions in tobacco control are increasing disparities for vulnerable and marginalized individuals. The use of tobacco is becoming increasingly associated with stigma. There is some evidence that those who smoke are more likely than non-smokers to report being targets of perceived discrimination in both health-care settings and the workplace. They are also more likely to report emotional and physical symptoms in response to perceived discrimination.[14] The stigma of tobacco use is not limited to those currently smoking; it may also be experienced by individuals suffering the health consequences of smoking, such as those with lung cancer or even family members of individuals who smoke.[12] Individuals who are addicted to tobacco and those who suffer tobacco-related disease have been negatively impacted by the tobacco epidemic. Through stigma, are they also becoming victims of tobacco control measures?

PARTING THOUGHTS

Tobacco use and addiction is a critical health issue and one that deserves urgent and concerted attention. The editors believe the most reasonable response to the tobacco epidemic is comprehensive tobacco control—a comprehensive, coordinated, and multi-level strategy involving all of the pillars of tobacco control; prevention, protection and cessation. These strategies have been considered responsible for the substantial gains observed in the domain of tobacco control. It was only a few decades ago when smoking was allowed on planes, cigarette vending machines were commonplace, and tobacco companies sponsored art and athletic events. Since that time, smoking rates have been halved and most public buildings are smoke-free in Canada.

But with almost half of lifetime users dying of a tobacco-related disease, and more suffering from chronic diseases induced by their tobacco use, it cannot be concluded that our current smoking rates ought to be the endpoint.[15,16] Can it be concluded that our current responses to the problem of tobacco are enough? If we do not do more, or do not act with greater urgency, what is the underlying statement regarding the value of the lives of those who are taking up, using, and addicted to tobacco? It is hoped that this chapter will encourage further contemplation and discussion in this meaningful field.

REFERENCES

1   'evil,' *n*. In Merriam-Webster's collegiate dictionary, 11th ed. Springfield MA: Merriam-Webster, Inc; 2004.

2   Austin W. The ethics of everyday practice: healthcare environments as moral communities. ANS Adv Nurs Sci. 2007;30(1): 81-8.

3   Bergum V, Dossetor J. Relational ethics: the full meaning of respect. Hagerstown MD: University Publishing Group; 2005.

4   Slade J. A disease model of cigarette use. N Y State J Med. 1985;85(7):294-7.

5   Husten CG. A call for ACTTION: increasing access to tobacco-use treatment in our nation. Am J Prev Med. 2010;38(3S);S414-7.

6   Gollust S, Schroeder S, Warner K. Helping smokers quit: understanding the barriers to utilization of smoking cessation services. Millbank Q. 2008;86(4):601-27.

7   SCENIHR (Scientific Committee on Emerging and Newly-Identified Health Risks), Scientific opinion on the Health Effects of Smokeless Tobacco Products, 6 February 2008.

8   World Health Organization. Constitution of the World Health Organization [accessed 2012 May 30]. Available from: http://www.who.int/governance/eb/constitution/en/.

9   McDonald P. A recommended population strategy to help Canadian tobacco users. Toronto: Ontario Tobacco Research Unit, Special Report Series; 2003.

10   Tajema B, Guydish J, Delucchi K et al. Staff knowledge, attitudes, and practices regarding nicotine dependence differ by setting. J Drug Issues. 2009;30:365-84.

11   Appolonio D, Malone R. Marketing to the marginalized: tobacco industry targets the homeless and mentally ill. Tobacco Control. 2005;14:409-15.

12   US Department of Health and Human Services. The health consequences of smoking: a report of the Surgeon General. Atlanta: US Department of Health and Human Services, Centers for Disease Control and Prevention, National Center for Chronic Disease Prevention and Health Promotion, Office on Smoking and Health; 2004.

13   Penz E, Manns B, Heberts P, Stanbrook M. Governments, pay for smoking cessation. CMAJ. 2010;182(16):1761-2.

14   Purnell J, Peppone L, Alcaraz K et al. Perceived discrimination, psychological distress, and current smoking status: results from the behavioral risk factor surveillance system reactions to race module, 2004-2008. Am J Public Health. 2012:102(5):844-51.

15   Chapple A, Zeibland S, McPherson A. Stigma, shame, and blame experienced by patients with lung cancer: qualitative study. BMJ. 2004;328(7454):1470-3.

16   World Health Organization. WHO report on the global tobacco epidemic, 2008: The MPOWER package. Geneva: Author; 2008.

17   Centers for Disease Control and Prevention. Cigarette smoking-attributable morbidity—United States, 2000. Morbidity and mortality weekly report; 2003 [accessed 2012 Jan 24]. Available from: http://www.cdc.gov/mmwr/preview/mmwrhtml/mm5235a4.htm.

CONTRIBUTORS

*Yoram Barak, MD, MHA, is an Assistant Professor of Psychiatry at the Sackler School of Medicine, Tel-Aviv University. He trained in medicine and psychiatry at the Sackler School of Medicine. In 1993 he became an Israel Medical Scientific Council Specialist in Psychiatry, and in 2004 was awarded a Master in Health Administration from Ben-Gurion University, Beer-Sheva, Israel. Dr. Barak is the past president of the Israeli Association of Old-Age Psychiatry, and is on the editorial board of the *Israel Journal of Psychiatry* and the *Open Psychiatry Journal.* He has published extensively in these areas, and is author or co-author of over 150 peer-reviewed journal articles.

*Megan Barker, MA, has worked for the Centre for Addiction and Mental Health since 2010 as the Continuing Medical Education Coordinator for the TEACH Project, a University of Toronto accredited Certificate Program in Cessation Counselling. In 2009 Barker graduated with distinction from the University of Guelph with an Honours Bachelor's degree in Criminal Justice and Public Policy and Women's Studies. In 2010 she completed her Master's degree in Criminology and Socio-legal Studies at the University of Toronto.

*Joan L. Bottorff, PhD, RN, is a Professor in the School of Nursing and Director of the Institute for Healthy Living and Chronic Disease Prevention at the University of British Columbia's Okanagan campus. She has led the Families Controlling and Eliminating Tobacco (FACET) research program, and is co-leader of an interdisciplinary research team, Investigating Tobacco and Gender (iTAG). Additional details about these programs of research are available at www.facet.ubc.ca and www.itag.ubc.ca.

*Michael Chaiton, PhD, is an Assistant Professor at the Ontario Tobacco Research Unit (OTRU), in the Dalla Lana School of Public Health at the University of Toronto, and Co-Head of the Population Research Initiative on Mental Health and Addictions (PRIMHA) at OTRU, where he is the project lead for the Ontario Tobacco Survey, a population representative longitudinal cohort study, and is the principal investigator on a Canadian Institutes of Health Research funded study on policy options for addressing tobacco retail availability.

Jotham W. Coe, PhD, is a medicinal chemist who worked from 1994 until 2009 on approaches for the treatment of depression, schizophrenia, ADHD and addiction. He is an inventor of varenicline, sold as Champix™ varenicline tartrate (Chantix™ in the United States), a pharmaceutical aid to smoking cessation. He was appointed Research Fellow in 2003. Prior to joining Neuroscience, Dr. Coe worked for six years in oncology, and since 2009 has studied inflammatory pathways. Coe received his AB degree in chemistry from Harvard College in 1981 and his PhD in 1988 from the Massachusetts Institute of Technology.

*Stephanie Cohen, MSW, RSW, received her Master's of Social Work degree from the University of Toronto in 1997. Since then she has served in clinical, educational, and managerial roles in the Nicotine Dependence Service at the Centre for Addiction and Mental Health. In 2009 Cohen became a member of the Motivational Interviewing Network of Trainers (MINT).

*Karina Czyzewski, BA, MA, completed her BA at the University of Alberta and her MA at the University of Toronto in Anthropology and Indigenous Health, focusing on the Residential School Truth and Reconciliation Commission, colonialism as a broader social determinant of health, and transformative education. Czyzewski has extensive volunteer and professional experience in anti-racism, mental health, addictions education and anthropology education, peer support, and community outreach. Most recently she has worked as the Aboriginal and Francophone Projects Coordinator at the Nicotine Dependence Service in Toronto and is a MSW candidate at the University of British Columbia.

Rosa Dragonetti, MSc, is Manager of the Nicotine Dependence Clinic and Tobacco Projects as well as the Eating Disorders and Addictions Clinic at the Centre for Addiction and Mental Health (CAMH). Among her project management duties are the STOP Program, the TEACH project, and PREGNETS. She has published several articles on gambling and tobacco, co-authored a chapter on assessment interventions for alcohol and tobacco addiction, has contributed to CAMH's Smoke-free Policy development and implementation, and was involved in several tobacco control initiatives including the Rainbow Tobacco Intervention Project, and the Provincial Cessation Task Group. She has delivered many workshops across Canada and internationally.

*Jolene Dubray, MSc, is a Research Officer at the Ontario Tobacco Research Unit (OTRU) at the University of Toronto. She obtained her MSc in Community Health and Epidemiology from Dalhousie University. At OTRU she has coordinated several evaluations related to the implementation and enforcement of

315

the Smoke-Free Ontario Act and provided statistical support to OTRU's Tobacco Informatics Monitoring System (TIMS) and Strategy Evaluation Reports. She has also lead research studies related to the impact of a total display ban of tobacco products on impulse tobacco purchases and patterns of cigarillo use among young adults.

*Charl Els, MBChB, FCPsych, MMedPsych (cum laude), Dipl. ABAM, MROCC, is a Psychiatrist and Addiction Specialist. He serves on academic faculty at the University of Alberta and the John Dossetor Health Ethics Centre.

*Roberta Ferrence, PhD, is Deputy Director of the Ontario Tobacco Research Unit at the University of Toronto, Professor at the Dalla Lana School of Public Health, and Affiliate Scientist with the Centre for Addiction and Mental Health. She has training in medical sociology and epidemiology. Her research focuses on tobacco smoke exposure, including the economic and environmental impact of smoke-free bylaws, indoor and outdoor air quality studies including waterpipe, and thirdhand smoke exposure. She has published more than 150 peer-reviewed papers and authored three books including *Nicotine and Public Health*.

*Marleen Filimon, MSc, is a psychologist who obtained her Master's in both Clinical and Cognitive Psychology and stands at the start of her career. Through work at several psychiatric hospitals in the Netherlands and in the counselling field for the United Nations in Haiti, she has extensive experience with mental health patients and the understanding of various addictions, including tobacco.

*Becky Freeman, PhD, has worked in the field of tobacco control for more than 10 years. She is an early career researcher at the School of Public Health, University of Sydney. In 2011 she was awarded her PhD for "Tobacco control 2.0: Studies on the relevance of online media to tobacco control." Freeman has held tobacco control positions in Canada and New Zealand with both government and non-profit organizations. Freeman is the Associate Editor of New Media for the international journal, *Tobacco Control*.

Tony George, MD, FRCPC, is Professor of Psychiatry, Chair in Addiction Psychiatry, and Co-Director of the Division of Brain and Therapeutics in the Department of Psychiatry at the University of Toronto. He is also Clinical Director, Schizophrenia Program at the Centre for Addiction and Mental Health. He graduated from Dalhousie Medical School in 1992, and completed his psychiatry residency and fellowship at Yale University School of Medicine, where he served on the faculty prior to coming to Toronto. Dr. George's research is funded by CIHR, NIH/NIDA, OMHF and CFI, and he is a Fellow of the American College of Neuropsychopharmacology (ACNP).

*Lorraine Greaves, PhD, is the Senior Investigator and former Executive Director of the British Columbia Centre of Excellence for Women's Health, and Clinical Professor, School of Population and Public Health, Faculty of Medicine, University of British Columbia. She is an international expert on women's tobacco use and has authored numerous books, articles, chapters, and reports on tobacco use during pregnancy and postpartum, gender equity and tobacco policy, Aboriginal girls' smoking, and women's cessation. She is the author of *Smoke Screen: Women's Smoking and Social Control* and lead author of *Expecting to Quit: A Best Practices Review of Smoking Cessation Interventions for Pregnant and Postpartum Girls and Women.*

*Natalie Hemsing, MA, is a Research Associate at the British Columbia Centre of Excellence for Women's Health. She specializes in research on tobacco use, addictions, and health promotion among girls and women. She has an extensive background in primary and secondary research on sex- and gender- based analysis, smoking prevention, cessation and tobacco policy among diverse populations, and systematic reviews and knowledge syntheses.

Marilyn A. Herie, PhD, RSW, is Director of the TEACH Project at the Centre for Addiction and Mental Health, a university-accredited interprofessional certificate program in tobacco cessation counselling for health practitioners. She is also Director of the Collaborative Program in Addiction Studies at University of Toronto, Assistant Professor (Status Only), U of T Factor-Inwentash Faculty of Social Work, and first author of *Substance Abuse in Canada*. Her interests include motivational interventions, clinical education, and knowledge transfer/exchange.

*Patrick Hlavac-Winsor, BFA (Hon), LLB, is currently completing an MBA at the University of Calgary and holds a BFA from the University of Victoria and an LLB from the University of Ottawa. In addition to serving as in-house counsel to Health CPR, he has worked as a litigator in private practice, has been involved in numerous non-profit engagements involving Calgary arts development, and is the Communications Director for YMCA Calgary.

John R. Hughes, MD, is Professor of Psychiatry, Psychology and Family Practice at the University of Vermont. Dr. Hughes is Board certified in Psychiatry and Addiction Psychiatry. He has over 400 publications on nicotine and other drug dependencies and is one of the world's most cited tobacco scientists. He has been a consultant on tobacco policy to the World Health Organization, the US Food and Drug Administration, and the White House. Dr. Hughes has received fees from almost all of the companies who develop smoking cessation devices, medications, and services, from governmental and academic institutions, and from public and private organizations that promote tobacco control.

*Jaclyn R. Kaye, MSc, earned her MSc in Education from the University of Edinburgh and her Honours BA in Cognitive Science from the University of Toronto. Prior to her work for the Ontario Tobacco Research Unit, she worked in public health administration for the Scottish Government and the Public Information Service for the Scottish Parliament. Her interests include education policy and curriculum development, and the promotion of science literacy. She resides in Edinburgh, Scotland.

Milan Khara, MBChB, CCFP, Dipl. ABAM, is an Addiction Medicine Physician with Vancouver Coastal Health, physician lead of the Vancouver General Hospital Smoking Cessation Clinic, and Clinical Assistant Professor in the Faculty of Medicine, University of British Columbia. He serves as Medical Advisor for QuitNow Services, a service operated by the British Columbia Lung Association, and is on the faculty of TEACH. Dr. Khara has authored a number of papers on smoking cessation, mainly relating to populations with substance use disorders and/or mental illness.

* Davida Kidd, MVA, is a Faculty member of the University of the Fraser Valley Department of Visual Arts in Abbotsford B.C. Davida has been a recipient of numerous international awards and grants for her work including a major Canada Council Project Grant in 2009, the Grand Prix/Solo Exhibition Award at the International Print Triennial Krakow, Poland in 2003 and a Statutory Award there in 2012. Davida's art practice addresses themes of Tug of War: between the psyche and the dream; the conscience and transgression; the personality by rapture.

*Diane Kunyk, RN, PhD, is academic faculty with the Faculty of Nursing and the John Dossetor Health Ethics Centre at the University of Alberta. Dr. Kunyk is the recipient of a number of awards including the Presidents' Doctoral Award of Distinction and funding including both SSHRC and CIHR grants. She was one of the original designers of both TRaC (Tobacco Reduction and Cessation) Education and Clinical projects. Dr. Kunyk is involved in research in the field of addiction, ethics and health policy.

*Rod McCormick, PhD, is a Mohawk Psychologist and Professor at the University of British Columbia. In addition to being a senior Aboriginal mental health clinician and consultant, Dr. McCormick is one of the most highly funded Aboriginal health researchers in Canada.

*Daniel McKennitt, BSc, MD, is from the Sandy Bay Ojibway First Nation, was raised in St. Albert, Alberta, and holds a Bachelor of Science degree as well as a Doctor of Medicine with Special Training in Research Certification from the University of Alberta. Dr. McKennitt has been deeply involved in Aboriginal health research and has authored several peer-reviewed publications on the topic. He is active in Edmonton's Aboriginal community, having formed the first ever Aboriginal health student group at the University of Alberta, and sits on various committees and councils such as Canadian Heritage, Canadian Red Cross, Alberta Advanced Education, and the Alberta Cancer Board. He is currently completing his residency in Public Health and Preventative Medicine at the University of Alberta.

*Sarah Muir, MPH, obtained her Master of Public Health from the University of Sydney, Australia, specializing in chronic disease health promotion. Prior to working at the Ontario Tobacco Research Unit, she completed an internship at Bridgepoint Health, Toronto, to assist with the development of a tobacco cessation program for their inpatients.

*Kerri-Anne Mullen, BSc, MSc, has been with the University of Ottawa Heart Institute since 2006. She manages the Ottawa Model for Smoking Cessation Network, assisting Canadian healthcare organizations to implement and evaluate clinical approaches to treating tobacco addiction. Mullen is completing her PhD (Population Health) at the University of Ottawa. Her research interests include health, healthcare, and economic impacts of health interventions. From 2009 to 2011, she held a CIHR fellowship in Population Intervention for Chronic Disease Prevention.

*Shawn O'Connor, PhD, is a recognized expert in the monitoring and surveillance of tobacco control outcomes. He was a founding member of the Canadian

Tobacco Control Research Initiative's National Advisory Group on Monitoring and Evaluation and was co-author of CTCRI's *Indicators for Monitoring Tobacco Control*. Dr. O'Connor has led the development of OTRU's Tobacco Informatics Monitoring System (TIMS) and its sister site, the Chronic Disease Informatics Monitoring System (CDIMS), innovative web-based data portals designed to enhance the use and adoption of risk-factor indicators by public health stakeholders. His recent research has focused on how cigarette package design elements are imbued with messages of lifestyle and (perceived) strength.

Pamela O'Donaghey, RN, BSN, is from the Boston Bar First Nation in British Columbia. She is currently working on her Master of Public Health from the University of British Columbia, and is an Addiction Nurse for Vancouver Coastal Health. O'Donaghey has a keen interest in Aboriginal health and tobacco dependence. She volunteers in her spare time and does contract work for Aboriginal organizations and communities.

John Oliffe, RN, MEd, PhD, is Associate Professor and Associate Director Research at the School of Nursing, University of British Columbia. His research focuses on masculinities and gender relations in the context of men's health particularly, smoking behaviour and cessation intervention, depression and masculinities, and the cardiac health of South Asian Canadian immigrants. He is currently involved with many national and international men's health studies, and has authored 80 peer-reviewed publications, 12 book chapters, and an edited book designing and conducting gender, sex, and health research. Additional details about his men's health research program are available at www.menshealthresearch.ubc.ca.

Sophia Papadakis, MHA, PhD, is Associate Professor, Division of Cardiology, University of Ottawa and Program Director for the Primary Care Smoking Cessation Program, Division of Prevention and Rehabilitation at the University of Ottawa Heart Institute. Dr. Papadakis holds a Ph.D. in Applied Health Sciences from the University of Waterloo and Masters in Health Administration from the University of Ottawa.

Anne Philipneri, BSc, MPH, is a research officer at the Ontario Tobacco Research Unit at University of Toronto and a PhD candidate in the program of Health Research Methodology at McMaster University. Philipneri played a key role in the design and development of the Tobacco Informatics Monitoring System

(TIMS), a web-based application that provides national and provincial data on key tobacco control indicators. Her research interests include monitoring and surveillance of tobacco use, examining effects of tobacco control policies, and social determinants of smoking.

Andrew Pipe, CM, BA, MD, LLD (Hon), DSc (Hon), graduated from Queen's University in 1974. He is Chief of the Division of Prevention and Rehabilitation at the University of Ottawa Heart Institute and Professor in the Faculty of Medicine at the University of Ottawa. He was instrumental in the development of the widely adopted Ottawa Model for Smoking Cessation at the Heart Institute. Dr. Pipe is currently involved in clinical research assessing new approaches to smoking cessation, strategies designed to facilitate exercise adoption, and novel initiatives to prevent cardiovascular disease. He has addressed audiences in over 30 nations and is frequently consulted on issues related to tobacco use and smoking cessation. In 2002 he was named to the Order of Canada.

Ron Pohar, BScPharm, is a Clinical Pharmacist specializing in mental health, geriatrics, and smoking cessation. He works with Edmonton's inner city residents and those with mental illnesses to assist in tobacco reduction and cessation. Pohar has extensive training in tobacco addiction and smoking cessation from the Centre for Addictions and Mental Health. He is a recipient of the Alberta Pharmacy Centennial Award of Distinction.

*Nancy Poole, BA, MA, is the Director of Research and Knowledge Translation for the British Columbia Centre of Excellence for Women's Health. She has extensive experience in research and knowledge exchange relating to improvement in policy and service provision for women with alcohol, tobacco, and other substance use problems. Poole is a Canadian leader in piloting online participatory methods for knowledge generation and exchange, including virtual networks and communities of inquiry/practice.

*Robert Reid, PhD, MBA, is Deputy Chief of the Division of Prevention and Rehabilitation at the University of Ottawa Heart Institute, and Full Professor in the Faculty of Medicine at the University of Ottawa. Dr. Reid is one of Canada's leading health behaviour change experts, particularly concerning smoking cessation, physical activity promotion, dietary change, and cardiovascular rehabilitation. He is the co-developer of the Ottawa Model for Smoking Cessation and for the past 15 years has conducted research on smoking cessation interventions among hospitalized individuals.

*Emilene Reisdorfer, RN, MPH, Ph.D(s), is currently studying in Psychiatric Nursing at College of Nursing, University of São Paulo at Ribeirão Preto (EERP-USP/Brazil). She earned her Master's Degree in Public Health at Federal University of Santa Catarina (UFSC/Brazil). She has experience in addictions and mental health in primary health care settings.

Hans Rollema, PhD, studied Pharmacy in The Netherlands and in 1976 received his PhD in Pharmaceutical and Medicinal Chemistry at the University of Groningen, where he was an Associate Professor at the School of Pharmacy. In 1992 he was recruited by Pfizer, Inc. and supported neuroscience discovery projects with microdialysis data. He was a member of the nicotinic partial agonist project team that discovered varenicline and became the preclinical point of contact. He has published around 90 scientific papers. After retiring from Pfizer in 2010, he started a biomedical consulting business.

Amit Yosef Rotem, MD, graduated medical school at the Faculty of Health Sciences, Ben Gurion University of the Negev, Israel. As a student, he initiated a unique HMO cooperation to deliver evidence-based services for smoking cessation which became the first Israeli academic centre for smoking prevention and cessation. During his residency in child and adolescent psychiatry, he developed educational methods to incorporate nicotine addiction into health curricula. Dr. Rotem trains and supervises new smoking cessation counsellors and works with high-risk teenagers in drug rehabilitation and smoking cessation clinics. He is a founder and active committee member of the Israeli Medical Association for Smoking Prevention and Cessation. Dr. Rotem has published clinical studies, reviews, and chapters on nicotine dependence and clinical psychiatry issues.

*Andriy V. Samokhvalov, MD, PhD, is a staff psychiatrist and scientist at the Addictions Program and the Social and Epidemiological Research Department of the Centre for Addiction and Mental Health (CAMH) and assistant professor at the Department of Psychiatry, University of Toronto. He has published a number of works in the field of addictions and psychiatry, with the most important areas of clinical and research interest in recent years being nicotine, alcohol, and opioid dependence. His clinical research and expertise in the field of tobacco addiction are supported by his active involvement treating hundreds of clients of the CAMH Nicotine Dependence Clinic.

*Gayl Sarbit, PhD, is a Knowledge Broker with the Families Controlling and Eliminating Tobacco (FACET) and Investigating Tobacco and Gender (iTAG) research projects. She brings extensive knowledge and experience in education and leadership to her role as a knowledge broker, which includes strengthening relationships between research team members and community partners to facilitate knowledge transfer, creation, and exchange, as well as supporting the translation of evidence into practice.

*Debra Scarf, RN, MN was a co- developer of the Alberta province wide tobacco education program for health professionals, Tobacco Reduction and Cessation Training (TRaC) and was a faculty for TEACH (a comprehensive course on smoking cessation). She was the tobacco lead for a large psychiatric facility that banned indoor smoking.

*Robert Schwartz, PhD, is Executive Director of the Ontario Tobacco Research Unit (OTRU), Associate Professor at the Dalla Lana School of Public Health at the University of Toronto, and Senior Scientist at the Centre for Addiction and Mental Health. He is Editor-in-Chief of the *Canadian Journal of Program Evaluation* and Principal Investigator of the CIHR Strategic Training Program in Public Health Policy. At OTRU, Dr. Schwartz directs a comprehensive evaluation and monitoring program which includes surveillance, monitoring, evaluation, performance measurement, and evaluation support and quality assurance. He has published widely about tobacco control accountability, public health policy, policy change, program evaluation, and government–third sector relations.

Peter Selby, MBBS, CFCP, FCFP, dipABAM, is the Clinical Director of the Addictions Program and Head of the Nicotine Dependence Clinic at the Centre for Addiction and Mental Health. He is an Associate Professor in the departments of Family and Community Medicine, Psychiatry, Faculty of Medicine, and the Dalla Lana School of Public Health at the University of Toronto, and is a Principal Investigator at the Ontario Tobacco Research Unit. His research focuses on tobacco addiction and innovations in translating evidence into practice in a variety of populations, especially in those who have high rates of tobacco addiction.

*David Sweanor, J.D., received his law degree from the University of Toronto in 1981 and was called to the bar in 1983. Since then he has worked in public health efforts, specializing in tobacco issues, and focusing on how legal and economic measures can impact population health. He has played a key role in Canadian and global efforts on tobacco taxation, advertising restrictions, package labelling, environmental tobacco smoke, smoking cessation, litigation, and product regulation. His current interests are in improving smoking cessation rates and substitution of less toxic nicotine delivery systems for those not ready to quit.

Serena Tonstad, MD, MPH, PhD, is head physician at the Department of Preventive Cardiology, Oslo University Hospital, Oslo, Norway and a professor in the Department of Health Promotion and Education at Loma Linda University in California. She is interested in a multifactorial approach to prevention of cardiovascular disease including lifestyle change and medications, and has over 210 publications in cardiovascular prevention including smoking cessation and treatment of lipids and obesity. She received her MD and specialty training in Preventive Medicine at Loma Linda University, and earned a PhD on treatment of familial hypercholesterolemia in children at the University of Oslo.

*Alison van Driesum is a third-year nursing student at Grant MacEwan University in Edmonton. She holds first-class standing in her BScN program and has received various awards such as the Jason Lang and Alexander Rutherford scholarships. Her long-term goal is to build a career in community health.

*David van Driesum, BPE, BScPt, was the Regional Vice President for Centric/LifeMark Health. He had 22 years of clinical and administrative experience in interdisciplinary rehabilitation, was a member of the Diagnostic and Treatment Protocols Working Committee for the Government of Alberta, the Physical Therapy Advisory Committee for the Workers Compensation Board of Alberta, and has served on numerous health-related advisory and steering committees. He had been a clinical and sessional instructor in the Faculty of Rehabilitation Medicine at the University of Alberta and participates in a number of roles for the College and Association of Physical Therapists of Alberta. David passed away right before this volume was published.

*Dennis Wardman, MD FRCPC MCM, is from the Key First Nation in Saskatchewan. After completing medical school, he was the first Aboriginal person in Canada to complete a fellowship in Community Medicine. Dr. Wardman had worked on the tobacco file for a number of years when he was employed with the First Nations and Inuit Health Program in BC. Presently he practices addiction medicine in various clinics in the Vancouver area.

For each contributor, disclosure of any potential competing interests was requested. This may include Conflict of Interest situations where the professional and/or personal interests may have actual, perceived, potential or apparent influence over their judgment and actions. The arbitrary cut-off of 3 years was used as a threshold for reporting. Contributors with an asterisk (*) did not declare any competing or related interests.